WORKPLACE CONCEPTS *for* ATHLETIC TRAINERS

WORKPLACE CONCEPTS *for* ATHLETIC TRAINERS

EDITORS

Stephanie M. Mazerolle, PhD, ATC, LAT
Assistant Professor
Director, Entry-Level Athletic Training Education
Department of Kinesiology
University of Connecticut
Storrs, Connecticut

William A. Pitney, EdD, ATC, FNATA
Professor
Department of Kinesiology and Physical Education
Northern Illinois University
DeKalb, Illinois

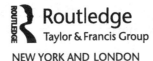

Routledge
Taylor & Francis Group

NEW YORK AND LONDON

Workplace Concepts for Athletic Trainers includes ancillary materials specifically available for faculty use. Included are Test Bank Questions. Please visit www.routledge.com/9781617119347 to obtain access.

First published in 2016 by SLACK Incorporated

Published 2024 by Routledge
605 Third Avenue, New York, NY 10158

and by Routledge
4 Park Square, Milton Park, Abingdon, Oxon OX14 4RN

Routledge is an imprint of the Taylor & Francis Group, an informa business

© 2016 Taylor & Francis Group

Library of Congress Cataloging-in-Publication Data

Workplace concepts for athletic trainers / editors, Stephanie M. Mazerolle, William A. Pitney.
      p. ; cm.
  Includes bibliographical references and index.
  ISBN 978-1-61711-934-7 (alk. paper)
  I. Mazerolle, Stephanie M., 1978- , editor. II. Pitney, William A., 1965- , editor.
  [DNLM: 1. Physical Education and Training. 2. Workplace. 3. Organizational Culture. 4. Sports--education. 5. Workplace Violence. QT 255]
  RA781
  613.7'1--dc23
                        2015028616

ISBN: 9781617119347 (pbk)
ISBN: 9781003526971 (ebk)

DOI: 10.4324/9781003526971

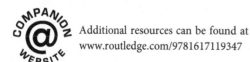

Additional resources can be found at
www.routledge.com/9781617119347

DEDICATION

To Camden and Beckett—my sons, who remind me daily to stop and take a moment to enjoy what really matters most in life. You challenge me to be the best I can be, no matter the role. To my husband, Phil, my constant supporter and friend, you accept my ambitions and remind me to stay true to my beliefs. To my parents, my champions, you've given me the love and support necessary to stay confident and grounded. I would be remiss not to thank and acknowledge my colleagues and students, as without their interactions and encouragement I would not be where I am today.

Stephanie M. Mazerolle, PhD, ATC, LAT

To Liam and Quin—2 young men who have kept me grounded; and to my wife, Lisa, who has helped me understand what matters most.

William A. Pitney, EdD, ATC, FNATA

CONTENTS

Section III Personal Skills to Foster Success and Commitment in the Workplace **165**

Workplace Concepts for Athletic Trainers includes ancillary materials specifically available for faculty use. Included are Test Bank Questions. Please visit www.routledge.com/9781617119347 to obtain access.

Acknowledgments

The development of this text would not have been possible without the mentoring and friendship of my co-editor William Pitney, so I thank you for being able to coach me, praise me, and challenge me to think big.

Stephanie M. Mazerolle, PhD, ATC, LAT

To my friend and colleague, Stephanie, who is not only a joy to work with, but also the finest scholar I know. Thank you for raising the bar for me. Working with you as a co-editor on this project has truly been my pleasure.

William A. Pitney, EdD, ATC, FNATA

We are appreciative of our contributing authors whose expertise has allowed us to put together a text that surpassed our vision. Finally, to Brien Cummings and the staff at SLACK Incorporated, we are indebted to your acceptance of our ideas and vision, and for making the publishing process enjoyable.

Stephanie M. Mazerolle, PhD, ATC, LAT and *William A. Pitney, EdD, ATC, FNATA*

ABOUT THE EDITORS

Stephanie M. Mazerolle, PhD, ATC, LAT is an Assistant Professor in the Department of Kinesiology within the College of Agriculture, Health, and Natural Resources at the University of Connecticut. She earned her Bachelor of Science degree in exercise science with a specialization in athletic training from the University of Connecticut; her Master of Science degree in athletic training and science education from Old Dominion University; and her Doctorate in Kinesiology from the University of Connecticut. Dr. Mazerolle has clinical experience as an athletic trainer in the high school and college settings and has been the program director at the University of Connecticut for the professional bachelor's program for 9 years. She currently serves as a section editor for the *Journal of Athletic Training* and is a reviewer and editorial board member for other journals including the *Athletic Training Education Journal* and the *International Journal of Athletic Training and Therapy*. She also is the Chair for the National Athletic Trainers' Association's (NATA) position statement for Work-Life Balance for the Athletic Trainer. Dr. Mazerolle has more than 50 peer-reviewed journal articles and more than 40 professional presentations. She currently serves as an exam writer for the BOC and is a member of the NATA Research and Education Foundation (NATAREF) Free Communication Review Committee and the NATAREF Scholarship Committee. She is recognized as a leader and scholar in the athletic training profession as it pertains to professional concepts and issues in the workplace. Dr. Mazerolle, in her leisure time, is an avid runner, and enjoys hiking, coaching basketball, and spending time with her husband and 2 sons.

William A. Pitney, EdD, ATC, FNATA is a Professor in the Department of Kinesiology and Physical Education at Northern Illinois University. He earned his Bachelor of Science degree in physical education with a specialization in athletic training from Indiana State University; his Master of Science degree in physical education from Eastern Michigan University; and his Doctorate of Education degree in adult continuing education from Northern Illinois University. He has practiced as an athletic trainer in the high school and college settings, as well as the outpatient rehabilitation setting. For the last 20 years, he has worked in higher education. Dr. Pitney has served as the editor-in-chief of the *Athletic Training Education Journal* and as a section editor for the *Journal of Athletic Training*. He is a fellow of the NATA and with more than 50 peer-reviewed journal articles, 4 textbooks, and more than 60 professional presentations, he is recognized as a leader and scholar in the athletic training profession. In his leisure time, he enjoys endurance bicycling, hiking, mountaineering, and spending time with his family.

CONTRIBUTING AUTHORS

Kirk Brumels, PhD, AT, ATC (Chapter 4)
Professor and Chair
Department of Kinesiology
Hope College
Holland, Michigan

Laura J. Burton, PhD (Chapter 6)
Associate Professor
Sports Management Program
Department of Educational Leadership
University of Connecticut
Storrs, Connecticut

*Jennifer Doherty-Restrepo, PhD, LAT, ATC
(Chapter 14)*
Clinical Assistant Professor, Program Director,
and Chair
Department of Athletic Training
Florida International University
Miami, Florida

*Christianne M. Eason, MS, ATC
(Chapters 1, 10, 11)*
Doctoral Candidate
Sports Management Program
University of Connecticut
Storrs, Connecticut

*Ashley Goodman, PhD, LAT, ATC
(Chapters 8, 9)*
Associate Professor
Athletic Training Program
Department of Health and Exercise Science
Beaver College of Health Sciences
Appalachian State University
Boone, North Carolina

*Matthew R. Kutz, PhD, AT, CSCS, CES
(Chapters 2, 13)*
Associate Professor
School of Human Movement Sport and Leisure
Studies
Bowling Green State University
Bowling Green, Ohio

John T. Parsons, PhD, ATC (Chapter 1)
Director
Sport Science Institute
National Collegiate Athletic Association
Indianapolis, Indiana

Stacy E. Walker, PhD, ATC (Chapter 12)
Associate Professor of Athletic Training
Department of Kinesiology
Ball State University
Muncie, Indiana

*Celest Weuve, PhD, ATC, CSCS, LAT
(Chapter 5)*
Associate Professor, Chair
Department of Athletic Training
Director
Athletic Training Program
Lincoln Memorial University
Harrogate, Tennessee

INTRODUCTION

Athletic trainers find themselves immersed in organizations that can critically influence the way they fulfill their professional obligations. Indeed, the workplace can offer many circumstances and situations that are challenging, particularly for those athletic trainers who are transitioning into clinical practice.

Workplace Concepts for Athletic Trainers provides students with clear and meaningful information that addresses concepts or issues that occur in the workplace. The topics selected are a reflection of those covered within the literature as problematic, yet identifiable and manageable. Each chapter begins with learning objectives and then includes a presentation of content related to the primary issue, how it manifests (sources, antecedents), and strategies and solutions to address the concern. Infused in each chapter are call-outs identifying important concepts. The conclusion of each chapter contains a summary and appropriate pedagogy to facilitate learning. This section, titled Activities for Reinforcement, includes questions for review, case vignettes, and discussion questions. The companion instructor's manual contains test questions that can be used to test students' knowledge acquisition. The text is appropriate both for undergraduate and graduate courses such as Administration and Organization, Professional Development, or Current Topics and Issues.

We have organized the chapters into 3 sections. Section I contains an overview both of employment organizations or workplaces, and leadership and management principles. We placed this content first to provide a broad overview of what is meant by the "workplace" and what leadership and management principles an individual will be exposed to in various organizations.

Section II presents various workplace issues and concepts ranging from work-family conflict to employee retention and attrition. On the one hand, these components can appear to present the negative dimensions of our work lives; on the other hand, we present tactics and strategies that organizations can employ to effectively address these various issues.

Section III presents personal skills an individual can tap to effectively address various workplace issues to foster success and commitment. Indeed, this section presents the positive dimensions of the workplace and provides individual tactics and strategies to employ to guide you toward a long and successful career as an athletic trainer.

I

An Overview of the Athletic Training Workplace

1

The Athletic Trainer in the Workplace

The Structure and Function of Work Organizations

John T. Parsons, PhD, ATC and Christianne M. Eason, MS, ATC

OBJECTIVES

After reading this chapter, the reader will be able to do the following:

1. Identify the 5 key features of a workplace.
2. Define social structure and explain where it comes from in a work setting.
3. Compare and contrast social structure from workplace culture.
4. Identify and explain the 3 layers of workplace culture, and provide examples of cultural artifacts from each layer.
5. Define workplace identity and distinguish it from personal identity.
6. Explain how workplace identity may be a source of negative emotion, and identify the potential consequences of that emotion.
7. Identify key structure features of the athletic training profession.

INTRODUCTION

"What is the workplace, and why is understanding it important for students of athletic training?" This seems like an appropriate and reasonable question to pose at the start of a textbook dedicated to guiding readers through a detailed exploration of workplace concepts. After all, athletic trainers are health care professionals, and their work is more about the people and patients they treat rather than the place in which they deliver their care. Right?

As it turns out, there are several different perspectives from which to consider those questions and consequently many ways to answer them depending on which perspective you choose. Several well-established academic disciplines exist that are dedicated to understanding the same workplace concepts that will be discussed in greater detail in subsequent chapters. The topics reflected

Mazerolle SM, Pitney WA.
Workplace Concepts for Athletic Trainers (pp 3-13).
© 2016 Taylor & Francis Group.

in the chapters of this textbook accurately reflect the landscape of perspectives and answers to the question of what is a workplace.

The answers to those questions begin with an understanding that a workplace is just another name for *an organization*. So to understand concepts salient to a workplace is also to understand concepts that are salient to an organization. Therefore, this textbook is essentially asking the athletic trainer to consider more deeply those concepts that are relevant to organizations and consequently to the process of organizing, for it is these processes that give rise to organizations themselves. For the remainder of this chapter, the reader should consider the terms *workplace* and *organization* as synonymous.

FEATURES OF A WORKPLACE

Workplaces can be talked about in terms of 5 interactive elements.[1] These elements are the following:

1. Social structure
2. Participants
3. Goals
4. Technology
5. Identifiable boundaries

Social structure refers to relationships between people in the workplace, and includes both formal and informal aspects of those relationships. Formal structure is typically established through official workplace policies and reflects organizational policies and formal reporting relationships of the kind that may be captured in an organizational chart. For example, a formal superior-subordinate relationship is likely to exist between a head athletic trainer and his or her staff athletic trainers. In contrast, informal structures are usually not captured through formal organizational documents, and in fact, may be "hidden" and largely unknown to the organization. Informal structures often reflect the social relationships that occur in the workplace and the power that often arises from these relationships. It is not uncommon for informal structures to contradict, and even overwhelm, formal organizational structures.

As an example, think of a class that you have recently taken. The dynamics of a classroom frequently mirror those that occur in more traditional workplaces. According to the formal structures common to a typical educational classroom, the leader of the class is the professor, who is formally authorized to assign homework, conduct examination, direct resources, and assign grades. If you had to represent this structure in a diagram, you might draw it so that the professor was at the top of the pyramid and the students were below.

However, the classroom, like all workplaces, also has an informal structure that reflects the structure of the class *as it actually is*, based on the actions and communication of the students. While the professor maintains his or her formal authority, we have all had experiences where a particularly bright and successful student is the one to whom students actually take their questions, in spite of the fact that that student has no formal authority to answer such questions. The informal authority given to that student by her classmates is a form of social power, which increases her capacity to influence the workplace.

Both formal and informal structures create certain expectations about what are expected and acceptable behaviors. Within the workplace, these behaviors are often referred to as *normative*. For example, normal behaviors in a superior-subordinate relationship between a head and staff athletic trainer include the head athletic trainer giving directions or assigning responsibilities to staff athletic trainers. However, it would be unexpected, and probably inappropriate, for staff athletic trainers to do the same to the head athletic trainer. To do so would be a violation of established normative workplace behaviors, and would likely lead to negative consequences, such as workplace conflict, or even formal disciplinary action. More about these workplace norms will be discussed in the next section of this chapter.

MISSION STATEMENT	<ul><li>Defines the present state or purpose of the organization</li><li>Answers 3 questions: Who (it does it for), What (it does), How (it does what it does)</li></ul>
VISION STATEMENT	<ul><li>Defines the optimal desired state</li><li>Provides guidance as to what the organization is focused on achieving</li></ul>

The second component of the workplace is *participants*. Participants are those people who contribute some form of activity to the workplace. Within a typical athletic training workplace, participants may include staff athletic trainers, team physicians, athletic administrators, student-athletes, visitors, and academic faculty. The personal and/or demographic characteristics of the participants can have a significant impact on the workplace itself, and can shape both the formal and informal structures discussed above. For example, an athletic training facility that is staffed by female athletic trainers is a potentially very different workplace from one staffed by males, even if the physical location of the facility and the experience and skill of the clinicians are exactly the same. One potential reason for these differences is the effect of *gender*, which is the socially constructed aspects of masculinity and femininity, and which are largely cultural in nature. Gender alone is capable of changing the dynamics of a workplace.[2]

The third component of organizations is *goals*. Defined simply, goals are the end product or outcome of workplace activity.[1] In the case of an athletic training workplace, the most obvious goal is improvement in the health and well-being of the patient. In fact, goals provide one way of comparing and contrasting workplaces and categorizing organization according to similarities and dissimilarities. In other words, established goals make the typical athletic training room more like a hospital than like a bank.

It is also worth noting that goals play an important part in the study of management and leadership. Leadership may be the most widely studied and the most widely misunderstood workplace phenomenon but most scholars agree that leadership and management are different. Whereas a manager may be responsible for executing a strategy in pursuit of established goals, it is a leader that is responsible for the identification of the goals and the strategy with which to pursue them.[3] In fact, many well-established theories of leadership include the development and accomplishment of goals as a critical factor in the evaluation of leadership ability.[4] Some leadership scholars go so far as to argue that leadership does not and cannot exist in the absence of established goals.[4] Typically, organizations will have several different types of goals. While some goals may overlap, they each perform a specific function within the organization. Table 1-1 provides a definition and example of each of the 7 organizational goals.

The difficulty in creating goals is that "effectiveness" is not a simple concept. Different individuals within an organization (coaches, athletic trainers, strength and conditioning coaches, sports information personnel) may view effectiveness in different ways. It is possible that individuals within an organization may have goals that conflict with one another. If a coach has an ultimate goal of making the playoffs and an athletic trainer has an ultimate goal of ensuring the safety and health of all athletes, what happens when the star player is diagnosed with a concussion or grade II lateral ankle sprain? To manage this complexity, leaders need a clear understanding of organizational goals and an even clearer understanding of how individual goals relate to the overall organizational effectiveness. It also creates an interesting question of whether athletic training

	TABLE 1-1	
	DEFINITIONS OF ORGANIZATIONAL GOALS	
TYPE OF GOAL	**DEFINITION**	**EXAMPLE**
Official goal	General purpose of the organization, often subjective and usually not measurable, express values	To provide a high-quality academic and athletic experience for all student athletes and proudly represent the university
Operative goal	Tells us what organization is actually trying to do, regardless of official goal	To make money
Operational goal	Can be measured objectively, and highlights how operative goal will be met	To sell more than 75% capacity to all home football and basketball games
Non-operative goal	Cannot be measured objectively (official goals and mission statements are typically non-operative)	To provide a fair return to all student athletes
Short-term goal	Goals set for a relatively brief set of time	To win the first conference men's basketball game of the season
Long-term goal	Goals the organization would like to set over a relatively lengthy period of time	To win the NCAA Division I men's basketball championship
Departmental or subunit goal	Goals set by individual departments or subunits within the organization	Prevent musculoskeletal injuries by implementing strength and stretching program

departments should be housed within sports organizations where they report to athletic directors or if perhaps there are better organizational reporting structures for athletic trainers, which we will address in the next section.

Technology has relevance to goals in that it refers to the tools, techniques, knowledge, and skills that support the work of the organization, which is typically pursued in support of organizational goals. This definition allows for more traditional forms of technology, like computers, electronic medical records, and various therapeutic modalities. But it also allows for a more abstract conceptualization of technology where the very practice of athletic training is a technology. In essence, athletic training, or any profession for that matter, is a technological system: a coordinated set of practices, skills, and techniques that are strategically and skillfully directed at the completion of goals.[5] In the case of a health care profession like athletic training, those goals relate to the health and well-being of patients.

The last characteristic is *identifiable boundaries*. Organizations have identifiable boundaries that are able to distinguish members from nonmembers. Members of organizations typically have an agreement, either explicit or implicit, with the organization through which they receive some benefit for their involvement. Athletic training is a group of people (or in some cases just one person) that makes up a department within an organization. In most traditional clinical settings (collegiate, professional, secondary schools), athletic training is a department within a sports organization. Like any other organization, a sport organization consists of the above elements but also includes the unique context of being situated within an athletic setting.

WORKPLACE CULTURE

A closely related concept to that of social structure discussed above is the idea of workplace *culture*. The most widely accepted definition of culture was provided by Schein,[6] who explained culture in the following way:

> *A pattern of shared basic assumptions that the group learned as it solved its problems of external adaptation and internal integration, that has worked well enough to be considered valid, and therefore, to be taught to new members as the correct way to perceive, think, and feel in relation to those problems.*[6(p12)]

The assumptions to which Schein refers will guide the behavior of participants in the workplace who are a part of that culture, even though the participants may not be consciously aware of them or able to articulate or explain them to others. This is a key distinction between culture and social structure that we discussed above.

For example, Schein has argued that there are 3 levels to workplace culture (Figure 1-1), each more deeply embedded within the organization than the last.[7]

ARTIFACTS	Any tangible, overt, or verbally identifiable elements in an organization that can be identified by individuals not part of the culture. • Dress code, furniture, décor, office jokes, etc
ESPOUSED VALUES	Stated values and member representation of the organization to themselves and others. • Mission statements, vision statements, philosophies, etc
ASSUMPTIONS	Deeply embedded behaviors that are usually unconscious and are often hard to recognize from within. • Sociocultural beliefs, individual differences, etc

At the most superficial level are *artifacts*, which are the things that can be observed when one encounters a new group. Artifacts can include clothing and dress, shared language and stories, and important rituals or ceremonies.

At the middle level is what Schein calls *espoused values or justifications*. Espoused values are lessons, beliefs, or strategies that the group arrives at together in response to repeated trial-and-error periods. Through these periods, the group develops a shared belief about things that work or lead to successful outcomes and those that do not. Individuals and leaders are particularly influential in shaping espoused values, especially if the group eventually perceives their recommendations as having been successful. In this way, a head athletic trainer has significant influence over the culture of his or her athletic training facility, just as a coach has significant influence over the culture of his or her team.

The last and deepest cultural levels are *basic assumptions*. Basic assumptions are so deeply located with an organization's culture that they are likely unknown to the members of that culture. This makes them very hard to understand, even though they are very influential in shaping the day-to-day behaviors of the members of that culture. In fact, assumptions are so ingrained in our daily decisions that we feel uncomfortable if we are forced to behave in contradictory ways, or if

Figure 1-1. Artifacts are the most easily recognizable component of workplace culture, while basic assumptions are so deeply embedded in the culture they are often hard to recognize.

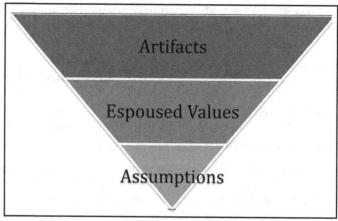

someone around us behaves in such contradictory ways. A well-known cultural researcher took advantage of this fact in order to learn more about the characteristics of culture. He designed what he referred to as "breaching experiments," so named because they were designed to "breach" or violate existing behaviors in order to reveal underlying cultural assumptions.[8]

A well-known example of a breaching experiment involves a common elevator. Think about the last time you rode in an elevator and imagine that the elevator stops and a new passenger boards the elevator with you. What is your expectation for where and how the new rider should situate himself or herself in the elevator? How would you begin to feel if the new rider did not behave in the way you expected? If you are at all like us, your expectation is that the new rider will board the elevator, establish a reasonable amount of space away from you, and then turn and stand so facing the elevator door.

But, what if instead of doing what was expected, the rider boarded the elevator, stood closer to you than necessary given the amount of room on the elevator, and instead of turning to face the door, looked directly at you for the remainder of the ride? Again, if you are like us, you would begin to feel very uncomfortable. You might be so uncomfortable that you would try to move away from the offending rider. You might even ask if there is a problem. Imagine your relief when the elevator ride is over!

These strong feelings of discomfort occur because the rider's behavior violates existing cultural norms and betrays a lack of understanding of the basic assumptions held by members of our society for how to behave in tight, intimate quarters. Those behaviors also violate our cultural understanding of personal space and privacy, which is called *proxemics*. It may be difficult for us to articulate exactly why this behavior felt so wrong to us, but the feelings they produce are still very real and very powerful, even when we can't fully explain them.

Culture serves several important roles within a workplace, but perhaps the most important is that it brings order and social stability to the workplace in what could otherwise be an ambiguous and confusing environment. Think about a typical college/university athletic training facility: While it is true that the culture of each facility has a unique local environment and participant demographics, underlying each facility is the steady cultural stream of the athletic training profession. In other words, what every athletic training facility has in common is an understanding of what it means to be an athletic trainer and to practice athletic training. In this way, the culture of the athletic training profession is a consistent touchstone across all clinical facilities, and helps to generate some level of familiarity and predictability across different facilities.

You may notice this same similarity when you've taken a trip in an airplane. Have you noticed that most flight attendants read the flight announcement in very similar ways, with similar tone or pacing? Or that pilots make announcements in ways that sound surprisingly similar to each other, even when they are pilots from different airlines? These are very simple examples of the power of a professional culture. The similarity and familiarity culture produces is important because in spite of our best attempts, workplaces tend toward complexity, ambiguity, and irrationality.[9]

This brings us to a final point about workplace culture. While some aspects of social structure can be changed relatively quickly, say by changing workplace policy, culture is much more difficult to change. This is largely because culture, with the values, practices, and assumptions that accompany it, are so deeply rooted within a particular workplace (or profession) that participants in that workplace are often completely unaware of existing cultural norms. They know only that those norms create a sense of stability and predictability that makes their life easier to manage. But we must also recognize that existing *socialization processes,* those systems that teach newcomers about the cultural norms of a workplace or a profession, are also difficult to change. For example, in many professions, including athletic training, the most significant contributors to a new athletic trainer's understanding of the culture of the profession are the established didactic (ie, classroom) and clinical education processes. Only recently have athletic training researchers begun to study those processes.[10-12]

WORKPLACE IDENTITY

Another critical concept for understanding the workplace is that of *identity*. There are 2 aspects of identity that are relevant to this discussion. The first is *personal identity*, which is your own sense of who you are or who you want to be or are becoming. The second is *workplace or organizational identity*, which is the identity that you occupy within the workplace and the one for which you are likely paid.[13] In some cases, personal and workplace identities align closely, and a person finds that at work they play a role consistent with how they perceive themselves in everyday life. However, in other cases personal and workplace identity are in conflict, which can be a source of great intra-personal and inter-personal conflict and emotion.

Complicating the situation is a contemporary appreciation for the fact that identities, both personal and workplace, can be fragmented as well as fluid.[14] This means that we may have several different personal and workplace identities that we may swap depending on the situation. The fluidity with which we move from identity to identity is also a product of *concertive control*, meaning that we feel social pressure to adhere to one identity or another, and our choice of identity may be dependent on the specific situation in which we find ourselves.[15] Preferred identities play an important role in influencing the conscious, and to some degree unconscious, choices that we make in our day-to-day lives. Identifying one's preferred identities can provide important insight into the choices we make on a day-to-day basis.[16]

It is also important to note that the interface between workplace culture and identity is a potential source of great emotion. For example, when the culture of the workplace prevents a participant from enacting his or her preferred identity, or forces the participant into an identity with which he or she is uncomfortable, negative emotion, such as stress and anxiety, can result.[14] Such *role strain* can lead to several negative employment outcomes, including burnout, absenteeism, and turnover. Another relevant example involves the idea of *emotional labor*. Emotional labor occurs whenever a person must conceal his or her true emotions and instead display the emotional countenance required or preferred by the workplace.[17] Some occupations are prone to high levels of emotional labor, including health professions, police and corrections officers, and service industry personnel.[17-19] Emotional labor has been linked to high levels of stress, anxiety, and burnout.[18]

THE SOCIAL STRUCTURE OF THE ATHLETIC TRAINING WORKPLACE

What is the "athletic training workplace"? There has been no single answer to that question, even though the athletic training profession places great importance on the setting in which athletic trainers work. Historically, 2 work settings captured the majority of the practicing athletic trainer population: 1) the traditional setting and 2) the clinical setting. The "traditional" setting is often further sub-organized into 3 categories, including secondary school, college/university, and professional. The college/university setting represents the single largest work setting for athletic training members of the National Athletic Trainers' Association (NATA), the national member organization for athletic trainers, with more than 19% of its 32,000 members working in that setting. More recently, alternative athletic training workplaces have emerged. As of October 2014, the NATA identifies 12 active settings in which its members work.[20]

Demographically, the profession is characterized as majority female and majority White, with more than 80% of NATA members identifying themselves as White, non-Hispanic, and slightly more than 53% identifying as female.[20] While these numbers are similar to the sex and ethnicity demographics of other health care professions, they have the potential to vary significantly from the larger environments in which athletic trainers work, where ethnic minority populations may be much larger. And while age is not a measured demographic variable, it is worth noting that more than 25% of NATA members are students, which suggests that professional demographics as represented by NATA membership skew young.

Work settings have served an important organizing mechanism for the profession, and especially through the organizational structure of the NATA. For example, many standing NATA committees are organized around existing work settings as a way of giving voice to the unique needs of the athletic trainers working in these settings. Examples of these committees include the College & University Athletic Trainers' Committee and the Secondary School Athletic Trainers' Committee. These committees also oversee the administration of setting-specific awards, honoring athletic trainers who have earned distinction through practice and service to the setting.

The athletic training workplace is usually composed of a head athletic trainer and associate or assistant athletic trainers. Staff hierarchy and numbers vary greatly nationwide and depend on various factors within the organization such as school size and administrative support. In some settings there may just be one athletic trainer. Regardless of the number of athletic trainers, this group of people (or one person) is a social entity within the organization. Athletic trainers perform tasks that are essential to the organization. The purpose of the athletic training department is goal oriented and is centered on patient care and well-being, which is driven by the NATA code of ethics and the Board of Certification (BOC) Standards of Professional Practice. The organization that the athletic training department is in has its own purpose and goals. In an ideal working environment, the goals of the athletic training department should be in line with the mission and vision statement of the organization. Unfortunately, the goals of the athletic training department are not always in line with that of the organization as a whole and may lead to disputes within the organization. The athletic training department is intentionally structured and comprises individuals with specific certifications. The boundaries of the athletic training department are clear and members are employed through an explicit agreement to be paid and an implicit agreement to keep patients healthy.

From an organizational structure perspective, most collegiate athletic training staffs follow the "athletic model" by which they are housed under the athletic department, and the head athletic trainer reports to an athletic director or assistant athletic director. This can become an unfavorable infrastructure as highlighted by Laursen,[21] as it may negatively affect patient care as well as the overall well-being of the athletic trainer working in such an environment. Unfortunately, many athletic trainers working under "athletic models" don't always feel like they have the authority to challenge a coach, and if they do, they place their jobs at risk, which may link to the quality-of-life issues athletic trainers experience. As professionals, we need to carefully think about entering into any organizational structure where the reporting structure could force an athletic trainer to choose between player safety and his or her job. This is not to say that all "athletic models" have such potential conflict, as there are numerous programs that run smoothly under this reporting structure. However, it is important to know when entering into such an organizational structure whether the athletic trainer has the ultimate say in medical decisions. Some universities have transitioned to alternative models in an effort to improve both patient care and athletic trainer quality of life.[22]

SUMMARY

The purpose of this chapter was to provide a broad overview of several foundational concepts to the understanding of the athletic training workplace. In addition, these concepts serve as a gateway to the student's appreciation for the relevance of the topics addressed in subsequent chapters of this textbook. While these concepts are not specific to the athletic training profession or to the settings in which athletic trainers work, they are essential for understanding workplace dynamics and the behaviors of the participants who are exposed to them.

Athletic trainers work in a variety of settings, though the "traditional" settings of secondary schools, colleges and universities, and professional sports are the most common. Key structural features, such as athletic training demographics, demonstrate that the profession is majority White, non-Hispanic, and female. Historically, the settings in which athletic trainers work have served as important mechanisms for "organizing" the profession, especially through the NATA, as demonstrated in the presence of setting-specific standing committees and awards. However, regardless of the specific setting, issues of structure, culture, identity, and emotion are all salient to understanding the workplace and finding within it both professional success and personal satisfaction.

ACTIVITIES FOR REINFORCEMENT

Questions for Review

1. Identify the 5 key features of a workplace.
2. What is meant by the term social structure? What roles does this play in an organization's culture?
3. What is the difference between workplace identify and personal identity?

Case Vignettes

Case #1

Greg is 1 of 4 assistant athletic trainers working at a large Division III college. The 4 athletic trainers within the sports medicine department report to the head athletic trainer, who then reports directly to the athletic director. Greg is only in his first year at this job but is already feeling unhappy in his role. He does not get along well with the head football coach, who is always second guessing his medical decisions. He recently found out that the head football coach went to the athletic director and asked that Greg be switched to another sport. His head athletic trainer, who has worked at the college for 12 years, has told Greg that next fall he will work with women's soccer instead of football. Greg feels as though he is not getting support from his head athletic trainer and is confident that he has done a good job managing the health and well-being of his football athletes. Greg sought advice from one of his fellow assistant athletic trainers and was told that's just the way things are around here: "The coaches get the final say in everything."

1. What impact could another organizational structure have on Greg's experiences during his first year?

2. What advice would you give to Greg to help manage this situation?

3. How could the leader of the sports medicine department (the head athletic trainer) help Greg resolve this situation?

4. What questions could Greg have asked on his interview that may have helped identify future problems and conflict?

Case #2

You are the director of Athletic Training Services at a large state university with more than 15 years of experience leading a large sports medicine department. Your reputation, and that of your sports medicine services, is impeccable. Your department is widely regarded as a model of best practice for how a sports medicine department should be organized. You have been asked to consult with a mid-sized university that is looking to enhance the culture and effectiveness of its sports medicine services. The medical director who contacted you has concerns that the culture of the athletic training room is contributing to dissatisfaction in the staff and a lower quality of patient care than he expects for his athletes. Though you have never consulted before, you believe that your knowledge and experience could be helpful. You accept the job and are beginning to prepare a plan to guide you when you perform the consultation.

1. Identify examples of relevant cultural artifacts that you will look for when trying to determine the kind of culture. How would you interpret these artifacts?

2. What techniques might you use to gain insight into the espoused values that are held in the sports medicine department you are visiting?

3. Is it possible for you to develop an understanding of the cultural assumptions of the sports medicine department in the brief consulting visit you'll be making? Why or why not?

4. What general advice might you give to the medical director for strategies that may lead to changes in culture?

Discussion Questions

1. How do you believe social media, as a form of technology, has influenced the athletic training workplace?

2. What is an example of a cultural artifact that you have observed in an employment setting?

3. In what way might the goals of an organization run counter to those of the professionals working within it?

REFERENCES

1. Scott WR. *Organizations: Rational, Natural, and Open Systems.* Fifth ed. Englewood Cliffs, NJ: Prentice Hall; 2003.
2. Acker J. Hierarchies, jobs, bodies: A theory of gendered organizations. *Gend Soc.* 1990;4(2):139-158.
3. Bennis WG. *On Becoming a Leader.* Reading, MA: Addison-Wesley Pub. Co; 1989.
4. Northouse PG. *Leadership: Theory and Practice.* 6th ed. Thousand Oaks, CA: Sage Publications; 2012.
5. Abbott AD. *The System of Professions.* Chicago, IL: University of Chicago Press; 1988.
6. Schein E. *Organizational Culture and Leadership.* 2nd ed. San Francisco, CA: Jossey-Bass; 1992.
7. Schein EH. The three levels of culture. In: *Organizational Culture and Leadership.* 4th ed. San Francisco, CA: Jossey-Bass; 2010:23-33.
8. Garfinkel H. *Studies in Ethnomethodology.* Englewood Cliffs, NJ: Prentice-Hall; 1967.
9. March JG, Simon H. *Organizations.* 2nd ed. Cambridge, MA: Blackwell Publishers; 1993.
10. Pitney WA. The professional socialization of certified athletic trainers in high school settings: A grounded theory investigation. *J Athl Train.* 2002;37(3):286-292.
11. Pitney WA. Organizational influences and quality-of-life issues during the professional socialization of certified athletic trainers working in the National Collegiate Athletic Association Division I setting. *J Athl Train.* 2006;41(2):189-195.
12. Pitney WA, Ilsley P, Rintala J. The professional socialization of certified athletic trainers in the National Collegiate Athletic Association division I context. *J Athl Train.* 2002;37(1):63-70.
13. du Gay P. *Consumption and Identity at Work.* Thousand Oaks, CA: Sage; 1996.
14. Giddens A. *Modernity and Self-Identity: Self and Society in the Late Modern Age.* Stanford, CA: Stanford University Press; 1991.
15. Goffman E. *The Presentation of Self in Everyday Life.* New York: Doubleday; 1959.
16. Tracy S. Becoming a character for commerce: Emotion labor, self-subordination and discursive construction of identity in a total institution. *MCQ.* 2000;14:90-128.
17. Ashforth BE, Mael F. Emotional labor in service workers: The influence of identity. *AMR.* 1990;18(1):88-115.
18. Tracy S. *Emotion Labor and Correctional Officers: A Study of Emotion Norms Performances and Unintended Consequences in a Total Institution.* Dissertation Abstracts International, 6107A, 2519 (University Microfilms No. AAI99-79409); 2001.
19. Tracy S. Locking up emotion: Emotion labor and correctional officers. Paper presented at: Annual Meeting of the International Communication Association; 2001; Washington, DC.
20. National Athletic Trainers' Association. Membership statistics. 2014. http://members.nata.org/members1/documents/membstats/index.cfm. Accessed November 25, 2014.
21. Laursen RM. A patient-centered model for delivery of athletic training services. *Athl Ther Today.* 2010;15(3):1-3.
22. Scheid D. Room for change. *NATA News.* 2011;10-14.

Leadership, Management, and Beyond

What to Expect in the Athletic Training Workplace

Matthew R. Kutz, PhD, AT, CSCS, CES

OBJECTIVES

After reading this chapter, the reader will be able to do the following:

1. Distinguish the differences between leadership and management and between leaders and managers.

2. Explain the role of different theories in describing leaders.

3. Describe and compare different theories of leadership.

4. Define followership and identify different types of followers.

5. Synthesize historical leadership research into key guidelines for leadership development.

6. Describe what it means to be an "effective" leader.

7. Explain how transformational leadership differs from transactional leadership, and which behaviors set them apart.

8. Explain how complexity is a necessary element in current and future leadership practice.

INTRODUCTION

In a very real and practical way, leadership is a topic that interests just about everyone around the world regardless of race, color, religion, or origin. Leadership is truly a timeless and global phenomenon. People have always had a vested interest in who is running their government, schools, businesses, religious institutions, and civic organizations. Because of this interest, leadership has become a popular topic. As such, thousands of urban legends and myths about leadership have been propagated by well-intentioned people. Separating the fact from fiction is an extremely time-consuming and arduous task for even the most serious leadership scholars. Therefore, in this

Mazerolle SM, Pitney WA.
Workplace Concepts for Athletic Trainers (pp 15-38).
© 2016 Taylor & Francis Group.

chapter we will attempt to achieve 2 primary outcomes: to outline some of the good information relative to leadership so that you can make well-informed decisions about how to develop it as well as identify it in others. Table 2-1 delineates some of those myths and their reality. Secondarily, to help sort through and organize much of the jargon related to leadership and help describe how leadership is applied and relevant to the workplace.

Athletic trainers find themselves in many different workplace settings. Even within a single setting such as a university, athletic trainers find themselves interacting with faculty in different academic departments, coaches, and administrators in athletic departments, and physicians and nurses in student health service departments. Because of all the different places where athletic trainers are employed, understanding leadership in the workplace is critical, particularly how leadership is practiced and developed. In fact, the athletic training literature suggests that a working understanding of leadership is a must for executing one's professional role.[1]

Leadership is one of the most researched topics in social and organizational behavior, but still the least understood social processes within organizations.[2] The fact is, leadership is a nebulous and polarizing concept. Defining leadership has proven to be a difficult task.[1] There are about as many definitions of leadership as there are people to define it. Leadership includes many nuances and idiosyncrasies and as a result there are thousands of descriptions to consider. However, most experts agree that leadership requires some aspect of influence that is described as the ability to affect the behaviors of others.[1] While there are many caveats, it is *influence* that is the ultimate outcome of leadership.

Athletic training literature defines leadership as the ability to facilitate and influence superiors, peers, and subordinates to make recognizable strides toward shared or unshared objectives.[3] Within this definition is the understanding that leadership is multidirectional and affects followers, peers, and those in influential or formal authority positions. Furthermore, it is suggested that leadership requires movement toward accomplishing predetermined objectives. Sometimes those objectives are set by the leader without input from others and other times they are determined in collaboration. Regardless of who sets the objectives, accomplishing them is an aspect of leadership. From an organizational management perspective, leadership is often described as the process of guiding and directing the behavior of people in the work environment.[2]

Evolution of Leadership

Leadership studies have come a long way from trait-based theories of leadership, which speculated leadership was a divine or innate trait that one was either born with or received from the gods. One of the major advances made in the understanding of leadership is that everything does not necessarily rise and fall on the leader. While it is true that the leader may have ultimate responsibility, it is not only the leader that has sole influence on the practice or process of leadership. Research in contextual intelligence calls this the "leader-follower-context nexus,"[4] where contextual intelligence is described as the "ability to adapt or respond appropriately to any number of different contexts, where the context is determined by environmental factors and stakeholder values."[1] In other words, leadership is a process, not a position; and that process includes followers, the context, as well as the leader.

Leader-Follower-Context Nexus

When exploring how leadership has evolved over time, it is necessary to note that antiquity tends to recognize the leader as the single and dominant variable in the process of leadership. Organizational scientists and workplace engineers are starting to realize, however, that this is simply not true.[5] This does not minimize the role of the leader, but it does acknowledge other

TABLE 2-1	
LEADERSHIP MYTHS	
LEADERSHIP MYTH	**LEADERSHIP REALITY**
1. Good leadership is all common sense.	"Common sense" is a very ambiguous term and not everyone with common sense is a good leader nor is there any evidence to support the notion that common sense is a prerequisite for other leadership behaviors.
2. Leaders are born, not made.	While there may be certain physical or personality-based traits that are innate and correlated with leadership (eg, height, people of above-average height tend to be perceived by others as more of a leader, also people of above-average height tend to have higher self-confidence) there is no evidence to support that people with these traits are always leaders—in fact there is ample evidence to support the notion that people without these traits can also become effective leaders.
3. The only school you can learn leadership from is the school of hard knocks.	Formal study and learning from experience are not mutually exclusive. Experience enhances formal study and formal study enhances experience and one is not necessarily a prerequisite for the other. Both are necessary. The advantage of formal study is that it offers a vantage point of viewing a leadership situation from multiple perspectives—an opportunity that is typically not available in a trial and error situation.
4. Leaders work smarter, not harder.	Leadership, like any other worthwhile pursuit, requires dedication and diligence to develop. Many leaders attest to the fact that their leadership accomplishments were some of the hardest work they have ever done.
5. Great leaders are always in the spotlight.	While it is true that many leaders do occupy the spotlight, the concept of "always" being in the spotlight is false. One of the things that is admired by many great leaders is they share the credit for any accomplishments with their team.
6. The best leaders can solve every problem or have all the answers.	The best leaders have a very clear understanding of their limitations. A major aspect of successful leadership is to develop a team that accommodates their own and the organization's weaknesses. Furthermore, the best leaders are generally very receptive and welcoming of input from others when it comes to problem solving.
7. The person with the title, most rank or the highest position is the leader.	Authentic leadership is based on action and getting things done. Ultimately leadership is about influence, which requires no title or rank. One does not need to be at the top of the organizational hierarchy to be an action-oriented influencer.
8. All great leaders are charismatic.	True, many popular leaders are charismatic, but charisma is not an unqualified prerequisite. Leaders are often followed and respected because of their hard work, integrity, dedication, and character.

(continued)

TABLE 2-1 (CONTINUED) LEADERSHIP MYTHS	
LEADERSHIP MYTH	**LEADERSHIP REALITY**
9. Mimicking a popular leader's style or behavior will make me a better leader.	Obviously, on critical reflection this is a silly sentiment. However, many people are victims of believing that if Abraham Lincoln, Mahatma Gandhi, Winston Churchill, Mother Teresa, Nelson Mandela, Joan of Arc, St Teresa of Avila, Bill Gates, Jack Welch or other popular leaders and chief executive officers behaved this way, then I should too. This sentiment does not stand up under scrutiny, as successful leadership often depends on many variables that were unique to each of these individuals' era and circumstances.

Adapted from Hughes R, Ginnett R, Curphy G. *Leadership: Enhancing the Lessons of Experience.* New York, NY: McGraw-Hill; 2015; and Smith G. *5 myths about leadership.* Burlington, MA: Linkage.com; 2008.

Figure 2-1. Leader-follower-context nexus.

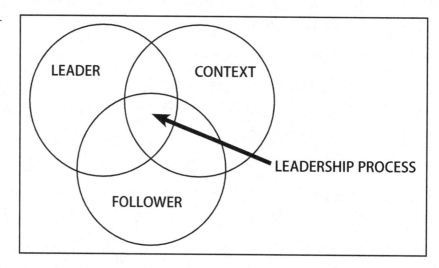

forces that influence how leadership is practiced in the workplace. Context and followers are 2 of those forces. Figure 2-1 shows the relationship of the leader-follower-context nexus.

Context

Context is a component that has a tremendous impact on the process of leadership, especially in the workplace. Context is the background of an event or situation; its meaning comes from the Latin word *contextere*, which means "to weave together." Therefore, context by implication consists of the threads that are interlaced together to fashion a specific situation or circumstance. Some of the "threads" of context include core values, cultural biases, political convictions, religious convictions, people's experiences, people's expectations, people's disappointments, and organizational climate. All of these threads get sewn together to create the context that influences the workplace. One of the ways to navigate the leadership process is to learn how to diagnose the context. Diagnosing the context requires a similar process to diagnosing an injury. To diagnose the context correctly it is necessary to take in relevant information from history about the workplace or industry, real-time observations relative to what is happening in the workplace today, evaluating workplace trends based on hands-on experience or close proximity to the workplace (or similar workplaces), and something akin to special tests like hands-on experience. Understanding and correctly navigating how context influences the leadership process has been called contextual intelligence[1,2,6] and has been reported as a "very important" behavior in the practice of athletic training.[7]

Followership

The other element in this interrelated nexus is *followers*. Followership is the process of being guided and directed by a leader in the work environment.[2] It is analogous to the concept of voluntary submission. The concept of submission is not nearly as nasty a concept as people might be led to believe. In his seminal work, *The Functions of the Executive*, by Chester Barnard,[8] a Harvard-educated organizational sociologist, offered this insight; ". . . the determination of authority lies with the subordinate individual."[8(p167)] Barnard believed that the paradox of submission was that the true authority was held by the follower because the leader could never realize their own authority unless freely given in the form of submission. In other words, the worker could always walk away, find a new job, or find evidence to support their desired course of action. Therefore, because submission could be withdrawn at any time, it in itself was a potent form of power within the workplace dynamic. This is the essence of followership in the contemporary workplace, especially one that involves health care professionals, such as athletic trainers.

Obviously, leader and follower roles differ significantly; someone has to make decisions and someone has to implement those decisions. However, traditional views of followers as passive or unable to coordinate or direct are highly inaccurate. Today's followers are knowledge workers, which stands in direct contrast to the concept of employees as subordinates. According to Avery,[9] knowledge workers are employees who create new information, or are skilled at using knowledge, or possess professional expertise. In other words, knowledge workers are employees who know as much or in some cases even more than their direct supervisor or employer. One example of this is an athletic trainer whose "boss" may be an athletic director. Obviously, as a health care professional the athletic trainer has more working knowledge of injury prevention and care than his "boss," who may know nothing about it.

Obviously the concept of followership has a very profound impact on the leadership process and flow within the workplace. When followers, especially knowledge workers, refuse to participate in the process as delineated by the leader it can cause havoc in the workplace. Therefore, not only should the leader be skilled at motivating followers, but followers themselves need to recognize the process and not make it overly difficult on those with formal titles or rank.

The ideal follower recognizes their interdependence with the leader, respects the leader, but learns to challenge them effectively.[2] Kelley[10] identified 5 types of followers in today's workplace, which are classified on a 2 dimensional continuum; activity to passivity; and critical to uncritical thinkers. These types include effective followers, alienated followers, "yes people" followers, sheep followers, and survivors.[2] Table 2-2 is a list based of the types of followers, based on Kelley's descriptions.

Timeline of Leadership Thinking

Leadership scholar Gayle Avery[9] identified the dominant leadership paradigms throughout history. Her work identifies 4 major paradigms with respect to leadership thinking and philosophy from antiquity to our modern era. The first paradigm she calls the classical or trait paradigm, the second transactional paradigm, the third visionary paradigm, and the fourth the organic paradigm. These paradigms represent popular schools of thought and their era of origin, which can simultaneously exist. For example, different health care organizations around the United States can be found that operate with each of the paradigms. Figure 2-2 is a timeline that follows the dominant leadership paradigms and their main tenets.

	TABLE 2-2 TYPOLOGY OF FOLLOWERS	
FOLLOWER TYPE	**BRIEF DESCRIPTION**	**ATHLETIC TRAINER EXAMPLE**
Effective followers	Active-critical thinkers. They are highly engaged autonomous thinkers who respect authority.	An associate or assistant athletic trainer or athletic trainer student who actively engages in the workplace and contributes time and energy to making the athletic training room and work environment a better place.
Alienated followers	Passive-critical thinkers. They are emotionally distanced from authority, think critically, but act very passively.	An associate or assistant athletic trainer or athletic trainer student who withholds good ideas, energy, and creativity and does not care to offer useful or helpful suggestions.
"Yes people" followers	Active-uncritical thinkers. These workers do not think critically, but are very active; they never challenge the ideas or wisdom of leaders. These are the most dangerous followers because of the likelihood of giving a false-positive reaction to leadership decisions.	An associate or assistant athletic trainer or athletic trainer student who eagerly engages in the workplace, but fails to offer any constructive criticism or new ideas.
Sheep followers	Passive-uncritical thinkers. These workers simply do what they're told without any critical thought.	An associate or assistant athletic trainer or athletic trainer student who does what he or she is told without complaining, but avoids challenging the status quo so as not to be perceived as problems or threats.
Survivors	Non-committal to being active or passive and critical or uncritical. Tend to be the least disruptive and live by the motto "better safe than sorry."	An associate or assistant athletic trainer or athletic trainer student who tries to stay out of the way and "under the radar."

Figure 2-2. Leadership philosophy timeline.

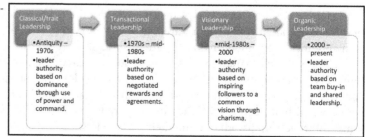

Classical or Trait Paradigm

Classical leadership describes authority that is maintained by a preeminent person or an elite group of people.[9] The authority that they wield is rooted in specific traits that are often considered innate or divine. In classical paradigms orders are rarely if ever questioned and subordinates implement directives out of fear of retaliation or respect for the leader. Within most classical or trait paradigms, the leader is usually autocratic. Autocratic leadership does not take into account the desires of others or consider the consequences their decisions may have on others. Unfortunately, within the contemporary workplace classical models of leadership are still extremely prevalent.

Within athletic training it is very possible (and even likely) that classical models still exist. For example, in athletic training rooms whose dominant culture is based on the athletic tradition of a head coach whose orders are not questioned, it is easy to adopt a "do-it-cuz-I'm-the-boss" attitude, which is based on a classical model. This model persists because it is "easy" to maintain and requires little vulnerability on the part of the leader.

Transactional Paradigm

In the 1970s classical models of leadership became irrelevant. It was also in the 1970s that the newer fields of management and organizational behavior gained popularity. Transactional leadership—more accurately called management—focused more on the individuality of followers as well as followers' skills, but still retained autocratic tendencies within the upper echelons of workplace hierarchy. The distinguishing characteristic of the transactional paradigm was that employer and employee entered into a contract or an agreement whereby the employer agreed to provide something, typically a salary, benefits, and training, in exchange for a certain amount of work, typically 40 hours a week, from an individual. One of the weaknesses of this model was that many employees did not feel a sense of ownership in their work nor were they incentivized to be innovative or creative.

Visionary Paradigm

One of the major drawbacks of the previous 2 paradigms (classical and transactional) was their inability to flourish in a VUCA world. A VUCA world is one that is volatile, uncertain, complex, and ambiguous.[11] In other words, the former paradigms worked only in times of stability, predictability, or when change was very slow,[9] which is unlike many work settings in athletic training. In the mid-1980s the visionary paradigm gained prominence, most likely because of the recognition of the phenomenon called globalization. Globalization is the integration of different world views, products, ideas, and cultures from around the world. It was then that people began to realize that the failure to navigate VUCA conditions in the workplace was attributed to too much management and not enough leadership.[12] This spawned the advent of the visionary leader. The visionary paradigm is characterized by leaders who are able to instill trust in their employees, demonstrate high levels of charisma, provide inspiration, and facilitate win-win problem solving. It was a valuable contribution to the process of leadership in a VUCA workplace.

Within the visionary paradigm the concept of transformational leadership came to the forefront of leadership thinking. Originally conceptualized by James McGregor Burns[4] in 1978, it wasn't until 1985 that Bernard Bass' book[13] *Leadership and Performance* popularized it. Later others, including Bass, began to describe 4 factors of transformational leadership.[14]

1. *Idealized influence* (or charisma) describes leaders as role models to be emulated.

2. *Inspirational motivation* is the capacity of the leader to inspire followers by communicating high but attainable expectations.

3. *Intellectual stimulation* is the capacity of the leader to facilitate creativity and innovation in followers.

TABLE 2-3 BEHAVIORS OF TRANSFORMATIONAL LEADERS	
TRANSFORMATIONAL BEHAVIOR	**DESCRIPTION OF BEHAVIOR**
Model the way	Leaders hold firm to the conviction that their attitudes and behaviors do in fact make a difference. Leaders identify how people prefer to be treated then create workplace standards based on those preferences. Furthermore, the leader serves as a living example and reminder of how those standards should be carried out in the workplace and beyond.
Inspire a shared vision	Leaders work tirelessly to create an ideal image of the future that everyone can see. They convince others within their workplace how their corporate and individual contributions are essential to accomplishing that ideal image. Leaders are able to excite and inspire others about the opportunities in front of them.
Challenge the process	Leaders are the main champion for disrupting the status quo. They are constantly looking for ways to improve and innovate and are willing to take experiments and risk toward that end.
Enable others to act	Leaders create and facilitate teams. They view their role as motivating and inspiring others to join in their efforts not for the extrinsic rewards, but the intrinsic reward that comes with a job well done. Leaders strive to help individuals feel as if they are valuable contributors to any desired outcomes.
Encourage the heart	Leaders work hard to keep morale high; part of that requires sharing in the rewards when goals are attained. Leaders identify and exploit the intrinsic motivation of each individual on the team and celebrate team and individual accomplishments. They strive to help people feel as if they are indispensable to the workplace or corporate mission.

Adapted from Kouzes JM, Posner BZ. *The Leadership Challenge*. San Francisco, CA: Jossey-Bass; 2007.

4. *Individualized consideration* represents a leader who is actively engaged in and supportive of the individual needs of followers. One of the underlying assumptions of transformational leaders is that it is wrong—or at least inefficient—to treat everyone the same.

However, it was Kouzes and Posner's seminal book,[15] *The Leadership Challenge*, that forever changed how transformational leadership is practiced. They introduced 5 behaviors of a transformational leader, which include modeling the way, inspiring a shared vision, challenging the process, enabling others to act, and encouraging the heart.[15] A summary of these behaviors are highlighted in Table 2-3.

Organic Paradigm

Once organizational leaders embraced the concept that leadership was needed for volatile and unpredictable situations and that management was useful in stable and predictable conditions, it wasn't long until the next phase of leadership thinking gained prominence. Coming into the

21st century was the organic paradigm of leadership thinking.[9] Since the VUCA world was a place without boundaries and rich in cultural and ethnic diversity, leadership needed to evolve to accommodate this new reality. Organic leadership includes cross-functional workgroups, team leadership, self-managing workgroups, leaderless organizations, and grass roots leadership emergence—rather than conventional promotions, extensive hiring practices, and seniority-based appointments. Most notably the organic paradigm is one that embraces the concept of organizational complexity.

COMPLEX VERSUS COMPLICATED WORKPLACES

Complexity-based models offer insights into workplace dynamics that are organic and knowledge driven.[16] Complexity is an important consideration for the workplace in the 21st century and beyond, especially in health care. There are few other industries more complex than healthcare. Complexity, as it pertains to the workplace, can be defined as the state or quality of being irreducibly interconnected and nuanced. The idea of a complex workplace is distinguished from one that is complicated.[6]

Since the discoveries of Sir Isaac Newton in the 17th century, most people—especially in Europe and North America—believed in a predictable, linear, and sequential world. Establishing or maintaining order and structure were priorities of leaders in every sector, which drove people to compartmentalize and categorize almost everything, consequently breaking apart their natural interconnectedness. In a sense, the world became complicated. Navigating that world required a view of the world where everything could be compartmentalized, isolated, or broken down to its smallest component part. The idea of a complicated workplace was prominent in classical, transactional, and visionary paradigms of leadership, and could be described relative to the number of parts (eg, stakeholders or departments) it had internally. It was believed that a complicated workplace could be understood by disassembling it and observing behavior in isolation—this thinking is still prominent in many management-based mindsets. As a closed system, a complicated workplace had little need to consider external variables. Therefore, even a traditional SWOT analysis (strengths, weaknesses, opportunities, and threats) had limited effectiveness, because the primary focus tended to be strengths and weaknesses—it lacked a 360-degree perspective.

On the other hand, a complex workplace, which also has many parts, includes external influences. Complex workplaces cannot be reduced to component parts. Instead of examining things in isolation, it is understood that workplace dynamics are best explored holistically. Therefore, problem solving and even leadership require a completely different mindset, which is why knowledge workers and team-based leadership are so important to this paradigm. The anthem of complex workplaces is that the whole is greater than the sum of its parts. Athletic trainers need to begin to consider their workplaces complex, as opposed to complicated. When that fundamental change occurs it should be followed by a different way of thinking when it comes to navigating complex workplaces. Table 2-4 is a comparison of complex versus complicated thinking. Non-Newtonian thinking is one way to appreciate the complexity of the workplace. That can be manifested in 2 ways, embracing chaos and 3-dimensional (3D) thinking.

The Role of Chaos in the Workplace

Different chaos theories have emerged in recent years offering a new way to understand the current leadership environment.[17] Few people have had more significant contribution in conveying the necessity of chaos than Margaret Wheatley.[18] Her main premise was that our understanding of organization and order are outmoded and that a true understanding of science reveals the world—and the workplaces in it—is much more chaotic than we would like to believe.[18] She concluded that many of our organizations mimic the chaos of the natural world. Therefore, workplace dynamics

TABLE 2-4 COMPLEX VERSUS COMPLICATED THINKING	
NATURE OF COMPLICATED THINKING	**NATURE OF COMPLEX THINKING**
Considers many independent parts	Considers many related parts
Outliers are eliminated and considered irrelevant	Outliers have a meaningful impact on decision making
Problems are reduced down to their smallest component parts	Problems are considered holistically and not reduced down to smaller component parts
Closed and unresponsive to outside influences (static)	Open and responsive to outside influences (fluid)
Problems are isolated and quarantined—kept secret	Problems are shared opportunities to change—shared
Component parts can be extracted and analyzed apart from the whole	Component parts are related and cannot be analyzed in isolation
Change is resisted because it means getting "new parts"	Change is welcomed because existing parts get more value

were not beyond our control or out of control, but merely signposts of our failure to understand the nuances of workplace dynamics.[18]

The term *chaotic*, however, poses a problem for many of us. "Chaos" is an unfortunate casualty of its name; it conjures up images of disorder, randomness, or confusion. To the contrary, what is often labeled chaos is a pattern that hasn't been recognized yet.[19] The irony of chaos is that while it is non-linear and unpredictable, it is patterned and non-random.[6] Typically we are in such close proximity to what needs to be solved that we cannot recognize the pattern that is taking shape. It is not until we step back and remove ourselves from the immediacy of a situation that we see its pattern. It is this phenomenon that is behind the axiom, "hindsight is 20/20." In other words, chaos is necessary in the workplace because it forces us—if we are determined to be resilient—to step back and take a look at the bigger picture or wait until the pattern emerges. Chaos is necessary in the workplace because it reminds us that not every outcome or pattern manifests immediately. Think of it in terms of the research hierarchy within an evidence-based practice model. You could use a case study to make a decision about an appropriate plan of action or you could use a meta-analysis. Chaos is more like the meta-analysis, which is a statistical method for contrasting and combining results from several research studies, it takes more time to develop, but has a much broader scope and reveals more nuances. It offers a more complete picture than a case study. Understanding that things (workplace and life) are chaotic reminds us of the necessity to navigate through the appearance of randomness or nonlinearity so as not to prematurely apply a solution, which will likely end up inappropriate or inadequate. Figure 2-3 is a graphic representation of how embracing chaos may impact the workplace. Note the differences between a traditional workplace hierarchy and organic hierarchy.

Three-Dimensional Thinking

In addition to correctly understanding chaos, there are other concepts that can help athletic trainers in the contemporary workplace embrace complexity. One additional concept requires

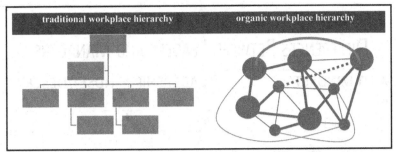

Figure 2-3. Workplace hierarchy comparisons. (Adapted from Kutz MR. Leadership factors for athletic trainers. *Athl Ther Today.* 2008;13(4):15-20.)

adjusting one's default *time orientation* to include 3D thinking. Simply put, 3D thinking is a way to approach decision making by simultaneously using hindsight, insight, and foresight.[6] Time orientation is the frame of mind a leader holds relative to the past, the present, and the future. There is a significant body of literature that stresses the importance of time orientation as it relates to leadership.[4,6] The general consensus of this body of literature implies that leaders use the past, present, and future differently and sometimes sporadically in their decision making. Three-dimensional thinking suggests that the time orientation—and the application of hindsight, insight, and foresight—become a focal point of workplace dynamics. **Hindsight** is the ability to use past experiences to their full advantage, and answers the question, how have my experiences contributed to where I am or want to be? **Insight** is about understanding what is currently influencing workplace dynamics, and answers the question, what is influencing my attitudes and behaviors about what I can do right now to move toward an ideal future? And finally, **foresight** is the ability to accurately articulate a realistic plan for the future. Operating in foresight requires one to be able to articulate an answer to the question, how would I describe the ideal future? The key is addressing each of these elements of time orientation proportionately and maybe even simultaneously. In other words, one should always consider all three and avoid disproportionately emphasizing one over another.

DIFFERENCES BETWEEN LEADERSHIP AND MANAGEMENT

Are there recognizable differences between leadership and management? If that question was asked 30 or more years ago, the answer would have likely been, "no," followed by an explanation that they are one and the same, or any differences were purely semantics. If that question was asked 20 to 25 years ago, the answer would have been, "the jury is still out." Today, if you ask that question, the likely answer is, "yes, they are different." Table 2-5 is a list of some of those differences.

Abraham Zaleznik,[20] Harvard business professor, proposes that leaders have distinct personalities that stand in direct contrast to the personality of managers. Albeit less extreme, Kotter[21] suggests that leadership and management are complementary, yet remain distinct. Likewise, athletic training literature[3] suggests that the 2 concepts are distinct, but should be integrated together. This begs the question, what has changed in the last several decades to warrant a shift in thinking away from the 2 being synonymous to being separate? While it may not be possible to address every issue relevant to that question, there are some reasons why the shift has occurred. Some more pertinent to athletic training include a new understanding about who can lead or demonstrate leadership behaviors and, perhaps most significant, the changing workplace dynamics. We will discuss in more detail each of these reasons in the following sections.

TABLE 2-5	
DIFFERENCES BETWEEN LEADERS AND MANAGERS	
MANAGEMENT MINDSET/ DESCRIPTION	**LEADERSHIP MINDSET/DESCRIPTION**
Views role as an administrator	Views role as an innovator
Maintain/accept the status quo	Upset/challenge the status quo
Tends to control people	Aspires to inspire people
Short-term view in problem solving	Long-term view in problem solving
Imitates desirable traits	Originates what is needed
Believes goals rise out of necessity and reality	Believes goals rise from desire and imagination
Seeks to minimize or mitigate risk	Embraces risk as an essential component of growth
Separates work activity from personal or private activities	Integrates work activity into personal and private life
Advocates for stability	Advocates for change
Embraces complication, thinks compartmentally	Embraces and engages complexity, thinks holistically
Is useful in times of stability, when change or opportunity is predictable	Is useful in times of instability, when change or opportunity is unpredictable
Influences by means of enforcing rules, policy, and procedure	Influences by means of transformational behaviors

Who Can Be a Leader?

Not long ago leadership (or management) was considered a privilege for only a select few. The prevailing wisdom in today's workplace is that everybody can lead something. Of course, there is still a distinction between formal leadership positions, like chief executive officer (CEO), owner, head athletic trainer, president, but generally speaking as leadership has become more associated with influence, the everyday rank-and-file employee is expected to influence something. Coinciding with this subtle shift—that leadership is influence and not a title or position—was a competency-based model of leadership. In other words, leadership was no longer a trait or gift someone possessed, but a set of behaviors someone demonstrated. This new understanding began to drive a wedge between the concepts of leadership and management. As more and more leadership behaviors were identified, it became possible for more and more people to develop them. This in turn led to more and more people being expected to practice them. In an effort to encourage the practice of these newly discovered leadership competencies (or behaviors), it became necessary to promote the idea that anybody and everybody can demonstrate them if given the proper training and opportunity.

In the contemporary workplace, while there are some exceptions to the rule, generally speaking it is commonly accepted that anybody can at least demonstrate leadership behaviors. It should be noted that it is still widely accepted that not everybody can be a leader—in the sense that they occupy a formal leadership position. What has not changed is that there still remains the need to have somebody in a position at whom the proverbial "buck" stops. In other words, you cannot have 2 head athletic trainers—or 2 managers—in the same workplace, but you can have 2 athletic trainers who are leaders in the same workplace.

Leadership Behaviors for Athletic Trainers

This competency-based model to leadership has found its way into athletic training. As a competency-based health care profession, it is a natural phenomenon. What are some of the athletic training behaviors that have been associated with—or deemed important for—athletic training practice? Athletic training research[7] has identified several leadership behaviors important for athletic training practice. Demonstrating these behaviors does not guarantee that you will become a director of sports medicine or head athletic trainer, but developing and demonstrating them can help facilitate the perception of leadership. Furthermore, there is some athletic training evidence to suggest that demonstrating leadership behaviors has a positive influence on different patient outcomes and clinical competency.[1] See Table 2-6 for a list and descriptions of leadership behaviors important for athletic training practice.[7]

Changing Workplace Dynamics

The other major contribution to the shift in thinking concerning differences between management and leadership is the changing context of the workplace. Three decades ago, phrases like, "don't take work home with you," or "don't bring your personal problems to work" were very common. The idea behind this was based in a *complicated mindset* that work-life and home-life could be separated or equally balanced. Today those sentiments almost seem ludicrous, especially in athletic training. Work-life-balance research has demonstrated that one's life cannot be sufficiently isolated between different contexts.[22] In other words, there is no equal "balance," in the contemporary workplace, work-life balance is out; and work-life integration is in. The idea that you can isolate aspects of life apart from another would be to perpetuate what Kanter[8] referred to as the myth of separate spheres. Try to tell a female athletic trainer who just had a baby, and also has 2 other school-age children, that the start of basketball season will not affect her home life. Furthermore, today's contemporary worker—athletic trainer or not—is essentially on-call 24 hours a day, 7 days a week. Smart phones, instant messaging, Skype® (Skype Technologies S.A.) and FaceTime® (Apple Inc.) were all science fiction in the 1970s. Today they are realities that require leadership skills to navigate. Some might be tempted to believe the best solution is to implement policies that no smart phones or personal emails are allowed at work, etc—in an attempt to reduce chaos or isolate a problem—but that is proven to not be effective. In a true sense of Darwinian survival—today's workplaces' complexity-based self-organizing ecosystems—smart phones, emails, etc have become essential to the contemporary workplace.

Further driving a wedge between management and leadership is that experience is evolving and being redefined. With the advent of evidence-based practice, experience isn't what it used to be, nor is it acquired the same way. No more does one need 30 years of experience to know the best treatment plan for a particular injury. Today, there is ample information available at our fingertips. The arrival of the VUCA world and necessity of non-Newtonian thinking has had a tremendous impact on the workplace, which continues to drive a wedge between management and leadership. None of these contemporary workplace concepts would be possible without the foundational work of early management scientists.

Management Science

In those early years of management science—at the turn of the 20th century—people like Frederick W. Taylor, the father of scientific management, advanced many ideas that are still used today. For example, Taylor promoted the idea that any responsibility ultimately rested with the manager and that subordinates are motivated only by extrinsic factors such as wages or the fear of discipline. Henry Fayol outlined 5 foundational tenets of management, which included planning,

TABLE 2-6

LEADERSHIP BEHAVIORS IMPORTANT FOR ATHLETIC TRAINING PRACTICE

LEADERSHIP BEHAVIOR	BRIEF DESCRIPTION
Advances knowledge	Contributes to professional advancement by promoting and participating in research or scholarship-related activities (peer reviews, abstracts, conferences, etc)
Advocates	Takes responsibility for actions of others and when necessary defends actions of others
Ambitious	Uses intrinsic and extrinsic resources to promote professional and personal development
Applies knowledge	Uses clinical evidence, research, and best practices in the promotion of the profession
Assertive	Proactive about new ideas, innovations, and change initiatives while maintaining respect for personal boundaries and rights of others
Change agent	Has the bravery to raise difficult and challenging questions that others may perceive as a threat to the status quo.
Collaborator	Effectively participates with other professionals within the local community and achieving goals.
Communicates well—verbally	Verbally articulates thoughts and ideas accurately, effectively, and succinctly to others
Communicates well—written	Writes thoughts and ideas effectively and succinctly
Communitarian	Expresses concern about social trends and issues and volunteers in social and community activities
Competent	Knows, understands, and is capable of performing the details and demands of tasks and roles specific to athletic training
Consensus builder	Exhibits interpersonal skill (eg, active listening, conflict management) and convinces other people to see the common good or a different point of view for the sake of the workplace
Contextual intelligence	Appropriately interprets and reacts to changing and volatile surroundings
Controls risk	Implements quality management strategies and risk management techniques to continuously improve care. Seeks to improve quality while simultaneously mitigating risk
Courageous	Has strong convictions and holds to convictions when faced with challenges
Credible	Is believable, honest, trustworthy, and ethical in dealings with others
Crisis management	Effectively handles unforeseen crises and limits or corrects problems in a reasonable amount of time; copes with conflict by providing effective strategies for conflict resolution

(continued)

TABLE 2-6 (CONTINUED)
LEADERSHIP BEHAVIORS IMPORTANT FOR ATHLETIC TRAINING PRACTICE

LEADERSHIP BEHAVIOR	BRIEF DESCRIPTION
Critical thinker	Makes practical connections, integrates concepts, and makes practical application of different actions, opinions, and information
Cultural sensitivity	Promotes diversity in multiple contexts and aligns diverse individuals by promoting opportunities for diverse members to interact
Dedicated	Has desire and energy in the discipline to achieve goals
Delegates effectively	Appropriately gives responsibility and authority to others in accomplishing desired tasks
Disciplined	Is consistent and steady in performing unpleasant or mundane tasks that produce long-term benefits
Effective use of body language	Uses nonverbal cues effectively and appropriately when communicating to others
Effective use of influence	Uses interpersonal skills, personal power, and influence to constructively and effectively affect the behaviors of others
Emotionally stable	Handles and manages stress associated with leadership roles. Exhibits a cool, calm, and relaxed demeanor even in the face of crisis or diversity
Empathetic	Demonstrates concern for the personal and professional lives of coworkers and patients. Takes risks on behalf of team members
Empowerment	Uses influence in interpersonal ability to promote and encourage personal growth of others
Ethical	Promotes team practices of ethical behavior in the treatment of patients and pursuit of organizational and personal goals and objectives
Flexible	Adapts to and copes well with unforeseen changes or volatile circumstances
Flexible leader	Demonstrates the ability to implement and transition between varieties of leadership styles when appropriate. Is able to identify when it is appropriate to transition between leadership styles/techniques
Future minded	Has a forward-looking mentality and sense of direction and concern for where the organization and others should be in the future
Identifies leaders/mentor	Identifies leadership attributes in emerging leaders and takes the initiative to facilitate their development
Improves morale	Facilitates and encourages a positive attitude and others toward their work and life
Influencer	Uses interpersonal skills to ethically and non-coercively affect the actions and decisions of others
Innovative	Produces plausible or useful ideas when asked or needed by others

(continued)

	TABLE 2-6 (CONTINUED)
	LEADERSHIP BEHAVIORS IMPORTANT FOR ATHLETIC TRAINING PRACTICE
LEADERSHIP BEHAVIOR	**BRIEF DESCRIPTION**
Intentional leadership	Assesses and evaluates own leadership performance and is aware of strengths and weaknesses. Takes intentional action toward leadership development. Has an action guide and delineated goals for achieving personal best
Mature	Handles scrutiny and criticism professionally and with tact
Mission minded	Understands and communicates how individual performance of others and self influences the perception of how the mission is being accomplished
Multicultural leadership	Can influence and affect the behaviors and attitudes of others in ethnically diverse contexts
Nurtures professional relationships	Builds relationships with other members of the health care community that are advantageous to others in the workplace
Open-minded	Willingness to discard old ways of doing things when evidence fails to support them
Organizationally savvy	Carefully observes the environment and people, participates in fulfilling the needs of the organization and industry, and interacts effectively with people in and outside the organization
Protector	Provides a secure environment, tending to others carefully, and prevents indiscretions
Resilient	Recovers from or adjusts easily to misfortune or change
Responsible	Has a strong sense of duty and dependability in different situations and roles
Risk oriented	Willing to accept a degree of uncertainty for the sake of implementing an idea or a needed value, or to see a goal accomplished
Time management	Makes use of processes and tools that increase efficiency and sets parameters for availability to others

Adapted from Kutz M. Leadership in athletic training: implication for practice and education in allied health care. *J Allied Health*. 2010;39(4):265-279.

organizing, commanding, coordinating, and controlling. His major contribution was the division of labor in the centralization of workplace governance. His ideas became known as the "command and control" style of management, which is still used extensively in the military and other bureaucratic organizations. Mary Parker Follett was also an early pioneer of management science. She introduced the notion that certain elements of management could be democratic and that employees may be motivated by things other than wages or punishment.

Peter Drucker introduced the concept of management by objectives (MBO), which included the idea that management and labor could work together to determine workplace objectives. His ideas were among the first to include collaboration between management and labor. However, the biggest contribution to the shift in thinking regarding leadership and management being the same or different coincided with a shift in workplace dynamics.

Integrating Management and Leadership in Athletic Training

While the 2 concepts (management and leadership) are generally accepted as distinct, both are necessary when operating an athletic training facility.[23] Leaders and managers project power, have influence and authority, and set goals. In other words, many of their outcomes can be similar. The differences become more obvious when you look at methods and motivation. For example, leaders tend to use vision casting, alignment, meaningful communication, self-reflection, and self-assessment to develop willing followers. On the other hand, management tends to use planning, organizing, controlling and coordinating, and consider to a lesser extent a follower's willingness.[1] Ronald Heifetz[24] states that leadership is necessary when problems are novel or new. The basis of his claim is that novel or new problems require creativity and innovation, something for which the managerial mind is not naturally equipped. On the other hand, he suggests that management is best suited to handle recurring problems because managers are experts at implementing policy and procedure. This in no way should be construed to imply one is better or more necessary than the other. Both are essential to a properly functioning workplace.

Within the athletic training context an integration of leadership skills and management skills is best for a highly functioning athletic training workplace.[1,7,23] For example, if an athletic trainer has a high degree of management skill and a lower level of leadership skill, the workplace suffers because of a propensity to maintain the status quo. On the other hand, if the athletic trainer has a high degree of leadership skill and a low degree of management ability, the workplace suffers because of a propensity to move forward too quickly or a failure to address uncertainty. The best scenario is for the athletic trainer to have a developed capacity to use leadership behaviors when appropriate and management techniques when necessary.

Leadership Research in Athletic Training

Leadership science is an emerging area within athletic training. As the profession continues to grow it is important that it become foundational to our practice and education of future professionals. Other health care professions such as nursing, physical therapy, pharmacology, and medicine have rich repositories of empirical evidence relative to leadership behaviors to inform their practice. While leadership science is a newer concept in athletic training, it is not absent. In 1994 Nellis[23] was one of the first to differentiate leadership and management within athletic training. In 2007 Laurent and Bradney[25] identified transformational leadership behaviors unique to athletic training program directors and the differences between program directors and head athletic trainers' leadership style. In 2008 Kutz and Scialli[26] identified specific leadership content that is necessary for inclusion in athletic training education, and in 2010 Kutz[7] identified specific leadership competencies important for athletic training practice.

TRADITIONAL LEADERSHIP THEORIES AND CONCEPTS

Leadership thinking has been evolving quickly with several fundamental changes occurring since the 1970s. Recently it has evolved to include a broader understanding of vision, teamwork, emergence, learning and development, and organizational complexity. There are many ways to categorize leadership and as a result several different theories have emerged. In this section we will identify and briefly describe some of the more pertinent leadership theories.

Trait and "Great Man" Theories

The trait theory of leadership is the one theory that has survived the longest. The basic tenet of this theory is that there are innate or learned qualities or distinguishing traits believed to contribute to effective leadership. In this model, traits are determined or discovered by in-depth exploration into the behaviors of iconic social, political, corporate, religious, and military leaders. A short list of such leaders include Joan of Arc, Mahatma Gandhi, Abraham Lincoln, Napoleon Bonaparte, Martin Luther King Jr, Jesus, Winston Churchill, George Washington, Bill Gates, Jack Welsh, the Dalai Lama, and Steve Jobs. This theory is propagated today, even though there is little empirical evidence to support it, by a plethora of books that tout the "leadership secrets of *so-and-so*." It was originally believed that people were born with these traits and that only "great" people possessed them.[27] It wasn't until the mid-20th century that researchers began to challenge the notion that there is no consistent set of traits that differentiate leaders from nonleaders.[27] Despite the lack of evidence, the trait theory of leadership has many ardent followers today. Some—this is a short list—traits that have been popularized as being possessed by great leaders include the following:

- Integrity
- Self-confidence
- Determination
- Intelligence
- Persistence
- Masculinity
- Extroversion

While few people would argue that leaders should possess some or all of these qualities, it is yet to be determined if these are universal and hold true in every situation or circumstance. One of the major weaknesses of this theory is the failure to produce a definitive list of traits and the apparent endless number of traits identified. Not only are these traits highly subjective, they fail to take context into account.

Contingency Theory

While there are other theories that can be considered contingency-based theories (eg, situational leadership theory or Path-goal theory), contingency theory is also standalone theory, developed by Frederick Fielder. In its most basic form, contingency theory is about fitting the leader's style to the appropriate setting. Whether they know it or not, it is the contingency model that influences certain people's ideas that only an athletic trainer with a certain disposition can work effectively with a particular sport or in a particular setting. In other words, if you believe that only strong and assertive personality types will be successful in a head athletic trainer role at a major university, then you are a contingency theorist. A contingency theorist tries to select leaders based on the fit between the leader's style and the setting's demands. In other words, success is *contingent* on the leader's style fitting the setting.[27]

Situational Leadership Theory

Situational leadership theory is one of the more popular approaches to leadership; it was developed by Hersey et al.[28] Having gone through several iterations over the last few decades, situational leadership, as the name implies, focuses on the specific situation in which a leader is asked to perform. The basic tenet is that an effective leader changes his or her style when necessary to accommodate the demands of a particular situation. In this theory the leader needs to be skilled at executing several different types of leadership behavior.

Within the situational leadership theory it is believed that the leader should demonstrate different amounts of **directive** and **supportive** behaviors based on an assessment of the follower's competency and commitment relative to a specific task. For example, if an employee is deemed incompetent but highly committed, the leader may adopt a directing style, which gives a high level of direction and a lower level of support. The situational leadership theory identifies 4 leadership styles:

1. **Directive style,** which is categorized by high directive and low support behaviors.

2. **Coaching style,** which is categorized by high directive and high support behaviors.

3. **Supporting style,** which is categorized by high supportive and low directive behaviors.

4. **Delegating style,** which is characterized by low support of and low directive behaviors.

An important aspect of this theory is the ability of the leader to accurately assess the competency and commitment of followers. In other words, the leader must be able to accurately determine if a given follower is able to perform the skills specific to a task (ie, competency or ability) and whether they have the right attitude regarding that task (ie, commitment or willingness). Therefore, all followers theoretically fit into 1 of 4 categories:

1. Willing and able (competent and committed)

2. Willing and unable (competent and uncommitted)

3. Unwilling and able (incompetent and committed)

4. Unwilling and unable (incompetent and uncommitted)

Applying the situational leadership style, it would follow that an employee who is unwilling and unable would need to be coached, whereas you could delegate to an employee who was willing and able.

Path-Goal Theory

Path-goal theory centers on a leader's ability to motivate followers. Among the main proponents of this theory are House and Aditya.[29] Path-goal theory is related to expectancy theory, which suggests followers are motivated when they believe they can do what is being asked of them or if they believe their efforts will be rewarded.[27] Within the Path-goal model, it is up to the leader to find the best way to motivate followers or groups. The basic idea behind the Path-goal model is for the leader to follow a specific sequence of actions:

1. Define goals for the follower.

2. Verify the path for the follower to take in accomplishing those goals.

3. Remove any obstacles in the path of the followers as they move forward.

4. Provide support to followers as they move along the path.

Servant Leadership

Servant leadership is a theory that originated with Robert Greenleaf[30] and has been a theory of interest for leadership scholars for at least 4 decades. Ironically, the basic tenet behind the servant leadership theory is that the leader takes on the role of a servant, which is counterintuitive to the traditional understanding of leadership. Servant leadership emphasizes the leader's responsibility to the needs and issues of his or her followers and requires a high level of empathy and a strong capacity to nurture followers. In essence, the authentic servant leader puts followers first and his or her own personal or organizational ambitions subsequent. The simplest description of servant leaders is one who places the interests and development of followers above their own. Finally, there is an extremely high ethical responsibility of the leader relative to how he or she handles all resources. While there is an ethical responsibility all leaders must adhere to regardless of the philosophy or theory espoused, servant leadership places ethics at a premium. Some characteristics cited of servant leaders include[31]:

- **Active listening**—sends and receives messages well.
- **Empathy**—attempts to see the world from another person's point of view.
- **Healing**—cares about the well-being of followers and tries to make them feel whole.
- **Community builder**—fosters the development and perception of community.
- **Commitment to the growth of people**—treats each person as unique with intrinsic value beyond their capacity to contribute.
- **Persuasion**—communicates in a clear and persistent manner in an attempt to convince others to change.

SUMMARY

Leadership is an extremely nuanced concept. For athletic trainers to be effective leaders, not only must they understand how leadership thinking has evolved from classical, to transactional, to visionary, to organic paradigms, they must also embrace the fact that leadership in the contemporary workplace brings with it a tremendous amount of complexity. The level of complexity requires a new way of thinking, which jettisons a view of leadership in the workplace as complicated and begins to embrace leadership from an organic perspective. Chaos in the athletic training work environment is not the enemy. To be effective leaders in our workplaces and our profession requires the athletic trainer of the future to be able to navigate and appreciate chaos and leverage it as a force for change. Embracing 3D thinking by simultaneously honoring the past, facing the reality of the present, and maintaining a vision of the ideal future is a prerequisite for leadership in today's workplace and beyond. Furthermore, it is necessary that athletic trainers begin to have meaningful discussions on the differences between workplace management (ie, the day-to-day operation of a facility) with the larger, more robust concept of leadership. This includes addressing the issue of who can be a leader and when and where can it be practiced. Leadership behaviors have been identified for athletic trainers that can be practiced anywhere and transcend formal workplace titles and roles. Finally, traditional leadership theories such as traits theory, contingency theory, situational leadership theory, servant leadership theory, and Path-goal theory should be understood and leveraged by athletic trainers to maximize efficiency in the workplace as we move toward a more holistic understanding of leadership.

ACTIVITIES FOR REINFORCEMENT

Questions for Review

1. What is the difference between transformational and transactional leadership?
2. What is the relationship between leadership and followership?
3. Compare and contrast trait leadership with visionary leadership
4. What are the primary differences between leadership and management?
5. What is situational leadership theory and why is it a popular way to view leadership?
6. What are the various styles found within situational leadership?

Case Vignettes

Case #1

Steve is the owner and manager of a community-based sports medicine clinic. His staff includes 2 physical therapists, a massage therapist, and 3 athletic trainers. Steve is a former physical therapist assistant (PTA) who let his PTA license expire while pursuing his athletic training degree. He now has a master's degree in athletic training, is Board of Certification (BOC) certified and state licensed as an athletic trainer. After he completed his athletic training degree, he opened his own clinic and hired a close friend and physical therapist, Jill. Jill was Steve's former supervisor—when he was a PTA—and was influential in encouraging Steve to hire an additional physical therapist and massage therapist, while Steve hired the 3 additional athletic trainers for the sole purpose of having outreach athletic trainers in the local high schools. Steve's business is going very well and he has been able to earn a solid reputation in the community as a quality health care provider and a fair and ethical business owner. Jill, a non-owner but senior partner, is very influential in how the day-to-day clinic is operated. She always has new and innovative ideas to share with Steve and the rest of the staff. In fact, her idea of hiring a massage therapist not only improved the clinical outcomes, but significantly increased revenue. Furthermore, the athletic trainers have proven to be a tremendous asset to the bottom line as well as reliable representation in the community. The one issue were Steve and Jill sometimes clash is the need to have at least one PTA on staff. Steve does not see the need for a PTA, but Jill insists it is necessary since—in her opinion—none of the other athletic trainers understand the nuances of treating patients in a formal clinical setting. Steve is of the opinion that they are very capable, but it is just not part of his business model and does not want to take them out of the community to serve in an "assistant" role. Jill thinks they can serve at least a couple hours a week on rotating or alternating days to help fill some of the assistant duties without compromising Steve's business model, and would be another way to boost revenue. Part of Steve's motivation for keeping his athletic trainers in the community is that he does not want them to perform "assistant" duties and rather than offend them by asking them to perform duties that he believes might be beneath them, he keeps them in an outreach capacity. Steve also does not want to open a can of worms with Jill, by implying or suggesting that certified athletic trainers (ATCs) are "equal" to physical therapists, something he knows is a "soap box" issue for Jill. When asked by Steve, the second staff physical therapist does not seem to care either way. He just goes about his business from day-to-day treating patients as they are assigned to him. For sure, he would appreciate the help if it were available, which is what he tells Jill, but tells Steve he does not think they are necessary for him to perform his duties.

1. What type of follower do you think the second physical therapist is, and in what way?
2. What type of follower do you believe Jill is?
3. What do you think is Steve's dominant leadership paradigm?
4. How might Steve better relate to and communicate with his staff?
5. What are some of the contextual variables that might be contributing to the difference of opinion between Jill and Steve?
   a. What events or experiences do you think informs Jill's position?
   b. What events or experiences do you think informs Steve's position?
6. If you were Jill, how would you approach Steve with your request?
7. If you were Steve, how would you communicate your concerns to Jill?

Case #2

Susan and Adam are senior athletic training students at a large university with a very public and dominant athletic program. In fact, a majority of their sport teams compete for national championships regularly. Both students have ambition to get their master's degrees in athletic training and become head athletic trainers at Division I universities. Both recently took the Board of Certification (BOC) exam and both were successful. Diane, the head athletic trainer at this university, is a typical autocratic leader who runs a tight ship and is noted for saying things such as, "It's my way or the highway in this athletic training room," and other things such as, "When I was a student we lived in the athletic training room and loved it—you should too." Diane is a respected administrator at the university and serves on several leadership committees with her local and national athletic trainers' association. Susan and Adam understand that a recommendation from Diane would go very far, both for admission into graduate school as well as any future job opportunities. Unfortunately, Diane is of the opinion that Susan and Adam are "good enough students," but "slackers" when it comes to being truly dedicated to athletic training. She believes that they repeatedly fail to put in the requisite amount of time necessary to be successful at the D1 level. Diane wants them to succeed and genuinely wishes them the best of luck, but secretly does not believe they have what it takes to put in the time required to be successful at a competitive D1 level; and because of that is hesitant to recommend them to her colleagues. Susan and Adam consistently argue that they meet or exceed every requirement put forth by the clinical education component of the athletic training program. Furthermore, Adam and Susan serve as officers in the athletic training student club, as well as volunteer in several leadership capacities for other extracurricular events and organizations. The other staff athletic trainers are not willing to say anything to Diane about her leadership style, nor are they willing to defend the students, because it always ends up in a lecture about how athletic training education used to be in the "old days" and that these new educational reforms are killing what athletic training really is. The program director for the athletic training program seems to always be getting on Diane's bad side, either by passing on news of new student "work hours" policies or trying to get Diane to understand that times have changed and that athletic training education is different from when they were athletic training students in the early 1980s.

1. According to Diane, what does it mean to be an effective leader?

2. What about Diane's leadership philosophy is problematic, and how would you approach it if you were the program director?

3. Susan and Adam are leaders in their own right and feel obligated to discuss the issue with Diane; how should they approach and communicate to Diane?

4. What are the major conflicts between the paradigms associated with Susan and Adam's leadership philosophy and Diane's leadership philosophy?

5. What type(s) of followers do you think the staff athletic trainers are, and in what way?

6. Put yourself in the shoes of the staff athletic trainers; would you speak up to Diane, why or why not?

Discussion Questions

1. Within your current athletic training environment, how do you see the leader-follower-context nexus working?

2. Which leadership theory sounds most appealing to you, and why?

3. If you had to explain the difference between management and leadership to a junior high class, what would you say about it?

4. Explain how chaos is not necessarily a bad thing and how it could be useful to bring about necessary change.

5. Which of the 4 prominent leadership paradigms do you believe is creating the culture within your current athletic training program, and why? Give examples.

6. Imagine yourself as the head athletic trainer: How would you reconcile the different types of skills needed for effective management of the facility and program (eg, staff and student schedules, coverage for teams practices, preceptor supervision, budgets, facility maintenance) and the skills needed for successful leadership of the staff and students (eg, motivation, inspiration, empathy, change)?

7. Using Table 2-6 (important leadership behaviors for athletic training practice), identify your top 5 leadership behaviors and your lowest 5 leadership behaviors.

   a. What did you do to develop your top 5?

   b. What specific action steps can you take to improve your lowest 5?

REFERENCES

1. Kutz M. A review and conceptual framework for integrating leadership into clinical practice. *Athl Train Educ J.* 2012;7(1):182-193.
2. Nelson D, Quick J. *Understanding Organizational Behavior.* Belmont, CA: Cengage; 2011.
3. Kutz M. *Leadership and Management in Athletic Training: An Integrated Approach.* Baltimore, MD: Lippincott, Williams & Wilkins; 2010.
4. Kutz M, Bamford-Wade A. Understanding contextual intelligence: a critical competency for today's leaders. *E:CO.* 2013;15(3):55-80.
5. Hughes R, Ginnett G, Curphy G. *Leadership: Enhancing the Lessons of Experience.* New York: McGraw-Hill; 2015.
6. Kutz M, Bamford-Wade A. Contextual intelligence: A critical competency for leading in complex environments. In Erbe ND, ed. *Approaches to Managing Organizational Diversity and Innovation.* Hershey, PA: IGI Global; 2014.
7. Kutz M. Leadership in athletic training: implication for practice and education in allied health care. *J Allied Health.* 2010;39(4):265-279.
8. Barnard C. *The Functions of the Executive.* Cambridge, MA: Harvard University Press; 1968.
9. Avery G. *Understanding Leadership.* London: Sage; 2004.
10. Kelley R. In praise of followers. *HBR.* 1988;66:142-148.
11. Johansen R. *Leaders Make the Future: Ten New Leadership Skills for an Uncertain World.* San Francisco, CA: Jossey-Bass; 2009.
12. Kotter JP. What leaders really do. *HBR.* 1990;68;103-111.
13. Bass B. *Leadership and Performance.* NY: Free Press; 1985.
14. Bass B, Riggio R. *Transformational Leadership.* Mahwah, NJ: Lawrence Erlbaum Associates Inc; 2008.
15. Kouzes JM, Posner BZ. *The Leadership Challenge.* San Francisco, CA: Jossey-Bass; 2007.
16. Uhl-Bien M, Marion R, McKelvey B. Complex leadership: shifting leadership from the industrial age to the knowledge era. *Leadership Quart* 2007;18(4):298-318.
17. Darling J. Global leadership: How an emerging construct is formed by complex system theory. In: Barbour JD, Burgess GJ, Lid-Falkman L, McManus RM, eds. *Leading in Complex Worlds.* San Francisco, CA: Jossey-Bass; 2012:189-208.
18. Wheatley M. *Leadership in the New Science: Discovering Order in a Chaotic World.* San Francisco, CA: Berrett Koehler; 1999.
19. Resnicow K, Vaughan R. A chaotic view of behavior change: a quantum leap for health promotion. *Int J Behav Nutr Phys Act.* 2006;3;25.
20. Zaleznik A. Managers and leaders: are they different? *HBR.* 1992;70:126-135.
21. Kotter JP. *A Force for Change: How Leadership Differs From Management.* NY: Free Press; 1990.
22. Munn S. Unveiling the Work-Life System: The Influence of Work-Life Balance on Meaningful Work. *Adv Dev Human Res.* 2013;15(4):401-417.
23. Nellis S. Leadership and management: techniques and principles for athletic training. *J Athl Train.* 1994;19(4):328-335.
24. Heifetz R. *Leadership Without Easy Answers.* Cambridge, MA: Harvard University Press; 1994.

25. Laurent T, Bradney D. Leadership behaviors of athletic training leaders compared with leaders in other fields. *J Athl Train.* 2007;42(1):120-125.

26. Kutz M, Scialli J. Leadership content important in athletic training education with implications for allied health care. *J Allied Health.* 2008;37(4):203-213.

27. Northouse P. *Leadership: Theory and Practice.* Thousand Oaks, CA: Sage; 2013.

28. Hersey P, Blanchard KH, Johnson DE. *Management of Organizational Behavior: Leading Human Resources.* Upper Saddle River, NJ: Prentice Hall; 2001.

29. House R, Aditya R. The social scientific study of leadership: quo vadis? *J Manag.* 1997;23(3):409-473.

30. DuBrin AJ. *Leadership: Research Findings, Practice, and Skills.* New York, NY: Houghton Mifflin; 2004.

31. Spears L. Tracing the past, present, and future of servant leadership. In: Spears L, Lawrence M, eds. *Focus on Leadership: Servant Leadership for the 21st Century.* New York: John Wiley & Sons; 2002:1-16.

SUGGESTED READINGS

DuBrin AJ. *Leadership: Research Findings, Practice, and Skills.* New York, NY: Houghton Mifflin; 2004.

Kutz M. *Leadership and Management in Athletic Training: An Integrated Approach.* Baltimore, MD: Lippincott, Williams & Wilkins; 2010.

II

Workplace Issues
and Concepts

II

3

Work-Family Conflict and Finding Work-Life Balance

Stephanie M. Mazerolle, PhD, ATC, LAT

OBJECTIVES

After reading this chapter, the reader will be able to do the following:
1. Distinguish between work-life conflict and work-life balance.
2. Discuss the theoretical models that explain work-life balance.
3. Explain how various practice settings can navigate work-life balance.
4. Describe how work-life balance influences success in the workplace.
5. Identify the factors that inhibit work-life balance.
6. Recommend different ways supervisors can promote work-life balance among employees.
7. Recommend various strategies to help individuals promote their own work-life balance.

INTRODUCTION

Work-life balance has become a central focal point for athletic trainers, primarily because of the potential implications it has had on retention within the profession. Fulfillment of a balance between work (professional) and non-work (family, personal) roles has been identified as a factor in maintaining quality of life.[1] Moreover, work-life balance is critical in retaining not only those working in the sport industry,[2-4] but also those working in the health care sector, such as physicians[5] and athletic trainers.[6-9] Concerns for finding balance are not only a growing concern for athletic trainers, but also all working professionals, including first lady Michelle Obama.[10] A recent *Parade* magazine article showcases the first lady's struggles with balancing a career, 2 children, and her husband's demanding schedule.

Discussions of work-life balance, however, must begin with an understanding of what it truly encompasses. Work-life balance involves effectively managing one's paid occupation with those

Mazerolle SM, Pitney WA.
Workplace Concepts for Athletic Trainers (pp 41-61).
© 2016 Taylor & Francis Group.

personal activities and responsibilities important to his or her existence in order to reduce conflicting experiences.[11] Balance, however, does not mean equity but rather satisfaction in and the ability to engage in work and personal activities in harmony. Conflict can arise from multiple factors that often manifest from a combination of organizational, personal, and/or sociocultural factors.[3,4] Organizationally speaking athletic trainers are susceptible to a reduced work-life balance because of demanding jobs that require long work hours, patient-care needs, and other duties including administrative tasks, supervision of athletic training students, and travel.[6,7] Other factors found to influence perceptions of work-life balance include wanting time to equally engage in parenting and work roles[12] and expectations related to gender norms.[13]

When athletic trainers experience conflict when attempting to balance their lives, they are at greater risk for job burnout, job dissatisfaction, and a reduction in their professional commitment.[7,14] Fortunately, many personal practices and organizational strategies are available to help athletic trainers balance their many roles, and reducing the possible impact conflict can have on their lives. The purpose of this chapter is to conceptualize the meaning of work-life balance and discuss its roots in role conflict; present various theories of work-life balance, identify sources of conflict, and describe the impact conflict can have on the athletic trainer. The chapter concludes with strategies and policies that can help create work-life balance for the athletic trainer.

WHAT IS WORK-LIFE BALANCE?

For many, the most important life domains are work and family, and juggling the domains of work and family have become an integral part of everyday life. The increased efforts of individuals to find balance has been stimulated by many factors, but mostly due to the change in the family make-up, which includes more dual-earning families and a shift in traditional gender roles.[15] In health care, the increased focus has been stimulated by the number of hours an individual works to maintain the role of the health care professional.

Work-life balance is an important topic discussed today by working professionals and is conceptualized as proper prioritization between work (ie, career and professional ambitions) and lifestyle (ie, health, pleasure, family, leisure, and spiritual/religious). Multiple terms are used interchangeably to describe the interface between one's numerous roles in life; however, conflict and balance offer dichotomous points where the roles function in either harmony or discord. As the concern for promoting a balance has grown, many researchers have attempted to gain a sense for those antecedents to conflict as well as those policies and strategies that can promote balance.

Historically, the concept of work-life balance has been termed as *work-family conflict* as it has been found to affect those working professionals who have families to support and care. The term *conflict* has been used, as theorists suggest multiple role occupation provides the backdrop for incompatibility.[16] Experiences of work-family conflict are much higher in the United States (US) when compared to other countries, simply because we work more hours.[17] Early research found that those who attempted to balance working full time and household and parenting roles were at greater risk for conflict,[14] thus the term *work-family conflict*. As the research has expanded, the concept has shifted and identified that regardless of relationship status, family make-up, and other nonwork-related roles, working professionals are at risk of experiencing conflicts in balancing their lives[18]; as a consequence the shift came to the term *work-life*, over work-family balance.

The contemporary definition of work-family conflict was established by Kahn et al,[19] who identified it as "a form of inter-role conflict in which the role pressures from the work and family domains are mutually incompatible in some respect."[19,20] Today, the term reflects the same concept of inter-role conflict; however, those roles have extended beyond just traditional family roles (such as parenting) and include elder care, child care, and personal hobbies and activities that can help define an individual (runner, horseback rider, etc). More important, the work-life interface is often investigated in a conflict perspective, where incompatibility of multiple role occupation will lead to issues. In contrast, a more equalized outlook acknowledges that multiple role engagement can have disadvantages (conflict) as well as advantages (balance/enrichment). Thus in the literature often the terms *work-life conflict* and *work-life balance* are used interchangeably, yet they are distinctly different as one infers the negativity of multiple role occupation, while the other the positive aspects.[21,22] Ultimately, work-life balance references the degree to which an individual is able to find happiness with his or her varying roles in life, and they can be viewed as in harmony.

Work-family conflict is the struggle to find the time to meet the demands of paid work and family and domestic responsibilities such as parenting and child care.
Work-life conflict is a more global concept that represents the challenges facing working individuals to balance their paid work, leisure activities, personal interests, and family obligations.

WORK-LIFE BALANCE THEORIES

Role Conflict

Role conflict at the grassroots happens because a person is viewed to have finite resources, yet will assume multiple roles that will compete with each; unavoidably resources spent in one role must come at the expense at another. Conflict then results because juggling time and resources becomes too stressful.

Role conflict refers to discordant demands placed on a person when assuming multiple roles within various different life domains. It is possible that role conflict can be transitory or long lasting, as situational experiences can influence its occurrence.[16] Work-life conflict is a common role conflict, as working individuals are often juggling multiple roles within the workplace as well as personal duties and responsibilities. Goode[16] hypothesized that multiple roles with boundless demands are more likely to cause role strain and conflict, as the resources necessary to meet the demands can be finite and limited. Kahn et al defined role conflict as the "simultaneous occurrence of 2 (or more) sets of pressures such that compliance with one would make more difficulty compliance with the other."[19]

Two main sources of role conflict as it pertains to work-life conflict have been described: time- and strain-based role conflict.[20] Inherently, completing responsibilities in one role requires time, thus the assumption of multiple roles creates the potential for conflict, as time spent on one activity reduces time available for others. Within the work domain hours worked, flexibility in work schedule, locus of control, and timing of work hours (day vs evening; weekend hours) are connected to time pressures, whereas age of children, dual-earning couples, and size of family describe family or personal aspects of time-based conflict. Strain-based conflict describes the pressures associated with each individual role, and the relationship it can have on the other roles. Simply, when one role becomes too difficult or demanding, the stress then spills over into the other roles, often limiting the resources and energy necessary to comply with the needs of the other roles.[20] Examples of strain in the home domain include spousal support, child care, and age and number of the children. Gender has traditionally been viewed as a strain, simply as it is assumed that women take greater responsibility in management of the domestic and parenting duties, regardless of

TABLE 3-1 ATHLETIC TRAINING EXAMPLES OF TIME- AND STRAIN-BASED CONFLICT	
TIME-BASED	**STRAIN-BASED**
Work	
• Long work hours (+40 per work week) • Travel responsibilities • Role overload and strain	• Coaches' expectations and demands • Multiple roles (patient care, supervision of athletic training students) • Compatibility with supervisor and family values
Home	
• Parenthood • Gender	• Spousal support • Child care resources

their work demands or employment. Juxtapose those with these examples of strain from the work domain, including role ambiguity, limited supervisor support, or role overload.

Role conflict theory holds that individuals who assume multiple life roles will experience strain and conflict because they are in competition rather than able to share time and resources. The theory creates distinction between roles and distinct borders that are not crossed; as time and energy needed to navigate the role is determined to be fixed rather than sharable. Individuals then spend time working on mitigating conflict and examining the cost each role has rather than focusing on the positive each role brings to their life.[23,24] Role conflict or the conflict theory is conceptualized as a psychological stressor that results because work and family responsibilities are irreconcilable.[16] The more roles one occupies, the more likely they are to experience increased stress and strain, and thus conflict ensues. Table 3-1 highlights time and strain based antecedents within the athletic training profession.

Enrichment Theory

The work-life interface is often described as the intersection of a person's professional life and his or her private/personal life, which is often viewed as in opposition rather than harmony. Work-family or work-life enrichment has emerged as a new definition of the interface, which attempts to create a positive platform for assessment, whereby effectiveness and satisfaction can be gained by multiple roles.[21] The model of enrichment, unlike the conflict theory, offers the notion that individuals who are engaged in work and family/life roles are valuable, productive members within each role offering productivity and positivity while immersed in each role. Sieber[25] and Marks[26] suggest that time, money, and energy are not infinite resources, and believe multiple role occupation can facilitate the development of these resources needed to succeed in each role. Many of the benefits of multiple role occupation focus on psychological well-being and improved satisfaction within each role (ie, life or job).[23]

Enrichment or facilitation can be used interchangeably and reflect the degree to which multiple roles can be a positive influence on one another. The enrichment theory centers on the positivity gained from spillover in each life domain (worker, parent, spouse, etc) and that one domain provides benefits and resources that can facilitate or improve engagement and performance in the other domain.[21] Enrichment has been found to occur in the sport industry, as found by Schenewark and Dixon,[22] who established a dual model of the work-family interface. That is, conflict is likely, but assuming the role of coach and parent may provide a positive influence within each role, despite also presenting challenges and obstacles to balance.[22]

Work-life conflict focused more on the negative influence multiple roles can have on an individual, whereas the enrichment theory focuses on the positive outcomes that result such as improved job and life satisfaction and improved overall mood.[27,28] The enrichment mindset really allows the individual to embrace all the positives that are offered in each role and that allows them to cope better, become more productive and efficient in performing their duties in each role. Simply seeing work, life, and family as allies allows for an improvement in work-life balance.[21]

Personality provides the platform for explaining work-life enrichment, where a person's disposition can influence experience; simplistically a more positive outlook leads to its occurrence. Individual antecedents have been identified as facilitators to enrichment, including extraversion and openness to experiences. Extraverts are characterized as outgoing, gregarious, and energized; their positivity often helps them succeed in the workplace because they interact and communicate with others.[29] Individuals classified as open also appear to embrace the work-life enrichment model, as they tend to be intelligent, creative, and broad-minded, allowing them to see possibility rather than the limitations of multiple roles and potentially conflicting responsibilities.[29]

> Work-life enrichment is the degree to which the work role (or vice versa) enhances the family role.
>
> Work-life facilitation is the degree to which the work role makes it easier to perform in the family role (or vice versa).

Integration/Separation Theory

Work-life integration and work-life separation theory is described as a dichotomous continuum in which integration represents no distinction between work and personal lives, whereas separation views each as independent of one another. Within this theoretical background, work is viewed with the purpose of providing an income for the family, and an individual gains satisfaction through a sense of accomplishment while earning a living. In opposition, home reflects one's involvement in close relationships, maintenance of domestic and household needs, and finding personal happiness.[30]

Work-life separation boosts a mindset whereby tasks are separated and defined by blocks of time. While engaged in work roles, someone with a separation attitude will not allow family or personal obligations to spill over. Work-life integration speaks to a mindset that allows for work or family roles to intersect the other; it is often described as having blurred lines between roles. In some cases, a person can have a work-first mentality that allows work to interrupt family, where family first allows family to interrupt work. Fundamentally, there is no distinction made between what belongs to the home/personal domain and what belongs to work. The notion of work and life separation and integration provide the platform for understanding conflict and creating a balance. In fact, both provide the opportunity for both conflict and balance to manifest.

Work-life integration often is described as meaning there are no borders to each role and daily activities can be managed and completed based on needs, practicality, and necessity. Work-life integration contrasts the issue that work and life are separate and must be balanced, which is subconsciously supposed to alleviate the stresses associated with work-life balance. Interestingly, the concept of work-life integration is more popular to millennials as they have grown into a world that blends roles (ie, social media). The increase in technology (iPhones and iPads) allows individuals to be engaged in working roles during their off time (at night, on vacation, etc).

In work-life separation there is an artificial separation between work and personal life, often defined by time and activities. Daily responsibilities are often arranged and executed based on time available or time expected to complete those responsibilities (ie, work day is 9 am to 5 pm). Work-life separation can, at times boost a negative mindset as an individual often has to exude time and energy keeping each role separate. However, the concept of separation may also support balance as the spillover that can occur is limited, especially if one domain is more stressful than the other.

Although the 2 concepts are distinctive, the reality is they can be used in unison based on the circumstances at the time. They offer individuals the flexibility to meet their demanding lives by engaging in multiple roles simultaneously or to disengage from those same roles that can become burdensome and overwhelming. In athletic training, in fact, both theories are used to combat high patient volumes, long work days, and the demands associated with the care of the student-athlete.[31]

Work-life separation and integration help provide context to the experiences of conflict, and also provide the foundation for strategies used to manage the domains of work and home life. In athletic training, separation can be used as an effective means to engage from the demands of health care, whereas integration can also help create more time in the day for spending time with family and managing domestic and household chores.[31]

Border Theory

An extension of the work-life integration or separation theory is the border theory. The theory attempts to describe the complex relationship that exists between work and personal life and how an individual falls on the continuum of separation and integration. In the theory first described by Clark,[32] borders are viewed as the demarcation between the roles of work and home and can be developed physically, temporally, and psychologically. Physical borders are those created by what can be viewed as "face time," the necessity of being present within the role.[32] Temporal borders are created when responsibilities divide the time needed for each role (ie, time for work). Rules created by individuals based on their thinking patterns and emotions regarding appropriateness for each role create psychological borders. Psychological borders are largely self-created, whereas the other 2 borders may manifest as the constraints of each role.

The border theory helps explain how an individual navigates managing work-life balance through the borders they maintain between work and home life. Borders, as mentioned above, also take on a degree of permeability, flexibility, and blending.[32] The degree of cross-over that can occur between domains explains permeability. Simply, an individual who works from home may have a home office, yet family members may be able to enter freely during the "workday." Flexibility is the extent to which a border can inflate or collapse depending on the demands within each role. For example, an individual may think about home when at work, or in contrast may think of work while at home. Blending can occur when an employee uses personal time to also enrich their home life (ie, serving dinner while taking a work-related phone call).

Multifactorial Theory

While the overall literature concerning work-family conflict has expanded exponentially, at the beginning of this century there was a lack of incorporation of multiple theoretical levels. Researchers appeared more interested in examining the concept from either individual, structural, or social perspectives. The multifactorial theory is founded on the premise that conflict, which is likely due to multiple role occupation, occurs from an interaction of multiple factors. Three factors have emerged from the work of Dixon and Bruening,[3,4] as facilitators to work-life conflict (Figure 3-1). In their model, Dixon and Bruening argued that individual responses and attitudes toward work-life balance have the capacity to influence organizational culture and climate from the bottom up, but that there is also a top-down influence.

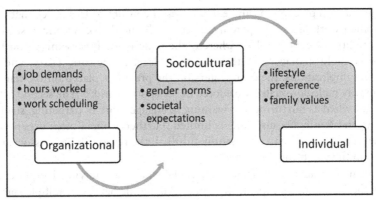

Figure 3-1. Multilevel work-life interface.

Organizational or structural factors embody those characteristics that are embedded within the job or workplace; they are inherently related to job performance and the expectations attached to the occupying role. The multilevel theory was developed from data garnered from a study investigating the work family interface of women National Collegiate Athletic Association (NCAA) Division I coaches, thus several of the foundational items are rooted in the sport culture. Essentially, the organizational level is shaped by work hours, work scheduling, job pressures and stressors, and the culture.[3,4] Hours worked is consistently a facilitator for conflict, and provides the framework for the organizational element to the theory. Like the coach, the athletic trainer is working in a multifaceted, high-paced employment setting that requires patient care, administrative responsibilities, travel, teaching/supervision of students, and a host of other potential duties related to their employment setting. Working in this type of environment is likely, therefore, to result in conflict.[7,8,33]

Although the work-family interface is described as bidirectional, often the discussions focus on the impact work has on family and thus hours worked and job pressures dominate the findings. Long, nontraditional hours (nights, weekends) surely affect an athletic trainer's ability to make choices regarding work, family, and life balance; however, it is also understood that individuals differ in their experiences of and ability to cope with work-family or work-life balance.[34] Research illustrates that individual differences exist with personality,[34] family values,[35] coping and support systems, and gender[36,37] in relation to work-life conflict. These individual differences ultimately navigate the occurrence of work-life conflict, and despite organizational constraints or barriers, individuals must make choices regarding the management of their roles, personally and professionally as it fits their lifestyles. In the Dixon and Bruening[3,4] model, individual factors account for personal preferences, values, and beliefs as a necessary piece to understanding work, family, and life interactions.

Appreciating individualistic values is needed to fully understand when conflict or harmony is experienced, as some individuals may value their work roles more than their family or home role, which can explain time and energy invested in each. Borrowing from the preference theory (as described next), a person is able to choose the roles and time spent in each role as it matches his or her core values and beliefs. Thus, conflict may emanate when the role requires too much time or resources, which limits the person's chance to engage in the other roles. For example, an athletic trainer who values his or her role at work and gains more satisfaction from that role, is more likely to experience conflict when responsibilities in the personal role (ie, parenting) begin to spill over into the work role.

The final piece to the multi-level perspective includes sociocultural factors, which describe the social impact on work-family conflict. Social and gender norms provide the underpinnings to this piece of the model, describing the way that expectations of masculine and feminine can have a critical impact on perceptions and experiences of conflict.[3,4] Despite changes in the workforce (more women working, single parents, or stay-at-home dads), American society is largely predicated on traditional gender roles—whereby the male is the breadwinner and the female is the domestic/household manager.[2] Within the multi-level framework, Dixon and Bruening[3,4] describe 2 critical implications: the first centers on the pressures placed on the female trying to survive the typically male dominated workforce in the sports world.[38] The second is that women, who are often described as nurturing and wanting to engage more in parenting, struggle to manage their careers and family because time is limited. Further, women often experience guilt and self-doubt when they are unable to successfully fulfill all the responsibilities associated with their roles, especially in the parenting domain.[6,39]

Although taken separately, each factor can explain how an individual experiences conflict, yet integrating the factors helps explain the complex dynamic between multiple role occupation. The multilevel model suggests examining the work and home lives of a person comprehensively can help gain a better understanding of conflict, its impact, and strategies to help cope with the competing roles.

Preference Theory

The preference theory speaks to the decision-making process regarding the selection and investment in productive and reproductive work.[40] Although this theory is heavily rooted in women's decision making about career selection and parenthood, it has implications for all working professionals because it provides insight into decision making as it pertains to engagement in work roles and home roles.

The preference theory speaks to the notion that individuals, in particular women, have the ability to choose their work-lifestyle preferences once genuine choices are open to them. Additionally, the theory contends that women's preferences are based on their personal needs and goals, which are likely independent of other factors such as societal contentions or organizational views. While Hakim did not argue that social and organizational constraints were nonexistent, she maintained that these factors were rapidly diminishing and that their influences on women's careers were outweighed by personal attitudes and preferences.[40]

Hakim describes 3 work-lifestyle preferences that articulate how women navigate their decision making regarding work and life. Home-centered lifestyle preference is rooted in very traditional thinking, where family life and domestic care are the main priorities and paid work is not preferred. It is estimated that a small portion of women fit this category, with ranges between 10% and 30% of all women. Work-centered preference is classified as a commitment to work, which drives decision making. Often women who fall into this category are childless and are employed in sports, politics, corporate settings, etc. The final classification is considered adaptive, which is contextualized by women who prefer to engage both in paid work and family with equal time and resources. A majority of individuals fall into the adaptive classification, as they are committed to their careers, but are not defined by it and value time for family and personal interests.

Preference theory actually predicts that men will retain dominance in the labor market owing to the minority of women who are work centered and willing to prioritize their jobs.[40] Preference theory has roused an academic debate that can be roughly divided into 2 groups: those who highlight personal preferences, and those who reestablish the role of sociocultural constraints. Those who disagree with the preference theory argue that it neglects the possibility that women will face different limitations on their careers at different stages of their lives. The main criticism of preference theory is its shortage of investigation into the relationship between gender-role preferences and employment behaviors and that there is no substantive evidence to show how preference actually influences women's employment. However, those who support the preference theory believe that women who have different fertility and career plans are also likely to have different attitudes toward work and home and that work-centered women are not particularly negatively affected by family responsibilities in their careers compared to home-centered and adaptive women.

A recent study by Kan[41] examined the major claims of preference theory and found evidence both in support of and in opposition to it by highlighting that women's preferences and career constraints interact with each other and play an important role in shaping careers. Most notably, it has shown that women with work-centered attitudes were more likely to engage in full-time work over a long period of time than other women.[41] Additionally, having children had a less negative influence on work-centered women's likelihood of maintaining full-time employment than on other women, highlighting that preference is a strong factor in shaping women's careers. It was also shown that women faced many constraints aside from child care responsibilities, including sex segregation in occupations, housework responsibilities, and limited wages;[41] thus stating that preference is an isolated causal factor in women's career paths is problematic.

In summary, preference theory states that women can be broadly classified as either home centered, adaptive, or work centered, and that it is these classifications that will influence their perceptions of work-life balance and career trajectories. In the sports industry, especially as reported by Bruening and Dixon,[42] it can be gathered that women tend to favor a more adaptive mentality regarding work-life balance. Women tend to experience conflict because of the need to fulfill parenting and mothering duties while engaged in their demanding athletic work roles. Emerging evidence suggests that female athletic trainers also favor this mentality, as they start to change practice settings or leave the profession to achieve this balance, something not afforded in the collegiate setting.[13]

SOURCES OF CONFLICT

The antecedents of work-life imbalance can be summarized using the context of the multilevel model described by Dixon and Bruening[3,4]: organizational, individual, and sociocultural. The model recognizes that conflict emerges not from one single factor, but rather from a mixture of interacting variables. Despite the plethora of information on the topic, globally and within athletic training, a majority of the literature specific to athletic training centers on the organizational factors leading to conflict. There are some emerging data that highlight additional sources of conflict as presented in Table 3-2. The following sections present the antecedents of work-life conflict, organized by using the multifactorial model previously discussed in the chapter.

Organizational Sources

Americans are working more hours per week on average than they did almost 10 years ago, but are also working more than other developed countries.[43] Hours worked, often conceptualized as role overload, has consistently been at the heart of the issue for athletic trainers when it comes to balancing their professional demands and home life.[8,18] Although several factors can influence the number of hours worked per week, several studies reveal that those athletic trainers working in demanding work settings (ie, professional sports, performing arts, NCAA Division I) are averaging more than 60 hours per week.[18] As outlined in the role conflict theory, as well as the multilevel framework, the more hours and resources needed to perform in one role depletes the time and resources to manage the others.[3,4,16] Eberman and Kahanov[44] reported both that men and women athletic trainers want to have more time at home, but because of work-related time constraints often neglect family obligations and responsibilities outside the workplace, findings that have been reported unfailingly throughout the athletic training literature, and often seem to be linked to the collegiate and secondary school settings.[7,18,44] Hours worked, however, is only one aspect of the organizational factors contributing to work-life conflict for the athletic trainer, sports professional, and health care worker.

TABLE 3-2		
ANTECEDENTS IN ATHLETIC TRAINING FOR WORK-LIFE CONFLICT		
ORGANIZATIONAL FACTORS	**INDIVIDUAL FACTORS**	**SOCIOCULTURAL FACTORS**
• Hours worked • Travel responsibilities • Work scheduling • Adequate staffing patterns • Coaching expectations and relationships	• Adaptive lifestyle preference • Kinship responsibility and needs • Family-friendly atmosphere	• Traditional role ideologies • Lack of social support

The unique demands of the profession are also a subsidizing factor to work-life conflict in athletic training. The demands include the need to be "present" to complete work-related roles, including patient care and practice and game coverage. The concept of "face time" was first coined within the multifactorial framework and is described as the necessity to be on the job at all times to showcase commitment and diligence to role requirements. Outside of the health care and sports industry, telecommunicating has become a popular method to afford some flexibility in the workday to accommodate for other demanding roles (ie, child care), a workplace policy that often is not feasible owing to the logistics of patient care. External to athletic training, flex-time and work scheduling have emerged as the secret to work-life balance, and thus those individuals who are afforded the availability to schedule their own workday are more likely to have better coordination of their roles and responsibilities as they can allocate time as necessary. Unfortunately, athletic training provides unique limitations when it comes to work scheduling and is often cited as problematic when it comes to finding a balance between work and life domains.[7,8,18]

Other aspects framing the demands of the profession include communication and scheduling conflicts with coaches for team practices as well as adequate staffing patterns for athletic training departments. Several investigations[7,8,12,18] have found that locus of control over work scheduling has become a concern for the athletic trainer, as often the coach is the one making the practice and game schedules. Last-minute scheduling changes or being the last to know are often discussed anecdotally and empirically as frustrating aspects of the profession and stimulate conflict.[7,18]

Compounding the issues with coaches is staffing patterns within athletic training, although this is a concern that arises mostly within the traditional sports settings (ie, college, high school), as many athletic training and sports medicine departments are understaffed and require an athletic trainer to provide medical coverage to multiple sports.[18] The shortage not only increases the role demands placed on the athletic trainer but it also increases the number of hours worked per week. Role demands have been found to be a catalyst for conflict outside the athletic training profession, as having too many roles at work, limited time to do them, and competing roles within the workplace creates the potential for increased stress and limiting time.[45]

Organizational support and work characteristics (job tenure, nature of job) have also been found to mitigate the occurrence of work-life conflict. Simply, those athletic trainers who have been perceived to be supported by the organization, their supervisor, and their co-workers are less likely to experience conflict.[4,31,45] Organizational support, which simply is the degree to which people feel and believe they are valued by their employer and profession, has been found to mediate the occurrence of work-family conflict. In fact, coaches and athletic trainers who believe their employer and supervisor can provide a supportive, family-friendly environment are more easily able to balance their roles.[12] Supervisor support and understanding were also found in the high school setting as an interceding factor for an athletic trainer to minimize work-life conflict.[46]

Individual Factors

Individual factors that can help determine experiences of work-life conflict can include family role involvement, family characteristics, personality, and marital and parental status. Role involvement involves the level of commitment and attachment one has to the family and the importance he or she places on being involved within that role. Family characteristics are an umbrella term used to describe the constructs of family life, including spousal role (working, stay at home), family climate (support, cohesion, sharing), and the demands related to meeting family needs.[45] Personality, referring to patterned feelings and behaviors of an individual, which lead to coordinated emotional and behavioral actions, has been found to be an antecedent for conflict. Two aspects have been repeatedly connected to work-life conflict, including internal locus of control and neuroticism.[45] Marital and parental status have long been linked to conflict, as it has been suggested that the work-life dynamics are fundamentally different for those who are married and/or have children.[45] The premise is heavily founded in role theory and the stresses that emanate from varying roles. It is suggested that being married and/or having children increases the demands of the person occupying the role.

Previous research has linked family role overload to conflict,[47] youth of children,[48] and number of children[49] to work-family conflict. Simply, the more demands required by family involvement the more likely conflict results as time, energy, and resources can become depleted. Unlike the past literature, relationship/marital status and family status have not been found to navigate conflict for the athletic trainer.[7,18] Conflict can simply occur for the athletic trainer independent of those demographic variables.

Personality traits have recently emerged as a new factor related to conflict, as those individuals who have an increased perceived control (internal locus) are less likely to experience conflict.[50] Neuroticism or negative affectivity have also been found to moderate conflict, as those individuals who are quick to react to stress and have limited coping mechanisms are more likely to experience conflict.[34,51] Other personality traits such as agreeableness, extraversion, and conscientiousness have been suggested as possible mediators of conflict, but research is limited. As outlined in Chapter 7 (burnout), the big-5 model of personality as become a staple for exploring the impact personality can have on professional issues. Conscientiousness has also begun to gain some momentum as a mitigating factor, as the trait describes someone who is a time manager and diligent to his or her roles and responsibilities.

Personality has yet to be fully explored in athletic training. Assumptions can be made, however, that athletic trainers are individuals at risk for conflict because they are selfless, conscientious, goal-oriented, and are committed to their roles as health care professionals. These are descriptions that are anecdotal in nature, yet can be drawn from the findings of many research studies that link hardiness and coping to burnout.[52,53]

Sociocultural Factors

Gender undoubtedly has been a fundamental catalyst to work-life conflict, mostly owing to traditional gender ideologies and stereotypes. Gender is often seen as a moderator as research has implicated gender ideologies in which work is viewed as more central to the male identity in contrast to women, who are often tied to the family role.[54] Cultural expectations are thought to navigate experiences of work-life conflict, as although women may engage in paid work, their alliances and devotion will still align with their family roles (caregiving and household labor). In some literature, hours worked has been linked to work-life conflict, but mostly among women workers as they likely want to have the chance to have equity in time spent working and parenting.[55,56] Role theory has often been the explanation for gender differences, as men and women differ in their identification with and expected role involvement in each life domain. Again, women are more likely to exert more energy and responsibility within the home domain, regardless of time spent working.[45] However, this does not mean that males do not have difficulty balancing work and life.

Recently it was reported that male athletic trainers find difficulty balancing work, personal, and home life; these struggles of finding balance appeared to affect males more so than females.[44] Although female athletic trainers do report difficulty with work-life balance, it appears as though males may struggle more with juggling multiple roles and the stressors each domain presents. Gender differences have not been reported in athletic training regarding experiences of work-life conflict;[7] however, it has been at the forefront of discussions regarding reasons for departing the profession. That is, female athletic trainers often leave their careers in athletic training because of their inability to meet their work and home life demands.[57,58] Although concerns related to work-life conflict affect male athletic trainers, they do not make the decision to depart, but rather persist or change clinical settings.[9,57] Emerging evidence does suggest that female athletic trainers do want an adaptive lifestyle that encompasses time for both roles—athletic trainer and mother—and this preference can influence experiences of conflict as well as career planning.[13,59] Gender ideology is an area that is relatively unexplored in athletic training, as it is in sports and other employment settings, and future research needs to investigate its impact.

A full appreciation of gender is limited as it is also likely that many women leave the labor force once they experience conflict or reduce the risk of conflict by removing themselves from time-intensive, demanding careers or roles.

> Work-life or work-family conflict is no longer just a working mother's issue as it's a conflict that affects all workers and their families.

Impact of Work-Life Conflict

Owing to the increase in research in the area of work-family conflict and work-life balance, scholars have attempted to understand the variables that cause conflict but also the impact it can have on a person. The harmful effects that have been reported include individual outcomes as well as organizational consequences (Table 3-3). Four major findings, burnout, job and life satisfaction, and turnover are associated with work-life conflict.[14] Although a host of outcomes can be directly linked to the occurrence of work-life conflict, these 4 constructs seem to receive a great deal of attention and are often reported in the literature. A comparison of these 4 outcomes as measured in other working professionals to athletic trainers is showcased in Table 3-4, highlighting the stronger impact it can have on the athletic trainer.

Job satisfaction often receives the most scholarly attention related to work-life conflict where a significant negative relationship is reported and the populations are diverse (teachers, nurses, retail employees, among others). The relationship is straightforward, as long working hours, work pressures, and other demanding work commitments that limit the abilities of individuals to escape from their professional roles the more stress they endure, and inevitably the more likely they will be to experience conflict. Thus, as work-life conflict manifests, individuals are more likely to begin to become dissatisfied with their job because it limits their opportunities to engage in other roles with the same effort, time, and resources.

Pitney[60] first reported that athletic trainers were concerned with their quality of life, simply not having enough time to balance their outside responsibilities because of long work hours due to high work (patient) volumes. Time, flexibility, and work overload due to insufficient number

TABLE 3-3

COMPARING THE OUTCOMES OF WORK-LIFE CONFLICT AMONG ATHLETIC TRAINERS WITH OTHER WORKING PROFESSIONALS

OUTCOME MEASURE	ALLEN ET AL, VARIOUS PROFESSIONALS	MAZEROLLE ET AL, ATHLETIC TRAINERS
JS and WLC	−0.23	−0.52
LS and WLC	−0.28	−0.11
JB and WLC	0.42	0.64
ITL and WLC	0.29	0.46
JS: job satisfaction; LS: life satisfaction; JB: job burnout; ITL: intention to turnover; WLC: work-life conflict.		

TABLE 3-4

OUTCOMES OF WORK-LIFE CONFLICT

INDIVIDUAL OUTCOMES	ORGANIZATIONAL OUTCOMES
Depression	Absenteeism
Hypertension	Organizational commitment
Substance abuse	Job dissatisfaction
Life and family dissatisfaction	Turnover intentions
Personal burnout	Job burnout
Physical and psychological strain	Job performance

of staff members has been reported as sources both of work-life conflict and job dissatisfaction,[7] linking the 2 constructs together. Athletic trainers are like other working professionals,[14] as they experience conflicts with balancing their work and personal roles, the factors stimulating the conflict become similar sources of disdain leading to dissatisfaction. In fact, it appears for athletic trainers that conflicts experienced between work and home have a greater effect on their assessment of their job as compared to other working professionals.[8,14]

Work-life conflict and job burnout have a positive relationship,[14] as feelings of conflict increase, so do the levels of burnout. As found with job satisfaction, job burnout demonstrates a stronger relationship for the athletic trainer when compared to weighted correlations from other professionals.[14] Fundamental to experiences of these organizational-based outcomes are hours worked and the demands placed on the individual; when they are overwhelming they create role conflict (ie, work to life), which stimulates experiences of dissatisfaction and burnout. The relationship to burnout is obvious, as burnout is a sequela of chronic stress due to repeated exposure to unrelenting demands, often in the work domain. The literature suggests that job satisfaction, burnout, and work-life conflict are intertwined as continued exposure to the stressful environment can lead to these outcomes because they often manifest from similar antecedents. For athletic trainers, long work hours coupled with travel and demands from patient care and coaches can lead to feelings of burnout, particularly as they are unable to spend time at home or engaged in personal hobbies or leisure activities.[8]

Life satisfaction and work-life conflict have a negative relationship, like that reported with job satisfaction. The negative affiliation between the 2 suggests that as one experiences greater levels of conflict, the more dissatisfied one becomes with one's life. Simply, this could speak to the greater demand for finding a balance, and when that balance is violated the individual becomes discontented. Life satisfaction as a construct is an overarching term that often encapsulates family life as well as marital and relationship status. For most working professionals a negative relationship is reported, and often women experience a stronger relationship compared to males.[14] Despite the existence of data, the association between work-life conflict and life satisfaction is not well understood. Athletic trainers do report a negative relationship between the 2 variables; however, it is small.[8] Athletic trainers appear to desire more time outside of the workplace,[8,61] but the full impact conflict has on life satisfaction is not well known. Likely, the explanation lies with the demographic composition of the profession, which as of now is characterized as young and mostly single athletic trainers.[7,8,57] Admittedly, those athletic trainers who do not have parental duties recognize the additional challenges having children places on them. Therefore, it is plausible that conflict may not affect their assessment of their overall life, as it may with an athletic trainer with family obligations and responsibilities.

Another plausible justification can be drawn from the theories of separation and integration, as previously discussed. Both theories offer some insights into the weak relationship between life satisfaction and work-life conflict. Separation allows the athletic trainer to disengage, so to speak, from each role allowing for time to focus on each role without the negative spillover and stress the other role can bring. Simply time away recharges the person, allowing for full satisfaction within each role. Integration, on the other hand, may also bring satisfaction to people, allowing them to juggle those demands without distinction. The permeability of the roles allows for time and energy to be shared between roles, thus reducing conflict and increasing satisfaction. In the end, work-life balance is individualized, and balance inevitably means finding satisfaction within each role by controlling the time allotted for each.

Career commitment, career intentions, turnover, and intentions to leave are often terms used interchangeably to reflect the degree of commitment a person has to his or her career, job, and profession.[62] Commitment and intentions, however, are distinctly different, indicating one's level of satisfaction and loyalty to a job, in comparison to one's pursuit of employment outside of his or her current job/profession. Work-life conflict can affect both commitment and intentions in a negative light. Researchers have found a positive relationship between the intentions to leave a job/profession, whereas conflict continues or increases the thoughts of leaving the profession/job increase. A negative relationship exists between career commitment and work-life conflict, as the conflict continues commitment decreases.[14]

A link between intentions to leave and work-life conflict has been established in athletic training,[8] and continual links are being made between experiences of work-life conflict and professional commitment and turnover.[6,8,9,58] Athletic trainers over time become overwhelmed and frustrated by the lack of time for outside obligations, family time, and leisure activities and because of a lack of balance begin to find positions or careers that allow this to happen.[63] Departure from the profession due to long hours and other underpinnings of work-life conflict have been reported since the early 1990s[64] and continue to be showcased as a facilitator for leaving the profession.[6,58] Female athletic trainers are leaving the profession before the age of 30, indicating a problem with motherhood and athletic training duties.[57] Although departure due to work-life conflict has been historically linked to females, growing evidence suggests that gender may not completely mitigate the relationship between the two.[9] Male athletic trainers do report issues balancing parental duties and athletic training roles, and do want to have the time to be at home and involved with household and domestic-related activities.[44,61]

The impact the work-life conflict can have on the athletic trainer extends beyond the 4 constructs just discussed. In fact, the implications of the work-life conflict can manifest comparably to job burnout in that emotional and physical symptoms can appear including depression, fatigue, absenteeism, and a reduced job performance.[14] Although the data are well established in other professions, limited information is available on the impact conflict has on the athletic trainer beyond those outcomes previously discussed. Continued research is warranted on the outcomes of conflict from an organizational and individual level, as well as longitudinally. The full impact of work-life conflict is understood only from a snapshot in time, rather than collected over time. Gathering longitudinal data can help gain a better understanding of the relationship of work-life conflict and its true impact on the athletic trainer.

RECOMMENDATIONS

Strategies to navigate work-life conflict can be classified as either individual or organizational. Individual strategies emanate from a person's own preferences and needs regarding their varying roles and responsibilities. These strategies recognize the individualistic aspect of finding work-life balance, as each person has different beliefs and needs and can place different values on each role they occupy. Organizational strategies are founded within the workplace, and may be formal or informal policies needed to help an employee find work-life balance. Research has begun to focus more on policy development and effective strategies to promote work-life balance rather than the causes of conflict.

Personal rejuvenation, advocacy, support networks, workplace cohesion and autonomy have emerged as fundamental aspects to work-life balance. These strategies, although specific to athletic training,[31,65] have also been discussed among various occupations and workplace settings. Self-reflection and goal setting are also found to be important in achieving balance,[66] mostly because work-life balance is not one size fits all.

Organizational Policies and Recommendations

Supervisors and administrators play a critical role in helping their employees find balance; this holds true in athletic training.[67,68] Head athletic trainers, athletic directors, and other administrators should not only educate their employees on available policies, but should also promote use of those policies and model appropriate work-life balance.[68,69] In athletic training, unlike other work/employment settings, very limited formal strategies exist to promote work-life balance, thus it is important for supervisors to informally promote it for their staff. Many corporations and organizations have a variety of policies that can facilitate work-life balance, such as flex-time, job sharing, parental leaves, and on-site child care.

Work-life policies should reflect the diversity of relationship and family status and be gender neutral.[66] Common work-life policies including job sharing, telecommunicating, work schedule flexibility, compression of workweeks, and child care and parental leaves. Many of these policies are human resource generated, and reflect a more traditional workplace, and thus do not meet the needs of the health care professional, medical care professional, or sports world. Policies that are helpful for the athletic trainer include medical coverage guidelines (hours of operation, practice schedule times, etc) and job sharing (teamwork to cover work-related responsibilities occasionally).

Job sharing traditionally is viewed as 2 individuals sharing 1 position, but splitting the time to complete the role (ie, each work 20 hours during week). In athletic training it is viewed as being a temporary substitute for when special occasions or situations arise during the workday. For example, one athletic trainer may cover a practice for a peer to allow them to attend a doctor's appointment or to go to a parent teacher conference. Continuity of care should not be disrupted, and the athletic trainer is able to attend to outside obligations with minimal conflict or disruption of daily responsibilities as an athletic trainer. Job sharing must be reciprocal and viewed as a means to promote increased time for outside needs and expectations without disruption to patient care.

Supervisors should support it and athletic trainers should use it as a means to promote work-life balance.[65]

Supervisors are encouraged to continually assess and evaluate their employees' workloads as means to ensure they are able to balance their responsibilities in the workplace as well as outside of it. An athletic trainer who is able to fulfill his or her work-life balance needs will be a more productive and satisfied employee, which will benefit the workplace atmosphere; an aspect also necessary for balance (a family-friendly, supportive one). A recent case study examining organizational aspects of work-life balance revealed that a workplace that includes a supervisor who advocates for his or her employees, values personal and family time, and promotes a flexible and reasonable workload for each athletic trainer is important for work-life balance.[70] Ultimately displays of organizational support[4] help athletic trainers feel valued and empowered to achieve their responsibilities and goals and are why supervisors must be supportive of their employees' needs.

Other important aspects to consider, especially for those in positions of leadership or management in athletic training, are allowing for workplace integration when appropriate and manageable as well as encouraging the use of personal or vacation time as a means to rejuvenate and de-stress.[65,71] Recognition of a staff member's efforts and completion of work tasks is also important; this can include a simple thank you or an unexpected day off. Moreover, providing autonomy over work scheduling or completion of job-related tasks is also helpful for the athletic trainer when trying to maintain work-life balance.[8,68]

The role of the supervisor is paramount to work-life balance, but the individual athletic trainer must make efforts to achieve it as well. In the workplace, the athletic trainer should capitalize on resources available for promoting work-life balance, engage in job sharing with co-workers, and take advantage of time away when presented and appropriate. Communicating with supervisor, co-workers, and other members of the sports medicine staff is needed to fulfill work-life balance.

Individual Strategies

Finding work-life balance is not a new concern for athletic trainers, but one that requires planning and thought. Achieving it often starts with the individual, whereby they need to reflect and determine personal and professional goals. Once individuals are aware of their priorities and are able to appreciate what roles they value or prefer to invest their time and resources in, they can then develop effective strategies designed to gain balance.

Athletic trainers should first and foremost establish professional boundaries and expectations within their role as a health care provider. Coaches, student-athletes, and other members within the sports medicine team should understand when it is appropriate to contact you (ie, no texts or calls before 6 am or after 9 pm). It is important to stick to these set parameters and clearly communicate those policies to your co-workers and others in the care of the student-athletes. Communication is fundamental to finding work-life balance, as it allows all members involved to understand expectations, needs, and policies that ultimately compete for time and energy, which leads to conflict. Without clearly communicated goals, expectations, and needs, it becomes hard for others to respect boundaries that can help promote work-life balance.

An athletic trainer must negotiate his or her role. That is, when time demands become too much, it is important to discuss it with a supervisor or administrator. This may lead to having to say "no" to additional responsibilities or reducing those expectations already being managed to help create more balance. The development of healthy lifestyle habits is a part of being able to say "no" to more responsibilities. Moreover, the need to exercise, eat right, and get enough sleep is critical to creating balance and preventing conflict.

Long work hours are commonplace in athletic training; however, there are times during the day that are flexible and can possibly be used for personal time. During those times, it is important for athletic trainers to prioritize that time for themselves, using it to workout, run personal errands, or catch up on administrative tasks. Regardless of the task, making time to complete them during the workday can increase the time available for multiple role demands. This approach can be viewed as workplace integration, whereby there are flexible lines drawn between the domains of work and life. In athletic training, this can be highly effective, especially for working mothers and fathers as a means to juggle the demands and unexpected aspects of parenthood and athletic training coverage.[65] It also can reduce the psychological strain multiple role occupations can have, as the pressure to keep the domains separate is removed, thus alleviating the stress of managing it.

Learning to disconnect is also critical for balance, that is, time away from stressful roles can help stimulate commitment and satisfaction. Disengagement must be reciprocal, meaning time must be spent away from athletic training and personal (parenthood, etc) roles. Pitney[71] illustrated the need for personal rejuvenation, which included time away from the daily grind. Others have extended the notion of time away[65] as a means to promote professional commitment and satisfaction for the role of the athletic trainer and should include a separation of roles. Simply, when engaged in the role of "mom," an athletic trainer should respectfully decline looking at emails, responding to texts, or thinking about what needs to be done at work. In contrast, when engaged at work, athletic trainers should focus energies on providing patient care, completing administrative paperwork, and providing supervision to their athletic training students (if applicable) and avoid worrying about domestic and household tasks (leaky faucet, dance recital, etc). Separation can provide the opportunity to disconnect from demanding roles, which allows for stimulation of renewed sense of commitment, satisfaction, and investment in the role.

Support networks, personal and work based, are important for the athletic trainer when managing multiple roles as they often provide encouragement, understanding, and at times assist with meeting the demands of a particular role. For example, on numerous occasions researchers[65] have cited social support as a means to maintain work-life balance. When a spouse or family member can help take a more active role in managing the household and domestic duties, it can alleviate the pressures for the athletic trainer when working long hours. Sharing the duties is one way of achieving work-life balance, particularly in the personal domain. As mentioned above, job sharing through teamwork is one way an athletic trainer can stimulate work-life balance despite limitations with work scheduling, something that can be paralleled in the home setting. A large portion of the data on work-life balance in athletic training are qualitative based, which has provided rich data on the experiences of athletic trainers striving for balance. The data highlight personal social support as key because it reduces the stress felt by athletic trainers as they endure longer work hours weekly, unorthodox work schedules, and travel.[65] Family support can be key too, as often athletic trainers must miss holidays or family functions because of game or practice schedules, thus having support and flexibility as to when those functions happen is helpful.

One's outlook is also important for finding work-life balance. The theory of work-life enrichment was shared in the beginning of the chapter; engagement in multiple roles can provide greater satisfaction as a person can gain skills and energy from the variety of each role. Having a realistic but optimistic attitude can allow for a reduction in stress and conflict, as it allows for adaptability when dealing with competing time and role demands.

SUMMARY

Work-life conflict has become a central issue for Americans. A recent report from the Center for American Progress and the University of California, Hastings College of the Law broadcast that 90% of U.S. mothers and 95% of U.S. fathers report work-life conflict. Conflict often manifests because of a myriad of factors, but work time is the most significant facilitator reported among all working professionals and most certainly for the athletic trainer. With the development of the National Athletic Trainers' Association (NATA)'s position statement on work-life balance and the continued discussions among educators and researchers, fulfillment of balance is more attainable. A blended approach is needed when it comes to implementing strategies to promote balance, which need to be initiated at the personal and organizational level and continued to be supported at each level. We encourage athletic trainers to review and discuss the NATA's Position Statement on Work-Life Balance as it can provide the foundation for policy development and implementation.

ACTIVITIES FOR REINFORCEMENT

Questions for Review

1. Describe the difference between work-life balance and work-life conflict.
2. List the factors that inhibit work-life balance.
3. Several theories lead us to understand work-family conflict. Compare and contract integration/separation theory with enrichment theory. Also, compare and contrast the border theory with the multifactorial theory.
4. What is meant by multilevel work-life interference?
5. What are the common sources of conflict that lead to work-life imbalance?

Case Vignettes

Case #1

Stacy is an assistant athletic trainer at a medium sized, Division I university and she is currently working with women's soccer and women's lacrosse. She has been working on average 55 hours per week, managing 18 women's soccer student athletes and 32 women's lacrosse student-athletes, and is supervising 2 athletic training students. In addition she is mentoring 2 graduate assistant athletic trainers who are covering swimming/diving and crew. Her role in clinical education adds about 10 hours a week to her work responsibilities. She has been in her role for 6 years and this was her first position post her graduate work. She is single and is enjoying her role, but is finding it hard to make time for herself and she hopes to get married someday and start a family.

1. What are Stacy's major sources for conflict?
2. How would her issues with work-life balance change if she were married or already had children?
3. What recommendations would you suggest for Stacy to help her manage her load and find a more balanced lifestyle?
4. How does her practice setting have an influence on her ability to find balance?

Case #2

Tom, an outreach athletic trainer, is contracted for 15 hours per week in the clinic and 25 hours per week in the high school. He has been employed with the company for 10 years. He is the sole athletic trainer working in his high school, which has football. He is married with 2 young children (ages 2 and 4), and a wife who works part time (25 hours per week). Most of his high school duties begin at 2:30 pm and he ends around 7:30 pm each day. He misses most dinners with his family, but sometimes is able to have lunch with his children. Tom's parents live in the next town over from him and are retired.

1. What sources of conflict are present for Tom as he attempts to balance his life?
2. How will his attempts to balance his roles change as his children grow?
3. What recommendations do you provide Tom to improve his work-life balance?

Discussion Questions

1. Which work-life balance theory do you believe offers the best explanation as to why individuals experience conflict between work and life?

2. What do you believe is the most important tact a supervisor can take to help an athletic trainer reduce his/her work-family conflict?

3. In what way would you help a coworker who was experiencing a great deal of difficultly balance work and life?

REFERENCES

1. Greenhaus JH, Collins KM, Shaw JD. The relation between work-family balance and quality of life. *J Vocat Behav.* 2003;63:510-531.
2. Pastore DL, Inglis S, Danylchuk KE. Retention factors in coaching and athletic management: differences by gender, position, and geographic location. *J Sport Soc Iss.* 1996;20(4):427-441.
3. Dixon MA, Bruening JE. Perspectives on work-family conflict in sport: an integrative approach. *Sport Manage Rev.* 2005;8:227-254.
4. Dixon MA, Sagas M. The relationship between organizational support, work-family conflict, and the job-life satisfaction of university coaches. *Res Q Ex Sport.* 2007;78(3):236-247.
5. Shanafelt TD, Boone S, Tan L, et al. Burnout and satisfaction with work-life balance among US physicians relative to the general US population. *Arch Intern Med.* 2012;172(18):1377-1385.
6. Goodman A, Mensch JM, Jay M, French KE, Mitchell MF, Fritz SL. Retention and attrition factors for female certified athletic trainers in the National Collegiate Athletic Association Division I Football Bowl Subdivision setting. *J Athl Train.* 2010;45(3):287-298.
7. Mazerolle SM, Bruening JE, Casa DJ. Work-family conflict, part I: antecedents of work-family conflict in National Collegiate Athletic Association Division I-A certified athletic trainers. *J Athl Train.* 2008;43(5):505-512.
8. Mazerolle SM, Bruening JE, Casa DJ, Burton LJ. Work-family conflict, part II: job and life satisfaction in National Collegiate Athletic Association Division I-A certified athletic trainers. *J Athl Train.* 2008;43(5):513-522.
9. Mazerolle SM, Goodman A, Pitney WA. Factors influencing retention of male athletic trainers in NCAA Division I setting. *Int J Athl Ther Train.* 2013;18(5):6-9.
10. The president and Michelle Obama on work, family, and juggling it all. http://parade.condenast.com/306214/parade/the-president-and-michelle-obama-on-work-family-and-juggling-it-all/. Updated 2014. Accessed July/21, 2014.
11. Work-life balance. www.worklifebalance.com. Updated 2014. Accessed July 21, 2014.
12. Mazerolle SM, Ferraro EM, Eason CM, Goodman A. Factors and strategies that contribute to work-life balance of female athletic trainers employed in the NCAA Division I setting. *Athl Train Sport Health Care.* 2013;5(5):211-222.
13. Mazerolle SM, Ferraro EM, Eason CM, Goodman A. Career and family aspirations of female athletic trainers employed in the NCAA Division I setting. *J Athl Train.* 2013. In press.
14. Allen TD, Herst DEL, Bruck CS, Sutton M. Consequences associated with work-to-family conflict: a review and agenda for future research. *J Occup Health Psychol.* 2000;5(2):278-308.
15. Greenhaus JH, Callanan GA, Godshalk VM. *Career Management.* 4th ed. Los Angeles, CA: Sage; 2010.
16. Goode WJ. A theory of role strain. *Am Soc Rev.* 1960;25(4):483-496.
17. Gornick JC, Meyers MK. *Families That Work: Policies For Reconciling Parenthood and Employment.* New York, NY: Russell Sage Foundation Publications; 2005:404.
18. Mazerolle SM, Pitney WA, Casa DJ, Pagnotta KD. Assessing strategies to manage work and life balance of athletic trainers working in the National Collegiate Athletic Association Division I setting. *J Athl Train.* 2011;46(2):194-205.
19. Kahn RL, Wolfe DM, Quinn RP, Snoek JD, Rosenthal RA. *Organizational Stress: Studies in Role Conflict and Ambiguity.* New York: Wiley; 1964.
20. Greenhaus JH, Beutell N. Sources of conflict between work and family role. *Acad Manage Rev.* 1985;10:76-88.
21. Greenhaus JH, Powell GN. When work and family are allies: A theory of work-family enrichment. *Acad Manage Rev.* 2006;31:72-92.
22. Schenewark JD, Dixon MA. A dual model of work-family conflict and enrichment in collegiate coaches. *J Issues Intercol Athl.* 2012;5:15-39.

23. Barnett R, Gareis K. Role theory perspectives on work and family. In: Pitt-Catsouphes M, Kossek E, Sweet S, eds. *The Work and Family Handbook: Multidisciplinary Perspectives and Approaches*. Mahwah, NJ: Lawrence Erlbaum Associates; 2006:209-222.

24. Murphy SE, Zagorski DA. Enhancing work-family and work-life interaction: The role of management. In: Halpern DF, Murphy SE, eds. *From Work-Family Balance to Work-Family Interaction*. Hillsdale, NJ: Lawrence Erlbaum Associates; 2006.

25. Sieber SD. Toward a theory of role accumulation. *Am Soc Rev*. 1974;39:567-578.

26. Marks SR. Multiple roles and role strain: some notes on human energy, time, and commitment. *Am Soc Rev*. 1977;42:921-936.

27. Wayne JH, Musisca N, Fleeson W. Considering the role of personality in the work-family experience: relationships of the big five to work-family conflict and facilitation. *J Vocat Behav*. 2004;64:108-130.

28. Voydanoff P. The effects of work demands and resources on work-to-family conflict and facilitation. *J Mar Fam*. 2004;66:398-412.

29. McCrae RR, John OP. An introduction to the five-factor model and its applications. *J Pers*. 1992;2(175):215.

30. Clark SC. Work/family border theory: A new theory of work/family balance. *Hum Relat*. 2000;53(6): 747-770.

31. Mazerolle SM, Pitney WA, Goodman A. Strategies for athletic trainers to find a balanced lifestyle across clinical setting. *Int J Athl Ther Train*. 2012;17(3):7-14.

32. Clark SC. Work/family border theory: a new theory of work/family balance. *Hum Relat*. 2000;53(6):747-770.

33. Pitney WA, Ehlers GE, Walker SE. A descriptive study of athletic training students' perceptions of effective mentoring roles. *Internet J Allied Health Sci Pract*. 2006;4(2):1-8.

34. Carlson D. Personality and role variables as predictors of three forms of work-family conflict. *J Vocat Behav*. 1999;55:236-253.

35. Carlson DS, Kacmar KM. Work-family conflict in the organization: do life role values make a difference? *J Manag*. 2000;26:1031-1054.

36. Kossek EE, Noe R, Colquitt J. Caregiving decisions, well-being and performance: the effects of place and provider as a function of dependent type and work-family climates. *Acad Manag J*. 2001;44(1):29-44.

37. Eby L, Casper W, Lockwood A, Bordeaux C, Brinley A. Work and family research in IO/OB: content analysis and review of the literature (1980–2000). *J Vocat Behav*. 2004;66:124-197.

38. Hewlett S. *Creating a Life: Professional Women and the Quest for Children*. New York: Talk Miramax Books; 2002.

39. Garey AI. *Weaving Work and Motherhood*. Philadelphia, PA: Temple University Press; 1999.

40. Hakim C. *Work-Lifestyle Choices in the 21st Century: Preference Theory*. New York: Oxford University Press; 2000.

41. Kan MY. Work orientation and wives' employment careers: an evaluation of Hakim's preference theory. *Work Occupation*. 2007;34:430-462.

42. Bruening JE, Dixon MA. Work-family conflict in coaching II: Managing role conflict. *J Sport Manag*. 2007;21:471-496.

43. Center for American Progress. https://cdn.americanprogress.org/wp-content/uploads/issues/2010/01/pdf/threefaces.pdf. Updated 2010. Accessed August 31, 2015.

44. Eberman LE, Kahanov L. Athletic trainer perceptions of life-work balance and parenting concerns. *J Athl Train*. 2013;48(3):416-423.

45. Michel JS, Kotrba LM, Mitchelson JK, Clark MA, Baltes BB. Antecedents of work-family conflict: a meta-analytic review. *J Org Behav*. 2011;32(5):689-725.

46. Pitney WA, Mazerolle SM, Pagnotta KD. Work-family conflict among athletic trainers in the secondary school setting. *J Athl Train*. 2011;46(2):185-193.

47. Frone MR, Yardley JK, Markel KS. Developing and testing and integrative model of the work-family interface. *J Vocat Behav*. 1997;50:145-167.

48. Bedeian AG, Burke BG, Moffett RG. Outcomes of work-family conflict among married male and female professionals. *J Manag*. 1988;14:475-492.

49. Kelly RF, Voydanoff P. Work/family role strain among employed parents. *Fam Relat*. 1985;3(34):367-374.

50. Noor NM. Work-family conflict, locus of control, and women's well-being: tests of alternative pathways. *J Soc Psychol*. 2002;142(5):645-662.

51. Rantanen J, Pulkkinen L, Kinnunen U. The big five personality dimensions, work-family conflict, and psychological distress: a longitudinal view. *J Indiv Differ*. 2005;26(3):155-166.

52. Hendrix AE, Acevedo EO, Hebert E. An examination of stress and burnout in certified athletic trainers at Division I-A universities. *J Athl Train*. 2000;35(2):139-144.

53. Kania ML, Meyer BB, Ebersole KT. Personal and environmental characteristics predicting burnout among certified athletic trainers at National Collegiate Athletic Association institutions. *J Athl Train*. 2009;44(1):58-66.

54. Cinnamon R, Rich Y. Gender differences in the importance of work and family roles: implications for work-family conflict. *Sex Roles*. 2002;47:531-541.

55. Duxbury LE, Higgins CA. Gender differences in work-family conflict. *J Appl Psychol*. 1991;76(1):60-74.

56. Gutek BA, Searle S, Klepa L. Rational versus gender role expectations for work-family conflict. *J Appl Psychol.* 1991;76(4):560-568.

57. Kahanov L, Eberman LE. Age, sex, and setting factors and labor force in athletic training. *J Athl Train.* 2011;46(4):424-430.

58. Kahanov L, Loebsack AR, Masucci MA, Roberts J. Perspectives on parenthood and working of female athletic trainers in the secondary school and collegiate settings. *J Athl Train.* 2010;45(5):459-466.

59. Mazerolle SM, Burton L, Cotrufo R. The experiences of female athletic trainers in the role of the head athletic trainer. *J Athl Train.* 2015; 50: 71-81.

60. Pitney WA. Organizational influences and quality-of-life issues during the professional socialization of certified athletic trainers working in the National Collegiate Athletic Association Division I setting. *J Athl Train.* 2006;41(2):189-195.

61. Naugle KE, Behar-Horenstein LS, Dodd VJ, Tillman MD, Borsa PA. Perceptions of wellness and burnout among certified athletic trainers: sex differences. *J Athl Train.* 2013;48(3):424-430.

62. Lee K, Allen NJ, Meyer JP, Rhee K. The three-component model of organisational commitment: an application to South Korea. *Appl Psychol.* 2001;50(4):596-614.

63. Bowman TG, Mazerolle SM, Goodman A. Career commitment of post-professional athletic training program graduates. *J Athl Train.* 2015; 50: 426-431.

64. Capel SA. Attrition of athletic trainers. *Athl Train J Natl Athl Train Assoc.* 1990;25(1):34-39.

65. Mazerolle SM, Pitney WA. Workplace environment: strategies to promote and enhance the quality of life of an athletic trainer. *Athl Train Sport Hlth.* 2011;3(2):59-62.

66. Mazerolle SM, Pitney WA, Goodman A, Eason CM. National athletic trainer's position statement: work-life balance recommendations. *J Athl Train.* 2014. In review.

67. Goodman A, Mazerolle SM, Pitney WA. Achieving work-life balance in the National Collegiate Athletic Association Division I setting, part II: perspectives from head athletic trainers. *J Athl Train.* 2015;50(3):89-94.

68. Mazerolle SM, Goodman A, Pitney WA. Achieving work-life balance in the NCAA Division I setting part I: the role of the head athletic trainer. *J Athl Train.* In press.

69. Mazerolle SM, Goodman A. An examination of work-life balance: a case study investigating the fulfillment of work life balance from the organizational perspective. *J Athl Train.* 2013;48(5):668-677.

70. Mazerolle SM, Goodman A. Investigating workplace culture and work life balance: a case study of a NCAA Division I university. *J Athl Train.* In press.

71. Pitney WA. A qualitative examination of professional role commitment among athletic trainers working in the secondary school setting. *J Athl Train.* 2010;45(2):198-204.

4

Role Complexities in the Workplace

Kirk Brumels, PhD, AT, ATC

OBJECTIVES

After reading this chapter, the reader will be able to do the following:

1. Define role complexity.
2. Differentiate between role stress and role strain.
3. Understand various role complexity typologies.
4. Identify sources of role complexity.
5. Explain how role complexity may be a benefit or detriment to job satisfaction of the role occupant.
6. Engage in discussions on how to lessen negative effects of role complexity.

INTRODUCTION

Organizations are complex centers of intertwined, patterned, and concerted activity that consist of individual employees who play a role in performing the functions that meet the collective mission, vision and objectives of the group.[1] We all exist in social organizations and with few exceptions will be considered part of an occupation or work organization when we accept employment.

As members of society, we are expected to behave and interact within certain parameters and norms. These boundaries vary greatly based on ethnicity, culture, geography, beliefs or group inclusion and are developed as laws, rules or socially accepted guidelines instituted in either formal or informal fashion. Individual knowledge and understanding of the role we are to undertake are ever changing, but are framed within rules, both written and unwritten.

Employment organizations also create a culture of roles and responsibilities. These roles are typically based on employment status within the organization and involve work obligations and

Mazerolle SM, Pitney WA.
Workplace Concepts for Athletic Trainers (pp 63-75).
© 2016 Taylor & Francis Group.

interactions with co-workers. With regards to the athletic training professional, employment organizations may include, but are not be limited to, hospitals, universities, private outpatient clinics, physician offices, colleges, performance clinics, high schools, military, corporations or the entertainment industry. As a member of society or employment organizations, each participant will be expected to behave or perform within predetermined or evolving roles with appropriate and often times predictable behavior patterns applied to personal conduct, interpersonal interactions, job responsibilities and/or philosophies.

Biddle and Thomas[2] sum up a role within an organization as being defined by: "social norms, demands, and rules: by the role performances of others in their respective positions; by those who observe and react to the performance; and by the individual's particular capabilities and personality." This definition of an employment role has its foundation in the work of Kahn et al,[1] who believe that people in an organization behave in 2 distinct *environments*: the objective environment and the psychological environment. Kahn states that the "objective environment of a person consists of real objects and events, verifiable outside his consciousness and experience," whereas "the conscious and unconscious representations of the objective environment constitute the psychological environment of the person."

Organizations consist of 2 distinct environments: objective and psychological.

Role complexities found among the multiple expectations of patients, students, and the employment organization have been examined in allied health care professions. The inherent stress of dealing with people who have health issues is often compounded by the stress of additional work-related obligations and responsibilities. Compounding of the time, effort, and energy required to fulfill all of the expected duties puts a stress on the role occupant and provides fertile ground for the potential growth of role complexities that may negatively affect job performance.

DEFINITIONS OF ROLE THEORY AND ROLE COMPLEXITY

Role theory is the examination, consideration, and study of how individuals exist and behave in the roles they fulfill and the environments they fulfill them in. It involves analysis of the complexities of role fulfillment and how internal and external factors affect the expected outcomes. Role complexity or complexities are terms used to describe the multiple difficulties that an individual has in performing his or her expected role according to established norms. Any and all sources or stressors that manifest into difficulty and complications related to performing expected responsibilities at work can individually or collectively be described as role complexities. However, to further delineate sources and causes of role complexities, research has been conducted into role theory and examination of associated role complexities or difficulties, with 2 major subcategories emerging: role stress and role strain. Additional facets of role complexity identified to describe situations or stressors that comprise role stress and role strain, but let's first examine these 2 major subcategories of role complexity.

Role Strain

Role strain is described as an internally felt role complexity that an individual feels while attempting to fulfill role obligations within his or her employment or social organization. Role strain is largely due to and comes from discontinuity in the "psychological environment" described by Kahn[1] and cannot be attributed to an organizational or structural problem. This type of role complexity is due to internalized and perceived complexities in fulfilling a role and is personal in nature. The role complexities that lead to role strain are rooted in the psychological environment and include perceived demands and internalized sensitivity toward co-workers, supervisors, administrators, patients, etc. This internalized sensitivity creates intrinsic role strain, which consists of subjective feelings such as frustration, irritation, tension, pressure, or anxiety regarding the responsibilities inherent in a particular position that possesses one or more of the aforementioned role stressors. Role strain may also become apparent to others when the external role stressors become internalized in ways that lead to negative outward emotions or behavior. Goode[3] defined role strain as the "felt difficulty in meeting one's role obligations." This seems to imply that once role stressors and difficulties are internalized and felt by the role occupant, they then create role strain that negatively affects job performance via internal or external conflict with job responsibilities. Hardy and Conway[4] have determined that the 5 most common psychological responses to role strain are identified as: anxiety, tension, irritation, resentment, and depression.

> Role strain is many times a by-product of the "psychological environment" of an organization.

Role Stress

Role stress, on the other hand, is the felt role complexity that has its source or origin in the "external environment" that surrounds and affects employees in their work setting. This may include the physical structure of the workplace, work conditions, reporting structures, expectations, work hours, work conditions, and expertise required. In continuing to apply Kahn's environment theory,[1] the physical environment is responsible for role stress because in those situations the social structure creates very difficult, conflicting, or impossible demands for the role occupant. Role stress has foundations in situations external to the person and originates in the social or work structure, and when not corrected may lead to internalized emotions or feelings. Owing to work arrangements or other external factors, an employee may experience role stress when responsibility expectations are unclear, conflicting, incongruous with expectations, philosophy, or morality, require more work than an employee can reasonably perform, or require a level of qualification and skill that is either too great or too minimal. Therefore, role stress can be created by role ambiguity, role conflict, role incongruity, role overload, and negative role qualification as an employee performs work responsibilities.

Based on the aforementioned researched and nuanced descriptions of role stress vs role strain, it is often difficult to determine whether felt role complexity is due to role stress or role strain. In fact, since these concepts are so closely related and in many cases intertwined, it may be more productive to describe and discuss role stress and strain as role complexity with the delineation of type of complexity occurring at the source level.

> Role stress is many times a by-product of the "objective environment" of an organization.

FACETS AND SOURCES OF ROLE COMPLEXITIES

Role complexities, including role stress and role strain, have become and continue to be more prevalent and problematic with multiple obligations present in the workplace. Hardy and Conway[4] have described the most common, influential, and frequently researched facets of role complexities that may lead to role stress or strain. Taking all the role conditions and typologies into account is important when studying role complexities in general and role stress and strain specifically.

Individual typologies alone may create role complexity in given situations, but many of the typologies are often discovered to intermingle, compound, and create overall role stress/strain. Therefore, it is essential to the understanding of role complexities that the individual sources of difficulty be studied individually and collectively as both sources may create stress for a role occupant.

The following typologies and definitions of role complexity are the result of the seminal work by Hardy and Conway.[4]

Role Conflict

Role conflict has been described by Hardy and Conway[4] as the "condition in which the focal person perceives existing role expectations as being contradictory or mutually exclusive." Failure to meet conflicting expectations from numerous sources is exacerbated by the prioritizing of the very same multiple responsibilities and obligations. According to Ruby,[5] the hierarchical delineation of job preference is made apparent by the amount of time a role occupant attributes to various tasks and responsibilities. Therefore, multiple responsibilities affect job performance, making it difficult to meet all the expectations and obligations, putting professional credibility and reputations in jeopardy.

Examples in athletic training may include situations in which an athletic trainer has multiple roles as part of an employment contract. Being hired by a hospital or outpatient sports medicine clinic to provide services to patients, as well as being contracted to deliver health care to a local high school or sports team, creates a situation where there are 2 separate and potentially conflicting reporting structures and expectations. Conflict may occur between expectations, time allocation, or specific responsibilities.

Role Ambiguity

Role ambiguity is described as situations in which the norms for a particular position are vague, unclear, ill defined, or consist of contradictory role expectations. Role ambiguity is often associated with poorly defined expectations, haphazard performance, and inconsistent discipline or performance evaluations. Consider, as an example, a novice athletic trainer working in a sports medicine center who has been asked by a supervisor to oversee the durable goods component of their operation. If the job expectation stopped there, and no further definition of "oversee" was provided, the athletic trainer may be unclear as to what his or her role is exactly. Is the role to order all necessary durable goods? Identify what durable goods the physicians want in stock? Is the role to work with patients to fit them with appropriate devices?

Athletic trainers who work without clear or detailed job expectations or responsibilities often are negatively affected by role ambiguity as the target for expectations move or change without communication between the employee and employer. This source of role complexity is a difficult one to overcome and without mediation efforts may certainly lead to poor job performance and satisfaction.

Role Overload

Role overload refers to a condition when an employee finds it difficult to perform job duties because they are either excessive or cannot possibly be finished in the time available. Coverman[6] describes role overload as "fulfilling several roles simultaneously"[6(p967)] and states that role overload leads to role conflict when one of the roles disallows the employee from performing the duties required of their other roles. Hardy and Conway[4] have defined role overload as when an individual is either unable to finish all of the required obligations or when an individual is able to finish all obligations, but not at a level of competence otherwise achieved if other duties were not present. Therefore, there are 2 components of role overload: quantitative and qualitative. Quantitative overload refers to the fact that the role occupant has too many tasks to perform and not enough time to perform them. Qualitative overload refers to work that is too difficult, complex, or intense and therefore the quality of work suffers. Qualitative overload is manifested in situations where the role occupant does not have the skills necessary to handle his or her job responsibilities.

At certain times of year, in certain employment positions, or upon addition of new responsibilities, athletic trainers may sometimes be heard stating "there are just not enough hours in the day to get everything done." Athletic trainers are not the only health care providers or employees who feel this way, but when they do, they are certainly feeling stress due to quantitative role overload. In addition, when the expectations of a position are such that the employee feels unprepared to complete the tasks owing to lack of competence or ability, then the stress can be attributed to qualitative overload and/or role incompetence, which will be discussed later.

Role Underload

Hardy and Conway[4] also discuss role underload, in which insufficient demands are placed on an individual's time and thus the individual is not challenged to perform to his or her level of capabilities or requirements of the job. When used as a reason for not offering a job to an applicant, the comment "you are overqualified for this job" is an attempt by the employer to negate the anticipated poor job performance due to role underload and expected manifestation of boredom, apathy, laziness, and underperformance.

Role Incongruity

Role incongruity describes situations where incompatibility occurs between either skills or personal values and the job requirements. It is not a well-researched or defined concept in the literature, but it refers to situations where the competence, ability, morality, self-perception, preference, or expectations of a professional might not align well with the requirements of a particular role.

Role Competence/Incompetence

Role competence/incompetence refers to an individual's overall ability to perform successfully in his or her current roles. Role incompetence describes a situation in which an individual does not have the necessary skills or knowledge to successfully perform the responsibilities inherent in a particular job. Role competence, on the other hand, describes a situation where the role occupant does have the social, mental, and physical abilities to perform well within his or her particular job. It has been agreed on by structural theorists that role competence is necessary to adequately perform a role, and to progress and develop both individually and socially. Role competence can be a learned behavior, developed through the socialization and acclimatization process at a place of employment.

Role Qualification

Role qualification can be examined as either underqualification or overqualification. In the case of role underqualification, the role occupant is overwhelmed by the amount of work responsibilities and obligations that need to be performed. These feelings are based on the fact that the professional is neither qualified nor able to perform the tasks in a timely manner. Role underqualification can also lead to feelings of role overload. Role overqualification occurs when individuals are overqualified and able to perform work much more difficult than what is being asked, causing underuse and frustration.

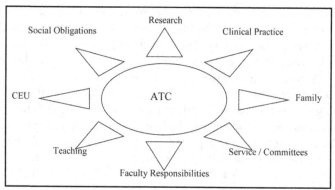

Figure 4-1. Theoretical role responsibilities/obligations. ATC: certified athletic trainer; CEU: continuing education units.

ROLE COMPLEXITIES IN HEALTH CARE PROFESSIONS

The balance between work, social, spiritual, family, and other obligations can often be described as tenuous, and can contribute to role complexities affecting satisfaction levels. Role complexities are a concern in many allied health professions, including athletic training, nursing, medicine, and physical therapy. Role complexities are present in all aspects of life. Research on role complexity issues and typologies has been performed previously in many health care settings, including athletic training.

Figure 4-1 is a theoretical depiction of the various influences that affect the lives and professional role complexities of athletic trainers in multiple settings. While this may not be inclusive of each job setting, it offers a visual representation of the many responsibilities that "pull" on the time, skills, and abilities of athletic trainers. There might be additional variables not depicted in Figure 4-1 that are specific to individual athletic trainers and their employment situations, but the idea is that each athletic trainers has multiple social and employment factors or entities that require attention. It is reasonable to assume that role complexities will be felt if these varied responsibilities are not kept in check. In conceptualizing these figures it is unfortunate that the depiction is 2-dimensional and static. Figure 4-1 assumes that each category has the same amount of influence on the life of the individual. In reality these pressures are not symmetrical or similar among individuals and the diagram should take on more of an active 3-dimensional look with each and every obligation or responsibility exerting pressure or pull on the time and roles of the athletic trainer.

Figure 4-2 more accurately depicts what happens to the overall role responsibilities that an athletic trainer may have. The amoeboid shape represents the ever-changing and continually moving aspect of role complexities. Given this phenomenon, the lines of responsibility often become blurred and imprecise. The "shape" of the professional role will be different for all athletic trainers, based on the role responsibilities and obligations that they may face. This "shape" may change on an hourly, daily, weekly, or yearly basis depending on the individual situation. It would be difficult to find 2 sets of responsibilities and obligations that are exactly the same among individuals regardless of how similar their employment situations may be, but several categories of employment situations for athletic trainers exist and are discussed.

Health Care Faculty

Faculty positions can create role complexity issues due to the teaching, research, and service responsibilities of traditional classroom and clinical instruction. Williams and Hadfield[7] found that athletic training education programs that have faculty who do not share clinical and teaching responsibilities produce graduates with a higher first-time passing rate on the national

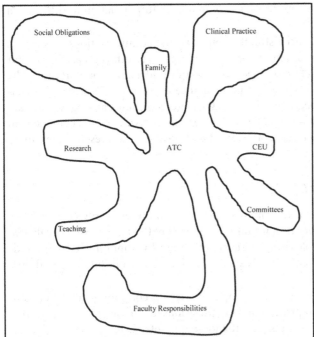

certification exam. It was felt that this was due to the fact that the faculty member would have more time to prepare for classroom teaching and perform academic duties than a joint appointee with responsibilities both to academics and clinical practice.

Health Care Clinicians

Role complexities certainly can occur with clinicians in traditional patient care roles who practice health care in various settings. In these clinical care settings, the role complexities originate from multiple sources including but not limited to patient care, continuing education, professional service, and student instruction. Dividing time between personal continuing education and mastery of skills along with the multiple responsibilities toward clinical education of health profession students can be fraught with difficulty. athletic trainers often possess multiple areas of responsibility, creating situations where role complexities may be present. The individual responsibilities of clinical work, patient care, administration of programs, supervision, continuing education, and clinical instruction are all areas that can contribute to overall role complexities.

Health Care Joint Appointees

Joint appointment health care professionals are those individuals that have responsibilities to 2 separate entities. This often involved several hierarchical reporting structures such as athletics and academics, clinical care and athletics, administration and athletics, academics and administration, or clinical care and administration. Role occupants in these work settings are often expected to perform and be evaluated by 2 separate but equal units. Position descriptions that create joint appointments are often constructed to meet demands of patients, educators, students, administrators, etc. Pressure on health care educators to maintain practice skills is encouraged as a way to improve the learning outcomes of the students in academic programs. In addition, many high school athletic trainers are employed by hospitals or sports medicine facilities with work obligations to the secondary school as well as their hiring agency. This may involve a split day with direct patient-to-practitioner care in the mornings and practitioner-to-population health care in the afternoons/evenings.

In order for joint appointments to be successful, the employee and administrations they report to must have the following: mutual accountability; the perception that both roles are important factors for the single identity; compatible role expectations; and understanding about how the clinical practice portion of the position will affect performance evaluations. Poor communication and unclear role delineation has been found to create role complexities among health care professionals. Joint appointments will most likely fail when an individual is accountable to 2 separate administrative bodies or when a lack of respect for clinical practice, research, teaching, or publishing exists.

Role Orientation in Joint Appointments

The issue in joint appointment positions is that one role expectation tends to receive priority from the role occupant, and thus the other responsibilities suffer. If both obligations are evaluated equally in performance reviews, then role complexities may arise. When multiple role demands exist, a common way of dealing with them is to create a hierarchy of responsibilities based on a determination of perceived importance.

Responsibilities to clinical patient care, research, teaching, service, continuing education, student advising, administrative duties, and professional organizations are among the many sources of potential role complexities for the joint appointee. If a joint appointee is to be successful, he or she must be able to manage the stress arising from multiple responsibilities.

When multiple role demands exist, a common way of dealing with them is to create a hierarchy of responsibilities based on a determination of perceived importance. This is called role orientation. The potential exists for individuals to possess a role orientation hierarchy among the roles of their joint appointment. Choices will be made regarding which of the roles will predominate and engage our time, talent, and attention.

Role orientation can be seen between expectations of a joint appointee, but it also has a tendency to exist when role overload occurs. When role occupants experience role overload, they begin to choose between multiple responsibilities, thus establishing role orientation and potentially creating escalating amounts of role conflict.

Knowledge and understanding of role typologies will help to evaluate employment environments and provide insight into attitudes toward work. Being able to identify role complexities is a first step in managing, controlling or mitigating them.

> Role complexities will exist in nearly all work settings. Being able to recognize and deal with them appropriately may mean the difference between job satisfaction and dissatisfaction.

IMPACT OF ROLE COMPLEXITIES ON JOB SATISFACTION

Role complexities in the health care professions have been shown to affect job satisfaction, thus providing a related body of knowledge to the current situation in athletic training. Acorn[8] determined that higher levels of role complexity facets had an adverse effect on job satisfaction. As higher levels of role ambiguity, role stress, and organizational conflict occur, there also is an increase in job-induced tension. Left unfettered these issues may manifest themselves and negatively affect job performance, patient care, and satisfaction with work.

These studies have shown how role complexities affect job satisfaction and propensity to leave within the health care professions. When role complexity is present it often affects job satisfaction with potentially devastating effects on the health care delivery system. Stressors due to constraints and restrictions of time, energy, money, and talent should be eliminated in an attempt to establish a framework where appropriate medical care is given to patients. Therefore, it is appropriate to measure these 2 constructs together because of the direct relational nature that role complexities have on job satisfaction. The challenging character of the job responsibilities for clinical athletic training professionals has the potential for leaving the athletic trainer feeling that there is too much work to do and not enough time or assistance to do it. It is important for practicing athletic trainers to take steps to alleviate negative effects of role complexity so they can enjoy the positive benefits of serving others as a health care professional.

SUMMARY

While too much complexity can prove negative and ultimately decrease job satisfaction, some complexity in the workplace may be beneficial as it increases awareness of negative work constructs and situations that facilitate creative problem solving to fix. Where and when existing role complexities change from a positive to negative component of the work/employee relationship is idiosyncratic for each employee and employer affiliation. Recommendations for lessening professional role complexities for certified athletic trainers were made and should be implemented to diminish the negative effects of role complexities for athletic trainers.

It can be suggested that athletic trainers, administrators, supervisors, and athletic training students need to be aware of the sources and results of professional role complexity in efforts to increase work efficiency, satisfaction, and longevity. A potential source of the problematic type of role conflict and ambiguity may be the lack of a structured set of responsibilities. Job responsibilities and performance expectations must be clearly defined by administrators and supervisors in an attempt to lessen the negative effect of these role conflicts and role ambiguity. Clear expectations and non-conflicting demands for time commitment and obligations are paramount to the job satisfaction of certified athletic trainers. Conversations regarding role expectations and obligations must take place between role occupants and their supervisors because employees must be aware of what is expected of them and how their performance will be evaluated if role stress from role ambiguity is to be alleviated. Creation, modification, or review of job descriptions and responsibilities are essential for each athletic trainer in an attempt to control potential sources of his or her individual role overload, conflict, and ambiguity. Only when expectations are known and potential difficulties discussed can the role occupant begin to eliminate sources of role complexity. This needs to be performed for each employee at each organizational setting, as each workplace may possess unique sources of role stressors.

> Role complexities can have either a negative of positive affect on employment. Appropriate management of role complexities is of paramount importance for healthy workplace environments.

The positive and negative factors associated with role complexities found in athletic training are important to understand and address as choices are made regarding student acceptance and process through athletic training education programs. It seems apparent that athletic training is similar to other allied health professions that have been studied with regard to role complexities (Fain,[10] Kopala,[11] Mobily[12,13]). Role complexity issues have and will continue to exist within the health care professions. Even though there has not been the volume of research conducted into role complexity for athletic trainers as compared to other health professions, there is no reason to believe that athletic training is any different. As more studies are undertaken to examine role complexities within athletic training there are both examples and reasonable expectations that they are and will be present in ways similar to those in other allied health professions. Although efforts should be made to eliminate or at least decrease the negative effects of these stressors, it would be erroneous to believe that these role complexities can be completely eradicated.

Coping strategies, conflict resolution, and understanding preferred role orientation are important skills and knowledge to develop. It also becomes imperative that individuals who have the interpersonal skills and characteristics to best handle the known complexities be recruited into the profession. This may prove to be difficult, but determining personal characteristics that are effective in navigating the role complexities found in the athletic training workplace and developing ways to measure this aptitude and ability is vitally important in lessening the negative effects of role complexity.

In addition, each student and employee should undertake a critical examination of characteristics and responsibility orientation of each potential employment opportunity as a way to lessen future role complexities. Making sure that the role applicant has a role orientation that is compatible with the open position is essential for a good working relationship. The opposite is also true when an applicant is looking for an employment position. Matching up personal skills with a job becomes an important step in the process of eliminating role complexities before they occur.

It seems that athletic trainers share role complexities with other health professionals. Role overload, role conflict, and role ambiguity were the role complexity typologies that are most reported for athletic trainers. Role overload is a concern for adversely affecting best practice in any field but it becomes more of a concern when individuals experiencing it are involved with patient care. Caring for others inherently creates a level of stress within the health care professional. Increasing this inherent stress in a health care position due to role overload creates an even more fragile situation. Emotional fatigue, tension, lack of attention to details, and mistakes are potential consequences of role overload, which may affect the quality of patient care and have potential legal ramifications if mistakes and oversights are made.

Clinical athletic trainers typically have minimal input into their work schedule and this may lead to some of the felt role overload. Responsibilities to multiple teams, athletes, and coaches may cause increased role overload and role ambiguity and affect the athletic trainers ability to perform well. Typically, clinical athletic trainers do not perform their duties within the normally accepted working hours for many other professionals. This is usually understood and accepted prior to accepting employment positions. However, the problem arises when the individual athletic trainer is not afforded ways to handle changes or additions to the time frame in which he or she works. The locus of control in these situations is external to the individual athletic trainer. This lack of control over the work schedule can potentially lead to the feeling of role overload for the clinical athletic trainer. There does not appear to be a standard set of guidelines with respect to how much work is too much work for the clinical athletic trainer. The accumulative effect of expanding responsibilities without additional assistance or workload reduction may be a source for role overload, and steps to alleviate this must be initiated.

There is often the assumption that the clinical athletic trainer will work long and hard enough to meet the needs and demands of the program, coaches, and athletes. The athletic program clinical athletic trainer often does not have the same workload boundaries, as their faculty or outpatient clinic athletic trainer counterparts. This lack of professional responsibility limitations may lead to workload creep as the athletic trainer provides service to expanding athletic program demands. Little thought is given to athletic support personnel when teams, programs, events, or practices are added and are often just included without taking other responsibilities away. This is unlike the policy for adding additional teaching responsibilities or hours to a faculty or clinic employee's workload. Many institutions or organizations assign workloads for faculty and teaching responsibilities for faculty according to student contact hours or hours per week. This creates a sense of boundaries with regard to workload. When teaching or clinical care duties are added there often is discussion regarding which responsibilities to eliminate in exchange. Careful examination of time spent on the job, staffing issues, and performance expectations should be undertaken in an attempt to lessen the felt amount of role overload for certified athletic trainers involved in patient care and to address the risk management issues inherent in the situation.

The educational process of future athletic trainers must address these role complexity issues. Skills and knowledge are important, but time management, prioritization of workload, life balancing skills, personnel management, co-worker tolerance, personal strengths, and decision-making processes are crucial to success in the field. Case studies, scenarios, clinical experiences, and internships are all methods that can be used to acclimatize the entry-level athletic trainer into the difficulties and complexities of the workplace. Part of the acclimatization and education process of athletic training students must consist of developing the culture in which the hours and responsibilities inherent in the profession of athletic training are many, but expected and accepted. Athletic trainers play an important role in our health care system and the job can be extremely satisfying and rewarding. Like many other jobs, there are positive and negative aspects to each employment situation. Role complexities exist in health care generally and athletic training specifically. It is a responsibility of the profession and its professionals to seek ways to diminish the negative effects of role complexities so that athletic training professionals can perform their job and provide the best health care possible to their patients. This implies a need for athletic trainers to possess, discuss, negotiate, and agree on a clear job description and underscores the need for performance evaluations with truthful discussions of how to improve job performance and growth. Each role occupant needs to be aware of role complexities, understand the various role typologies, and seek strategies, resources, and support for managing them in an effort to engage in healthy professional development.

ACTIVITIES FOR REINFORCEMENT

Questions for Review

1. What is the difference between role stress an role strain?
2. What are the various role complexities and what are the primary causes of each?
3. In what way does role complexity affect job satisfaction?

Case Vignettes

Case #1

Tammy Tricep is an athletic trainer employed at Ruffed Grouse High School (RGHS) in Aspen, Colorado. Tammy was hired by Pheasant Valley Orthopedics and Rehabilitation Clinic (PVOR) to fulfill a contract obligation for athletic training services at Ruffed Grouse High. In addition to her job responsibilities at RGHS, Tammy also has administrative oversight of 6 other athletic trainers who provide medical service to neighboring high schools each afternoon and at home contests. All athletic trainers hired at PVOR also assist with patient care, wellness course offerings, and prehabilitation programs for patients undergoing surgical intervention. Tammy reports to Freddy B. Femoris, the practice manager of the rehabilitation clinic, and Melinda Moosejaw the athletic director at RGHS. At times Tammy feels like both jobs could be considered full time based on the amount of physical and emotional time she exerts in doing both jobs well. Her working conditions at the clinic are exceptional with great benefits, fantastic facilities, and detailed job expectations. However, she struggles with her personal emotions relating to how well she is doing in managing 6 other individuals. Tammy's responsibilities at the high school are made difficult by poor budgets, inadequate facilities, difficult coaches, and unclear expectations relating to coverage of events. Tammy has received constructive feedback and evaluations from Freddy, whereas the majority of conversations with Melinda revolve around what Tammy has done wrong or could do better.

1. Please discuss the potential role complexities that Tammy could be experiencing both at the clinic and the high school.

2. Discuss and recommend suggestions for Tammy to use to eliminate some of the negative role complexities she is experiencing in her work setting.

Case #2

Tommy Tricep is an athletic trainer with 3 (of course) specific areas of responsibility in his role as head athletic trainer for the Holland Harbor professional women's soccer program. Tommy has just graduated and is excited about any job, but specifically this opportunity to work in professional sports. In addition to being responsible for medical coverage for the 25 members of the squad, Tommy was told he was also responsible for team travel and equipment needs, including ordering, upkeep, and laundry. As a new hire, Tommy did not exactly know the level of time needed to meet the expectations but was excited to begin his employment. Tommy gets along well with his head coach, Patricia Pitch, and the players of the team and since he was hired in the off season, Tommy invested a lot of his time in the medical care of the team and felt like he was making a difference. As the season drew near, Tommy was approached by Patricia and team General Manager Bobby Boots regarding equipment needs and travel expectations for the upcoming season. Not wanting to eliminate any of the momentum and benefit relating to provision of health care and availability to the players, Tommy began to extend the hours of his work day to fulfil the additional responsibilities related to travel and equipment management. Unfamiliarity regarding the travel industry, team meal planning, and managing equipment issues began to create emotional and physical issues for Tommy and his attitude toward his job.

1. Please discuss the potential role complexities that Tommy could be experiencing both at the clinic and the high school.

2. Discuss and recommend suggestions for Tommy to use to eliminate some of the negative role complexities he is experiencing in his work setting.

Discussion Questions

1. Think about a work setting in which you would like to eventually gain employment. What role complexities exist in this type of setting? What steps can you take now to better understand the complexities and alleviate them?

2. What role complexity subcategory is most challenging for you to deal positively with? Which one provides the greatest challenge to you and your personality?

3. What role complexity do you enjoy working through? Do you find yourself personally and professionally challenged by a particular role complexity?

REFERENCES

1. Kahn RL, Wolfe DM, Quinn RP, Snoek JD. *Organizational Stress: Studies in Role Conflict and Ambiguity.* New York, NY: John Wiley & Sons; 1964.
2. Biddle BJ, Thomas EJ. *Role Theory: Concepts and Research.* New York, NY: John Wiley & Sons; 1966.
3. Goode WJ. Theory of role strain. *Am Sociological Rev.* 1960;25:483-495.
4. Hardy ME, Conway ME. *Role Theory: Perspectives for Health Professionals.* 2nd ed. Norwalk, CT: Appleton & Lange; 1988.

5. Ruby J. Baccalaureate nurse educators' workload and productivity: ascription of values and the challenges of evaluation. *J New York State Nurs Assoc.* 1998;29(2):18-22.

6. Coverman S. Role overload, role conflict, and stress: addressing consequences of multiple role demands. *Social Forces.* 1989;67(4):965-982.

7. Williams RB, Hadfield OD. Attributes of curriculum athletic training programs related to the passing rate of first-time certification examinees. *J Allied Health.* 2003;32(4):240-245.

8. Acorn S. Relationship of role conflict and role ambiguity to selected job dimensions among joint appointees. *J Prof Nurs.* 1991;7(4):221-227.

9. Acorn S. Joint appointments: perspectives of nurse executives. *Canadian J Nurs Admin.* 1990;3(4):6-9.

10. Fain JA. Perceived role conflict, role ambiguity, and job satisfaction among nurse educators. *J Nurs Educ.* 1987;26(6): 233-238.

11. Kopala B. Conflicts in nurse educators' role obligations. *J Prof Nurs.* 1994;10(4):236-243.

12. Mobily PRC. *Socialization, Academic Role Orientation and Role Strain of University Nurse Faculty* [dissertation]. Iowa City, IA: University of Iowa; 1987.

13. Mobily PR. An examination of role strain for university nurse faculty and its relation to socialization experiences and personal characteristics. *J Nurs Educ.* 1991;30(2):73-80.

5

Workplace Bullying

Stephanie M. Mazerolle, PhD, ATC, LAT;
William A. Pitney, EdD, ATC, FNATA; and
Celest Weuve, PhD, ATC, CSCS, LAT

OBJECTIVES

After reading this chapter, the reader will be able to do the following:

1. Define workplace bullying.
2. Recognize and identify workplace bullying.
3. Differentiate between workplace bullying, discrimination, and harassment.
4. Understand the consequences of workplace bullying
5. Identify effective strategies to help prevent or deal with workplace bullying.

> Bullying is nearly invisible. It is nonphysical, and nearly always sub-lethal workplace violence.

INTRODUCTION

Approximately 27% of Americans have experienced workplace bullying and another 15% have witnessed its occurrence.[1] Workplace bullying has often been described as a silent workplace issue that appears to affect women more than men.[1]

Growing concerns regarding workplace bullying in health care have stimulated research in the area, revealing that nurses have a long-standing history with workplace bullying,[2] but more recently its occurrence has been identified in occupational therapy[3,4] and medicine.[5] Athletic trainers often interact with a diverse group of individuals, and recent evidence highlights that

Mazerolle SM, Pitney WA.
Workplace Concepts for Athletic Trainers (pp 77-90).
© 2016 Taylor & Francis Group.

14.7% of athletic trainers employed in the collegiate setting have experienced bullying.[6] Despite limited information on the prevalence of workplace bullying in other practice settings, it is important for an athletic trainer to recognize the signs and symptoms of workplace bullying and understand the methods to prevent or reduce its negative effects.

This chapter will discuss the concept of workplace bullying, focusing on the early signs of bullying, identify who gets bullied and how it manifests in the workplace, and what its ramifications are. Additionally, the chapter will identify ways to prevent it as well as how to manage a case of bullying if it does arise.

DEFINING WORKPLACE BULLYING

Workplace bullying is a subtle but purposeful act that is directed toward an individual or group of individuals in the workplace. Bullying in the workplace often involves the abuse or misuse of power, and is distinct from other forms of workplace incivility as it is a repeated, ongoing pattern of behavior toward a victim, or "target."[2] Many working definitions exist, but often are concomitant by the negativity it creates within the workplace. Maguire and Ryan[2] describe workplace bullying as . . .

> *a behavior that goes beyond simple rudeness and incivility. While workplace bullying may include overt aggression or threat of violence, like other forms of aggression experienced . . . it frequently involves subtle or covert acts, rather than direct violence.*[(p120)]

Acts of bullying are viewed as unwanted, negative behavior that can be instigated by one or more individuals (perpetrators) over a prolonged period of time.[1] Workplace bullying is composed of offensive behavior that is ". . . vindictive, cruel, malicious, or humiliating attempts to undermine an individual or groups of employees."[7(p255)] The Task Force on the Prevention of Workplace Bullying[8] has labeled bullying as an:

> *offensive abusive, intimidating, malicious or insulting behavior or abuse of power conducted by an individual or group against others, which makes the recipient feel upset, threatened, humiliated or vulnerable, which undermines their self-confidence and which may cause them to suffer stress.*[8(p5)]

Workplace bullying is a silent issue that when it occurs is generally persistent, systematic, and at times can be subtle enough that it goes unrecognized. Table 5-1 provides examples of bullying from the perpetrator-initiated negative act. Bullying in the workplace can have serious negative consequences for those who are the target, but because of its commonalities with other workplace issues, can be missed.

Categories and Distinctions of Bullying

Acts of bullying in the workplace are designed to create an environment that belittles others through humiliation, sarcasm, rudeness, overwork, violence, and other unethical treatment. It is a distinctive issue in the workplace that is very different from one-time aggressive or discriminatory acts (ie, harassment, discrimination). The following descriptions differentiate bullying:

- **Repetition:** Unlike other workplace issues, bullying entails recurring and frequent acts. It is suggested that bullying abuse occurs on a near daily basis, in one form or another.[9,10]

- **Duration:** Workplace bullying is a long-term phenomenon and often a key feature of the act. Reports document bullying acts that last 6 months, but it may last longer.[11,12]

TABLE 5-1
EXAMPLES OF WORKPLACE BULLYING

Lateral bullying actions	Yelling at co-workers
	Refusing to help others in need of assistance
	Interactions that are rude, sarcastic, patronizing, or condescending
	Gossiping or spreading rumors
	Creating isolation or exclusion
	Withholding information intentionally
	Unwarranted or constant criticisms that are destructive or inappropriate
Supervisory or power bullying	Unfair assignment of work tasks and workloads
	Constant negative criticisms
	Exclusion from workplace meetings or information necessary to perform work duties successfully
	Failure to recognize workloads or efforts compared to others
	Belittling, demeaning, or patronizing employee in front of others
	Increase in workloads, excessively, in comparison to others

- **Escalation:** Bullying is a silent workplace issues; it intensifies over time because it likely goes undetected. Initially the target is uneasy at work, but as it progresses he or she is unquestionably aware of the acts toward them.[13]

- **Harm:** Experiences of bullying leave the target feeling impaired physically, emotionally, and mentally. Over time bullying acts become destructive on the target's overall health and well-being.[14]

- **Recognized intent:** Bullying has been viewed as purposeful—the intentions of the bully are intentional and directive. Individuals on the receiving end of bullying acts believe they are intentional and are not accidental.[15,16]

- **Hostile work environment:** Bullying creates a workplace environment that creates hostility, unease, and negativity. Individuals on the receiving end of bullying acts work in fear and dread, and this can influence their productivity and willingness to be at work.[13]

- **Power disparity:** Most acts of bullying showcase a power disparity; although it can occur peer to peer, a marked difference exists between the bully and the intended target.[13] Bullies are often power seekers and want control over everything.

- **Distorted communication networks:** Reducing communication to avoid revealing the bullying behavior is important to the bully. The bully fears individuals rallying together to discuss the behaviors.[17]

Bullying acts may occur in everyday life; however, when they occur regularly they can lead to harm and humiliation. Rayner et al[15] described 5 categories of bullying behavior:

1. Work-related bullying that may include changing your work tasks or making them difficult to perform (overwork)

2. Social isolation

3. Personal attacks or attacks on your private life by ridicule, insulting remarks, gossip

4. Verbal threats during which the victim is criticized, yelled at, or humiliated in public in the workplace (threat to professional status)

5. Destabilization

A threat to one's professional status can manifest through verbal attacks that include belittling one's opinions or efforts in front of others. A threat to one's professional status can extend into a person's workload, assignment of work, or creating expectations for one's role in the workplace. Social isolation develops when the target is prevented access to opportunities given to others, such as training, continuing education, or other pertinent information related to the workplace or completion of work-related jobs. Personal threats involve name-calling, insults, and teasing that are directed toward the target, and are unwanted, and designed to make them uneasy and uncomfortable. Overwork happens when the target is given impossible deadlines, performance is evaluated with a stricter set of rules/expectations, and he or she is placed in more stressful situations. Destabilization occurs when the target is unrightfully removed of responsibilities/title, is given meaningless tasks, or not recognized for efforts or completion of tasks/assignments. Table 5-2 provides athletic training examples of the 5 categories of bullying behaviors described by Rayner et al.[15]

WORKPLACE BULLYING, NOT HARASSMENT OR DISCRIMINATION

Harassment is defined as an offensive behavior that is intended to upset or disturb an individual, and can be repetitive in nature. Sexual harassment is the most common form of harassment seen in the workplace.
Discrimination is the negative treatment of a person and/or group, and is intended to deny social participation. Discriminative behaviors are meant to isolate or segregate based on certain prejudices (race, age, etc).

Both bullying and harassment involve actions that attempt to degrade, intimidate, or victimize an individual, but they are not one and the same—bullying is a relationship issue, whereas harassment is a human rights issue. Although both workplace issues are seen as unwanted or unwelcome, harassment is often linked to classes or identifiable groups such as gender, race, and people with physical disabilities, among others. Furthermore, individuals are often more likely to recognize acts of harassment over those of bullying as they are more subtle, and generally extend over a period of time.[16] Acts of harassment can occur in a single incident.

Discrimination, which is fully covered in Chapter 6, manifests when a person is treated differently (favorably or unfavorably) because of their gender, age, race, or disability. Discrimination in the workplace can develop before entering the organization (access discrimination) or after being hired (treatment discrimination). Access discrimination occurs when a person is denied access opportunities to enter a position or organization based on variables related to age, sex, or other protected classes (ie, not hiring a female for a football position). Treatment discrimination simply indicates that an individual is not given the same rewards, opportunities, or other benefits as others in the workplace because of a given reason (ie, female athletic trainer hired at a lower salary than a male athletic trainer with same qualifications).

Currently there are no laws governing bullying in the workplace; however, in 1964 the United States Congress passed Title VII of the Civil Rights Act, which denies discrimination in the workplace based on race, color, religion, and sex. Since the passing of the Civil Rights Act, other laws

TABLE 5-2

CASE ILLUSTRATIONS OF WORKPLACE BULLYING IN ATHLETIC TRAINING

CATEGORY	EXAMPLE
Professional standing	Taylor heads into a meeting with her coaching staff to discuss the updated injury report. In the meeting is the head coach, assistant coach, and the team's strength and conditioning specialist. While reporting who can't play in tomorrow's contest, the head coach tells his staff and the strength coach to disregard Taylor's assessments as she is young and has mismanaged many of the team's injuries. He continues by saying he is getting a second opinion from the team's physician before listening to her final injury report. The head coach is new this year, but has continued to treat Taylor this way during each team meeting.
	Lisa, while working in the clinic, over hears a physical therapist say to a patient that she does not agree with her management of a few other patients' cases. The physical therapist also indicates that Lisa is only an athletic trainer, and doesn't have the necessary training to really manage her patients effectively. A few weeks later, Lisa hears the same physical therapist tell the same patient that she really doesn't think Lisa should be employed by the clinic, as she is not really doing a good job. Over the course of a few weeks, the same physical therapist continues to talk behind Lisa's back, but loud enough for Lisa to hear her comments.
Personal standing	Sarah's coach comments frequently on her appearance. He often says thankfully that she is an ugly duckling, and that it's better that way so she is not a distraction to his players. Daily he comments on her plain style, acting as though he is complimenting her.
	Mike and Brad have been employed at their current university for 5 years now. Mike has been promoted to the associate head athletic trainer position, yet Brad thought he was deserving of it. Since the promotion, Brad has been spreading gossip about Mike, mostly untrue statements, but focused on his recent divorce and custody battle.
Overwork	Berkley is assigned 3 morning treatment sessions (7 am to 10 am); however, his co-workers have to cover only one morning treatment session per week. He is also the only athletic trainer at one of those morning sessions; each of the other mornings has a minimum of 2 staff members. The schedule has remained the same, despite Berkley's discussions with his supervisor over the last 3 months.
	Harper is contracted for 25 hours per week at her high school. For a month now, she has been averaging 35 hours per week. Her athletic director only recognizes that she works 25 hours, not the 35 hours and when asked about her hours, her athletic director distorts the total hours, acknowledging only her contracted 25 hours.

(continued)

TABLE 5-2 (CONTINUED)
EXAMPLES OF WORKPLACE BULLYING IN ATHLETIC TRAINING

CATEGORY	EXAMPLE
Destabilization	Maggie has been working with the field hockey team for 2 years. The coach is very successful, but has very high expectations for his staff, players, and Maggie. Coach "J" has been known to make comments on Maggie's decision making regarding treatments and management of various injuries. His comments are always made in front of others, usually the assistant coaches and players, if around, and include "Are you sure you what you are doing?", "I could tape better than that," and "How long have you been an athletic trainer?"
	Gloria and Angela have both been working long hours because of several post-surgical injuries. Steve, their supervisor, has recognized Gloria's long hours in 2 different staff meetings. Angela, working the same number of hours, has not been recognized by Steve and over the last 2 months has also been asked to cover extra morning treatments to help fill "holes" in the schedule. The trend continues over the next few weeks, in which Steve praises Gloria and assigns more work to Angela.
Isolation	Payton and Amy share an office with Sue and have comparable work schedules. Payton and Amy have begun to work out before they start their workday in addition to having lunch or coffee together regularly. They never invite Sue, and during the slow periods of the day while doing paperwork often share inside jokes or talk about their outside work plans that exclude Sue.
	John overhears 2 co-workers discussing a meeting held earlier in the day regarding a new concussion policy. When he asks about it, they indicate it was an informal meeting and that he shouldn't worry about it. The following week, he learns that the staff meeting had been changed, but he never received the email. His supervisor ensures him he sent it, but it could have been an oversight. Over the next 2 weeks, John learns of other policy changes made at the hospital, but hasn't received any emails about them.

and updates have been enacted, including the Fair Employment Law, which directly addresses harassment in the workplace. As it stands now, bullying is not recognized within the legislation related to workplace behaviors and acceptable practices.

PERPETRATORS

Perpetrators refers to those who commit the act of bullying, and who often do it to exert control over others in the workplace. Table 5-3 provides a list of characteristics displayed by workplace bullies or perpetrators. Bullies use a variety of mechanisms, some subtle and others not so much, to control their targets.[1] In some cases, bullies are viewed as master manipulators. The Workplace Bullying Institute[18] suggests that a bully can use 20 different means to gain control in

TABLE 5-3	
CHARACTERISTICS OF PERPETRATORS	
TYPE	**QUALITIES SEEN**
Charismatic	Self-assured
	Occupies an important role in organization
	Gives off an impression of reliability and trustworthiness
Deceptive	Compulsive liar
	Distorts reality
	Keeps people "off-balance" through half-true statements
	Intentional misleading
Manipulative	Uses gossip for gains
	Drawn to power
	Subjective sense of right and wrong
	Uses guilt to make others feel sorry for them
	Selectively unfriendly or uncooperative
Ruthless and unpleasant	Impatient
	No remorse or conscience
	Humorless, joyless, or emotionally cold
	Impatient
	Compulsively criticizes

the workplace, including deceit, intimidation, isolation, diversion, undermining, and criticism. It is important to remember that bullies can be co-workers or supervisors, but regardless of their role within the organization, they can use tactics to gain control over the individual.

TARGETS

According to the Workplace Bullying Institute,[18] targets of bullies are those who pose a perceived threat to the instigator. Moreover, targets often have better job skills than the bully and have more social skills and emotional intelligence as well. In sum, targets tend to be those who are ethical, empathetic, and honest.[18] Targets of bullying also tend to occupy a lower-level job position (eg, assistant athletic trainer vs head athletic trainer) and have less job security (eg, perhaps they are on a probationary period for employment).[19]

The bully views competence as competition, and wants to take advantage of the capable worker. They will attempt to sabotage the work of the target to help cope with their insecurities and help improve their own self-worth. Bullies look for the co-worker that is passive, shy or reserved, and non-confrontational. Targets often possess honesty, ethical decision making, and loyalty.[20,21]

Workplace Bullying in Health Care

Workplace bullying is an established concern for the nursing profession.[20] In nursing, bullying is a silent epidemic, as bullying can occur between 21% to 46% in the nursing profession;[22,23] the greater numbers, however, may indicate witnessing its occurrence rather than being a direct recipient of a bullying act. It appears as though senior-level nurses or nurses serving as a supervisor are those who are bullying and are often using public humiliation, isolation/exclusion, or criticisms to create a negative workplace environment.[24,25]

Many theories exist as to why bullying is prevalent in nursing; however, many are just supposition. Motivations for the bully in nursing have been suggested to include experience (the super nurse), resentfulness (develops grudges), envy, gossip, and favoritism.[26] Many of the bullying attacks in nursing manifest as personal attacks (personal attributes, dress, etc), criticisms of professional competence and skills, and delineation of workloads and roles in the workplace (ie, grunt work).[27] In nursing, workplace bullying extends beyond just workload assignments and professional competence, but also to interpersonal conflicts that include personal judgments and dislikes of others.

Although interpersonal conflicts exist in the workplace and are even expected to occur, they appear to be increasing or at minimum are being more frequently recognized. As presented in other chapters within the text, issues pertaining to discrimination, burnout, and work-life conflict are occurring within athletic training.[28-32] Only recently has the topic of workplace bullying been examined in athletic training, which reveals that it is occurring within the college and secondary school settings.[6,33]

Athletic trainers, in comparison to nurses, may not experience workplace bullying at the same rate. For example, only 14.7% of athletic trainers in the college setting reported workplace bullying,[6] and even fewer (7.8%) athletic trainers in the secondary school setting reported workplace bullying.[34] Prevalence of bullying does not discriminate between male and female athletic trainers, and coaches are often the perpetrators.[6,34] Unlike in the nursing literature, athletic trainers appear to be bullied by administrators, coaches, and then supervisors.[6,34] In the recent work by Weuve and peers, athletic trainer to athletic trainer bullying did not seem to materialize, but rather males who were coaches were identified most frequently as the perpetrators.

Consequences of Workplace Bullying

Workplace bullying can have negative consequences both for the target of bullying and the organization in which the bullying occurs. Thus, as future employees and organizational leaders, it's important for all of us to understand the consequences at both levels.

Individual Level

Workplace bullying can have detrimental effects on the target not only mentally and emotionally, but also physically (Figure 5-1). A host of problems have been associated with workplace bullying, including depression, anger, insomnia, gastrointestinal (GI) distress, headaches, panic attacks, change in appetite, low self-esteem, and increased use of drugs and alcohol.[35]

Targets of workplace bullying have been reported to have higher levels of absenteeism, reduced productivity, and increased levels of health care costs due to their increased levels of stress and unhappiness.[36] Like other workplace issues, such as burnout, experiences with workplace bullying increase the level of stress felt at work, which then leads to a variety of stress-related responses. Such symptoms include frequent or persistent headaches, hypertension, chronic fatigue, and GI issues.[2,6,35] Murray[20] reported that nurses who were affected by workplace bullying demonstrated

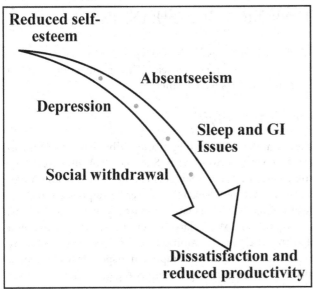

Figure 5-1. How workplace bullying affects the employee. GI: gastrointestinal.

signs of depression and anxiety, and in some cases if the bullying was experienced for a prolonged period of time the target developed post-traumatic stress disorders.

Other self-reported effects of workplace bullying include lower levels of self-esteem, increased anxiety, disruption of normal sleeping patterns, irritability, difficulty concentrating, and panic attacks.[20,35] Namie also reports that individuals who are experiencing workplace bullying will withdraw from family and friends, display aggressive behaviors, and engage in self-destructive behaviors such as overeating, increased alcohol consumption, gambling, and increased use of drugs and prescribed medications.[37] In rare instances individuals who are being bullied at work will turn their experiences into a positive experience, using faith and religion, exercise, or spending more time with family and friends as a means to cope.[37] Withdrawal and self-destructive behaviors, however, are more commonplace than the emergence of positive coping mechanisms.

In athletic training[33] increased stress and anxiety as described above were also found as a consequence of being a target. However, athletic trainers who were targets of workplace bullying also reported feelings of inadequacy and increased distrust,[33] meaning they second-guessed their skills and abilities and tended to second-guess whom to trust and confide in when problems arose.

Organizational Level

Bullying can affect not only the individual, but also the organization. Workplace bullying can lead to unsafe conditions, increased medical errors, and an overall negative reputation for the organization.[38] In general documented outcomes of workplace bullying include a toxic work environment (poor teamwork, low staff morale), decreased retention (ie, high turnover rate), increased health care costs, and counterproductive behaviors,[38] all of which can result in poor quality of patient care.[7] For health care providers, workplace bullying is more alarming as those targets of bullying can lose interest in their role, reducing their level of care, but also have been found to project their negative feelings and experiences onto their patients. In some cases, nurses who have been bullied have bullied their patients.

DEALING WITH WORKPLACE BULLYING

Many strategies exist to deal with bullying experiences in the workplace. Most center of the ideology of conflict resolution, but in extreme cases a target may leave the organization to avoid the bullying acts or because they feel their coping efforts were unmet.

Personal/Individual Strategies for Bullying

Be proactive. Once you have established that you are the target of a bully, it is important to seek advice and support in lieu of staying the course or avoiding it. Staying silent, unfortunately, allows the bullying to continue, and in some cases escalate.[20] Support can be gained from human resources, a supervisor, or peer/co-worker. Identify whether your employer has a policy and compliant resolution procedure for workplace bullying. This information can help you establish a plan, which is necessary to combat workplace bullying. The Workplace Bullying Institute[37] provides a detailed description of a target action plan that includes 1) naming it, 2) healing and developing a plan, and 3) exposing the bully. To expose the bully, the most important aspect is to document what is occurring. The idea of taking control or action can help the target regain some power over the bully and this includes keeping a daily journal or diary that chronicles the encounters, the frequency, patterns, and content of the bullying act (www.bullyonline.org). One must also collect substantive and quantifiable evidence, particularly since workplace bullying in the United States is not recognized or addressed by the Equal Employment Opportunity Commission. This evidence can then be used to build a case for appropriate intervention by a supervisor. Targets of bullying should keep a journal, chronicling their experiences including the situation, the date and time of the incident, as well as any artifacts that can be collected to validate the claims against the bully. Because workplace bullying can be difficult to quantify or define, it is important to provide examples of the acts. Gathering any evidence, such as emails or text messages, can help support the case.

Using workplace counseling services, often through employee assistance programs, can aid in managing bullying behaviors in the workplace. The workplace benefit program is intended to help employees deal with personal problems that can adversely affect their job performance, health, and overall well-being. The assistance programs are often in place to provide counseling services related to a variety of issues including work relationship issues, emotional distress, substance abuse, and depression. Often a free service, the counseling is confidential and privacy is maintained. At best, the target can gain advice, knowledge, and skills to manage their experiences with the bully.

Organizational Strategies to Prevent Bullying

Organizations would do well to have clear codes of professional conduct with zero tolerance for bullying behavior.[38] Indeed, workplace bullying is a managerial and leadership problem. When management styles are audacious and leaders are weak and unable, or unwilling, to intervene, the climate created in the workplace is such that it fuels aggressive behavior and promotes workplace bullying.[38] Cohen[39] notes that it is easy for managers to slip into a habit of ignoring unacceptable workplace behaviors; so long as the behaviors go unchecked, the greater the problematic effects on employee health, retention of staff, and effective health care delivery.[39] Having the courage to create, implement, and act on policies governing workplace behavior is critical.

Managers should foster an environment of open communication so employees feel free to report mistreatment.[40] Moreover, managers should work on supervision strategies so they avoid micromanaging, thus allowing their employees to feel trusted.[40]

Other prevention strategies have been used by health care organizations, including mentor programs with front-line nurses and students, assertiveness training for nurse employees, and planned responses to aggression—meaning individuals were taught how to cope with negative acts in the workplace.[41]

SUMMARY

Workplace bullying is a subtle, repeated, and purposeful act involving misuse of power that is directed from a perpetrator toward a target. These acts involve intimidation and aggressive behavior that make the target feel threatened. Perpetrators are often described as master manipulators that attempt to gain control over a target. Workplace bullying targets are often very competent and often have better job skills than a bully—the bully views competence as competition and attempts to sabotage the targets work. Workplace bullying has been a concern in nursing, which has an identified prevalence between 21% and 46%. Research in athletic training has thus far revealed substantially less prevalence with 14% of athletic trainers in the college setting and 7.8% in the secondary setting having been bullied. Organizations and individuals can proactively prevent bullying from occurring. Organizations can facilitate open lines of communication and enforce codes of conduct; individuals can expose the bully, document the incidents, and work with a supervisor to address the issue.

ACTIVITIES FOR REINFORCEMENT

Questions for Review

1. What actions from perpetrators are viewed as bullying?
2. Describe some consequences of bullying in the workplace.
3. What are some personal strategies one can use to deal with bullying behavior?
4. Explain what an organization can do to prevent bullying behavior.

Case Vignettes

Case #1

Sadie is the women's soccer athletic trainer at a mid-major university. Over the summer her institution introduced a concussion protocol that was approved up the chain of command and distributed to all coaches. Since the beginning of the soccer season she has had 2 athletes held out because of a concussion and the protocol was followed with grumblings but without incident. During yesterday's match another player suffers a head-to-head contact with a player from the other team. The athlete complains of a headache, nausea, and mild dizziness but is aware and able to get off the field on her own. According to the protocol the athlete is diagnosed with a head injury, and the coach is told the athlete will not be returning to the game (protocol). The coach begins to argue with Sadie but she stands her ground by continuing to refer to the protocol. The coach eventually goes back to coaching and Sadie finishes the game without incident. When talking to the team after the game, the coach is obviously upset and tells the athletes that they are to report injuries to him prior to going to the athletic training room. Sadie does not approach the coach after the game but documents the situation and sends an email report to her supervisor. First thing in the morning the coach comes to Sadie's office to "discuss" the protocol. The coach quickly escalates the situation to an argument regarding Sadie's decision to hold out his players and losing games because his players are hurt. Eventually, the coach, who is about 8 inches taller, towers over Sadie and is screaming and pointing his finger in her face.

1. Based on the account just previously described, would you say Sadie is a victim of workplace bullying?

2. If this behavior continued, what type of workplace bullying would Sadie be enduring?

3. What recommendations do you have for Sadie at this stage to help her manage the angry coach?

4. Who should Sadie speak to about the situation regarding her decisions for return to play and the coach's reaction?

Case #2

Amy is an athletic trainer at a large urban high school with a very successful athletics department. She has been employed by the high school for 5 years without incident. During the volleyball season, one of Amy's athletes suffers a third-degree ankle sprain. Based on the athlete's progress through his rehabilitation program he ends up missing 4 weeks of the season. During those 4 weeks Amy has several discussions with the head coach (who is new this year) regarding the athlete's progress. The head coach insists Amy is being overcautious and "it's only a sprained ankle." After the athlete begins returning to activity, Amy notices another athlete applying a wrap to his thigh. When Amy asks the athlete what's wrong the athlete says he hurt himself and the doctor said he should wrap the thigh when he plays and icing can help too. When Amy asks the athlete why he didn't come to her, he replies his parents wanted him to go to the doctor directly. After this incident Amy asks a few questions and finds out that the coach has told the athletes and their parents that if they are hurt they should go to Dr. Smith for care instead of Amy. This activity continues throughout the season in spite of conversations Amy has had with the coach and the athletic director.

1. What type of workplace bullying is Amy suffering?

2. What is the first step that Amy should take when dealing with her coach and athletic director?

3. How might this situation differ if it were in a different employment setting, such as a college or professional sport setting?

Discussion Questions

1. How can workplace bullying eventually be costly for an employer?

2. If an athletic trainer is bullied in the workplace, how might that ultimately reduce the quality of patient care delivered by the target?

3. What do you believe is the most critical workplace bullying prevention strategy an organization can use?

4. Should anti-bullying laws be federally mandated? Why or why not?

REFERENCES

1. Namie G. Workplace Bullying Institute 2014 Survey. http://workplacebullying.org/multi/pdf/WBI-2014-US-Survey.pdf. Accessed November 30, 2014.

2. Maguire J, Ryan D. Aggression and violence in mental health services: categorizing the experiences of Irish nurses. *J Psych Mental Health Nurs.* 2007;14(2):120-127.

3. Fuimano-Donley J. Are you committing lateral violence? Advance Healthcare Network. 2011. http://occupational-therapy.advanceweb.com/Features/Articles/Are-You-Committing-Lateral-Violence.aspx. Accessed November 30, 2014.

4. Fuimano-Donley J. What is 'lateral violence'? Advance Healthcare Network. 2011. http:// occupational-therapy.advanceweb.com/Archives/Article-Archives/What-Is-Lateral-Violence.aspx. Accessed November 30, 2014.

5. Quine L. Workplace bullying in junior doctors: questionnaire survey. *BMJ.* 2002;324:878-879.

6. Weuve C, Pitney WA, Martin M, Mazerolle SM. Experiences with workplace bullying among athletic trainers in the collegiate setting. *J Athl Train.* 2014;49(5):696-705.

7. Lee YJ, Bernstein K, Lee M, Nokes KM. Bullying in the nursing workplace: applying evidence using a conceptual framework. *Nurs Econ.* 2014;32(5):255-267.

8. Task Force on the Prevention of Workplace Bullying. Dignity at work: the challenge of workplace bullying. 2001. www.kjei.ie/publications/employment/2005/bullyingtaskforce.pdf. Accessed November 30, 2014.

9. Rayner C, Hoel H, Cooper CL. *Workplace Bullying: What We Know, Who Is to Blame, and What Can We Do?* London: Taylor & Francis; 2002.

10. Tracy SJ, Lutgen-Sandvik P, Alberts JK. Nightmares, demons and slaves: exploring the painful metaphors of workplace bullying. *MCQ* 2006;20(2):148-185.

11. Namie G. Workplace bullying: escalated incivility. *Ivey Business Journal.* 2003;68(2):1-6.

12. Namie G. The WBI 2003 report on abusive workplaces. 2003. www.bullyinginstitute.org. Accessed October 19, 2014.

13. Einarsen S, Hoel H, Zapf D, Cooper CL. The concept of bullying at work. In: Einarsen S, Hoel H, Zapf D, Cooper CL, eds. *Bullying and Emotional Abuse in the Workplace: International Perspectives in Research and Practice.* London: Taylor & Francis; 2003:3-30.

14. Lutgen-Sandvik P, Tracy SJ, Alberts JK. Burned by bullying in the American workplace: prevalence, perception, degree, and impact. *J Manag Studies.* 2007;44(6):837-862.

15. Rayner C, Hoel H, Cooper CL. *Workplace Bullying: What We Know, Who Is to Blame, and What Can We Do?* London: Taylor & Francis; 2002.

16. Workplace Bullying Institute. Employer resource council: 20 subtle signs of workplace bullying. http://www.workplacebullying.org/2013/11/10/erc. Accessed September 3, 2015.

17. Lutgen-Sandvik P. The communicative cycle of employee emotional abuse: generation and regeneration of workplace mistreatment. *Manag Communication Quart.* 2003;16(4):471-501.

18. Namie G, Namie R. Workplace Bullying Institute. http://www.workplacebullying.org/individuals/problem/who-gets-targeted. Accessed November 30, 2014.

19. Corina LM, Magley VJ. Patterns and profiles of response to incivility in the workplace. *J Occup Health Psychol.* 2009;14(3):272-288.

20. Murray JS. Workplace bullying in nursing: a problem that can't be ignored. *Medsurg Nurs.* 2009;18(5):273-276.

21. Kane A. Who is a workplace bully's target? 2015. Available at: http://legalcareers.about.com/od/careertrends/a/Who-Is-A-Workplace-Bullys-Target.htm. Accessed August 31, 2015.

22. Yildirim D. Bullying among nurses and its effects. *Int Nurs Rev.* 2009;56:504-511.

23. Leiper J. Nurse against nurse: how to stop horizontal violence. *Nurs.* 2005;35:44-45.

24. Vessey JA, Demarco RF, Gaffney DA, Budin WC. Bullying of staff registered nurses in the workplace: a preliminary study for developing personal and organizational strategies for the transformation of hostile to healthy workplace environments. *J Prof Nurs.* 2009;25:299-306.

25. Hoel H, Giga SI, Davidson MJ. Expectations and realities of student nurses' experiences of negative behaviour and bullying in clinical placement and the influences of socialization processes. *Health Serv Manage Res.* 2007;20:270-278.

26. Dellasega CA. Bullying among nurses. *Am J Nurs.* 2009;109:52-58.

27. Hutchinson, Vickers MH, Wilkes L, Jackson D. A typology of bullying behaviours: the experiences of Australian nurses. *J Clin Nurs.* 2010;19:2319-2328.

28. Mazerolle SM, Pitney WA, Casa DJ, Pagnotta KD. Assessing strategies to manage work and life balance of athletic trainers working in the National Collegiate Athletic Association Division I-A setting. *J Athl Train.* 2011;46(2):194-205.

29. Mazerolle SM. Bruening JE, Casa DJ. Work-family conflict, part I: antecedents of work-family conflict in National Collegiate Athletic Association Division I-A certified athletic trainers. *J Athl Train.* 2008;43(5):505-512.

30. Pitney WA, Mazerolle SM, Pagnotta KD. Work-family conflict among athletic trainers in the secondary school setting. *J Athl Train.* 2011;46(2):185-193.

31. Hendrix AE, Acevedo EO, Hebert E. An examination of stress and burnout in certified athletic trainers at Division I-A universities. *J Athl Train.* 2000;35(2):139-144.

32. Mazerolle SM, Borland JF, Burton LJ. The professional socialization of collegiate female athletic trainers: navigating experiences of gender bias. *J Athl Train.* 2012;47(6):694-703.

33. Weuve C, Pitney WA, Martin M, Mazerolle SM. Perceptions of workplace bullying among athletic trainers in the collegiate setting. *J Athl Train.* 2014;49(5):706-718.

34. Pitney WA, Mazerolle SM, Weuve C. The perceptions and experiences of workplace bullying among secondary school athletic trainers. *J Athl Train.* In review.

35. Namie G, Namie R. Workplace bullying: how to address America's silent epidemic. *Employee Rights and Employment Policy J.* 2004;8(2):315-333.

36. Elias A. *Workplace Bullying.* Oxford: Ruskin College; 1997.

37. Namie G. Workplace Bullying Institute. 2013. http://www.workplacebullying.org/2013/09/10/wbi-2013-ip-i/. Accessed November 30, 2014.

38. Skehan J. Why do we still eat our young? Strategies and interventions to decrease workplace bullying. *Prof Case Manag.* 2014;19(4):196-9.

39. Cohen S. From sheep to lion: confronting workplace bullying. *Nurs Manage.* 2014;45(7):9-11.

40. Trad M, Johnson J. Bullying among radiation therapists: effects on job performance and work environment. *Radiol Technol.* 2014;86(2):122-31.

41. Stagg SJ, Sheridan D. Effectiveness of bullying and violence prevention programs: a systematic review. *Workplace Health Saf.* 2010;58(10):419-424.

Discrimination in the Athletic Training Workplace

Laura J. Burton, PhD

OBJECTIVES

After reading this chapter, the reader will be able to do the following:

1. Explain discrimination within the context of the athletic training workplace.
2. Identify groups of individuals at risk for discrimination within athletic training practice settings.
3. Describe explicit and implicit discrimination and differentiate both types within the athletic training workplace.
4. Recognize and explain various types of workplace mistreatment.
5. Describe the outcomes associated with workplace discrimination.
6. Explain how discrimination can be reduced in the athletic training workplace.

INTRODUCTION

Issues of discrimination in the athletic training workplace must be addressed from a legal perspective as well as mistreatment that may not rise to the level of illegal action. The workplace context may also have an impact on how discrimination or workplace mistreatment is manifested and how it is addressed within the organization.

This chapter will address the concept of discrimination and how to recognize discrimination in the workplace. In addition, this chapter will include discussion of the understanding of both explicit discrimination and the pervasiveness of more implicit discrimination that manifests through workplace mistreatment. The consequences or workplace outcomes associated with discrimination will be examined followed by a brief discussion of the legal remedies available

Mazerolle SM, Pitney WA.
Workplace Concepts for Athletic Trainers (pp 91-106).
© 2016 Taylor & Francis Group.

to those experiencing such discrimination. The final section of the chapter will discuss how to address issues of workplace discrimination and provide practical implications that athletic trainer professionals can implement to reduce incidents of discrimination and incivility. Throughout this chapter, a focus will be put on intercollegiate athletics, secondary school athletics, and clinical facilities (eg, physical therapy practices, hospital outpatient settings) as these 3 employ the greatest percentage of individuals holding athletic training certification credentials.

WHAT IS DISCRIMINATION?

Prior to examining discrimination in the athletic training workplace, it is critical to define the construct of discrimination and briefly address the theoretical frameworks that help us to understand discrimination. This section of the chapter will also explore some of the outcomes of discrimination in general understanding, and then later in the chapter we will link these outcomes to specific athletic training workplace outcomes.

Discrimination occurs when an individual or group is denied equal treatment that they desire. Discrimination against groups is delineated by the Equal Employment Opportunity Commission to include race, sex, age, and ability.

RECOGNIZING DISCRIMINATION IN THE WORKPLACE

As a result of social, legal, and other organizational pressures, overt discrimination is no longer tolerated and has declined in the workplace.[1-3] Employees who are subject to overt sexism, sexual harassment, racism, ablism, or heterosexism (in some states in the United States [US])[1] can take legal action against their harasser(s). Title VII of the Civil Rights Act is the law that prohibits employment discrimination based on sex, race, color, national origin, sex or religion. Title VII applies to the following: organizations with at least 15 employees, employment agencies, labor unions, state and local governments, and the federal government.[4] Further, Title IX can protect individuals from sexual harassment for those employed by organizations that receive federal funding (eg, intercollegiate athletics). Though there has been a noted decline in overt discrimination, it has not been completely eradicated from workplaces in which athletic trainers are employed or where students learn the skills for the profession of athletic training.

Two forms of discrimination have been identified: access discrimination and treatment discrimination.[5] Access discrimination denies an individual access to a profession, job or organization because of membership in a social category.[4] This type of discrimination takes place when people are seeking out employment opportunities. An example of access discrimination is a woman who is more qualified than a male applicant is denied a position as an athletic trainer for a Division I football team. The second type of discrimination, treatment discrimination, occurs after an individual is already employed in the workplace. Treatment discrimination is defined as members of a specific social category having less-positive work experiences and receiving fewer rewards or opportunities than they legitimately deserve based on job-related criteria.[4] An example of treatment discrimination would be a lesbian who is performing better than her colleagues receiving a lower performance evaluation.

Existence of Access and Treatment Discrimination in Sport Organizations

Cunningham[4] provides an overview of examples of access discrimination in the sport and recreation context. Women, racial minorities, gays and lesbians, and people with disabilities have all experienced discrimination in attempts to obtain positions in sport organizations. Despite limited research in the area specific to sports, it is likely that religious minorities (eg, Muslims) also face these types of discriminatory practices.

Within the domain of athletic training, much of the work in regard to access discrimination has examined the experiences of women in the field.[6] Though not directly examined, the lack of women leading athletic training programs, specifically high-profile Football Bowl Subdivision (FBS) intercollegiate athletic departments (19.5%)[7] and professional sports medicine programs, indicates that women may face access discrimination when seeking these positions. Researchers in the field of athletic training should attempt to directly examine this type of discrimination to better understand if access discrimination is a constraining force for women and other minorities groups in intercollegiate and professional sports.

Considering treatment discrimination, Cunningham[4] noted that such discrimination is widespread in the context of sports. Women, racial minorities, and gays and lesbians have been denied opportunities for advancement in sport careers, receive fewer rewards when attempting to improve their professional skills, and are more likely to leave a sport-related profession. Further, gays and lesbians also report facing more negative attitudes from others when working in sport organizations.

ACCESS DISCRIMINATION
Access discrimination denies an individual access to a profession, job or organization because of membership in a social category.

TREATMENT DISCRIMINATION
Treatment discrimination is defined as members of a specific social category having less-positive work experiences and receiving fewer rewards or opportunities than they legitimately deserve based on job-related criteria.

In athletic training, the experiences of women working in intercollegiate athletics support other findings in the context of sport, as women face issues of treatment discrimination in their work.[6,8] When exploring the experiences of younger women working in Division I athletic programs, researchers noted that young women reported being denied opportunities to work the more high-profile, revenue-producing sports of football and men's basketball. In addition, male coaches were critical of the work performed by these women, often questioning their injury evaluations and treatment plans.[6] There has been limited research examining the experiences of other minority groups (eg, racial/ethnic minorities, gays and lesbians) working in the field of athletic training. This research would help us to better understand the prevalence of treatment discrimination in the athletic training workplace and how to remedy such discrimination.

Harassment by Sex and Sexual Harassment

Sex discrimination is defined as behavior that treats someone unfavorably because of that person's sex. One aspect of sex harassment is sexual harassment. The Equal Employment Opportunity Commission (EEOC) defines sexual harassment as a form of sex discrimination that violates Title VII of the Civil Rights Act of 1964. As noted on the EEOC website (www.eeoc.gov), "harassment can include sexual harassment or unwelcome sexual advances, requests for sexual favors, and other verbal or physical harassment of a sexual nature." Victims of sexual harassment and perpetrators of sexual harassment can be of either sex and harassment can be either opposite-sex or same-sex harassment. Sexual harassment can take 2 forms: quid pro quo harassment or hostile environment.

Requesting sexual favors in exchange for something else is considered quid pro quo harassment. An example of quid pro quo harassment is when a supervisor promises a subordinate an excellent performance evaluation if a sexual favor is fulfilled.

Hostile environment occurs when "an employee is subjected to repeated unwelcome behaviors that do not constitute sexual bribery but are sufficiently severe and pervasive that they create a work environment so hostile that it substantially interferes with the harassed employee's ability to perform his or her job."[9(p137)] Consider, for example, a female athletic trainer who dreads having to give an injury report to a coach because each time she does, he consistently makes inappropriate comments about her great "figure" and how if she would go out with him he would show her a "great time." The result for her is problems communicating the content of the report because she is so self-conscious and fearful of his advances. In this instance, we could argue that the circumstance is interfering with her job.

> A hostile work environment in athletic training is one in which an athletic trainer is subject to repeated unwelcome behavior that creates an environment that substantially interferes with the harassed athletic trainer's ability to perform his or her job.

Within the athletic training workplace, research published in 1998 and 10 years later, in 2008, indicated that female athletic trainers did experience sexual harassing behaviors. Velasquez[10] provided an extensive review of sexual harassment within the context of athletic training. Shingles and Smith[11a] noted that 64% of the women participating in their study had reported experiencing sexual harassment. The harassment reported by these women included both physical and verbal forms of harassment and was perpetrated both by athletes and coaches. In 2 incidents, charges were brought forward against the universities by whom these women were employed.[11a] In addition to the disturbing findings regarding the incidence of sexual harassment reported, Shingles and Smith[11a] noted "the majority of women athletic trainers interviewed did not know if they were being harassed."[11a(p106)] Further, many of the women also did not recognize that sexual jokes or innuendos and comments about one's appearance are classified as creating a hostile environment and are therefore sexual harassment behavior.[11a] Based on these findings, the authors noted the importance of evaluating athletic training clinic education and continuing education to determine whether the concepts of sexual harassment and assault were being adequately addressed. The most recent education competencies,[11b] specifically psychosocial strategies and referrals now includes content pertaining to recognizing personal/social conflict including sexual harassment that would be grounds for a referral.

An additional type of discrimination based on sex is pregnancy-based discrimination. An amendment to Title VII, the Pregnancy Discrimination Act requires that women who are "pregnant or who are affected by related conditions be treated the same as their colleagues who have comparable abilities or limitations."[4(p271)] Though there is no current research within athletic training that has examined this issue directly, implications of work-family balance and the burdens faced primarily by women with children working in the athletic training workplace have been examined.[12,13]

Contrapower Harassment

An important type of harassment that must be discussed in the context of athletic training is contrapower harassment. Benson,[14] credited with the term *contrapower harassment*, defined it as a type of sexual harassment that would occur when the victim of the harassing behavior has formal power over the harasser. Further, Benson[14] has noted that though contrapower harassment focuses on the organizational positions of those involved (eg, professor is harassed by a student), "gender-based sociocultural power is at the root of this type of harassment."[15(p43)] Power is an important issue to consider when describing discrimination in the workplace, and specifically when considering contrapower harassment. Studies exploring issues of contrapower sexual harassment have shown that faculty, those with formal power, experienced sexually harassing behavior perpetrated by students.[16] Within the context of intercollegiate athletics, as an example, we must consider not only formal sources of power (eg, head athletic trainer, coach, athletic director), but also informal sources of power (eg, star athlete for the most popular team on campus). Also, in the professional sports setting, an athletic trainer may have formal power as a member of the sports medicine staff for the professional organization, but an athlete would hold more informal power within the organization. Further work examining issues of contrapower harassment would help to uncover if athletic trainers are experiencing this type of harassment in the athletic training workplace.

> Power is important to consider in intercollegiate athletics. Not only must we consider formal sources of power (eg, head athletic trainer, coach, athletic director), but also informal sources of power (eg, star athlete for the most popular team on campus).

Race Discrimination

Title VII defines race discrimination as discrimination in any aspect of employment (eg, hiring, firing, pay, job assignments, promotions, layoff, training, fringe benefits, and any other term or condition of employment) based on the race of an individual[17] (EEOC). Though there continue to be reported cases of race discrimination, including a reported 33,579 in 2009,[4] there is limited research within the field of athletic training that has directly examined this issue.

Sexual Orientation and Gender Identity Discrimination

As of 2014, there is no federal law that protects individuals from employment discrimination based on sexual orientation; however, on July 21, 2014, President Barack Obama signed an executive order prohibiting federal contractors from discriminating on the basis of sexual orientation or gender identity. As of the publication of this book, 19 states and the District of Columbia do have state laws protecting individuals from sexual orientation and gender identify discrimination.[18] There is no research within the field of athletic training that has directly examined the experiences of athletic trainers identifying themselves as lesbian, gay, bisexual, or transgender (LGBT). In examining the experiences of young female athletics trainers, issues of perceived sexual orientation did contribute to how these athletic trainers were treated within their workplace.[6] However, recent research examining the attitudes of athletic trainers regarding LGBT athletes indicated that the majority of athletic trainers held positive or somewhat positive attitudes toward LGBT athletes responding to a survey regarding attitude toward LGBT athletes. Future research should examine directly the workplace climate for those identifying as LGBT to identify issues of discrimination.[19]

Workplace Mistreatment

Though there is a noted decline in overt discrimination within the workplace, in general, a more subtle and pervasive form of discrimination is manifested in the form of uncivil behavior through workplace mistreatment.[20] Incivility, sexual harassment, and racial/ethnic harassment are forms of interpersonal deviant behavior because individuals perceive these behaviors as insulting, degrading, or intimidating and they violate standards of interpersonal respect.[1] Further, 2 additional forms of workplace mistreatment include bullying and aggression. When considering these forms of workplace mistreatment in terms of intensity, physical aggression (eg, being kicked) is the most intense form and incivility the least intense (eg, being ignored), with bullying and nonphysical aggression falling somewhere in between on the continuum.[21] Next there will be a detailed discussion on aggression, bullying, and selective incivility, and considerations on how these can manifest in the athletic training workplace as forms of workplace discrimination.

Workplace Aggression

Overt physical or nonphysical behavior that harms an employee is considered workplace aggression.[21] It is defined as "efforts by individuals to harm others with whom they work, or have worked, or the organizations in which they are presently, or were previously, employed."[22(p395)] One type of workplace aggression that needs to be highlighted, as it is considered the primary source of workplace aggression,[23] is supervisor aggression. Supervisor aggression is defined as "employees' perceptions of the supervisor's intentionally harmful behavior against them."[24 (p1148)] Supervisor aggression represents an especially damaging form of workplace mistreatment as supervisors maintain control over things valued by employees (eg, feedback, resources).[24] When considering the athletic training workplace, supervisors could include a head athletic trainer, head coach, and/or athletic administrator, or sports medicine director (eg, physician). There is no research that has examined whether supervisor aggression is manifest within the athletic training workplace or whether a perception of multiple supervisors (eg, head athletic trainer and head coach) increases the likelihood or severity of supervisor aggression. More work is needed in this area to better understand this issue in the athletic training workplace.

Workplace Bullying

Bullying in the workplace is defined as "repeated and persistent negative acts toward one or more individual(s), which involve a perceived power imbalance and create a hostile work environment."[25(p1214)] Workplace bullying is the result of situations in which a target is exposed to repeated abusive and offensive workplace acts that occur over time and from which the target has difficulty defending himself or herself.[21] Bullying can included a number of different behaviors, such as rumors directed toward the victim, attacking the victim's private life, verbal aggression, excessive criticism or monitoring of work, or withholding information or depriving the victim of responsibility.[25] These types of behaviors constitute bullying when such behaviors are repeated, persistent, and continuous. Bullying involves a power imbalance between bully and victim, yet that imbalance does not have to be supervisor (as bully) and employee (as victim). Power imbalance can also be the result of societal, situational, or individual consequences. When considering some workplace contexts for athletic trainers, power imbalance could be the result of athlete (as bully) and athletic trainer (as victim), in addition to bullying by those in formal positions of authority.

Bullying can included a number of different behaviors, such as rumors directed toward the victim, attacking the victim's private life, verbal aggression, excessive criticism or monitoring of work, or withholding information or depriving the victim of responsibility.

Selective Incivility

Selective incivility can simply be described as a general rudeness at work and has been formally defined as "low-intensity deviant behavior with ambiguous intent to harm the target, in violation of workplace norms for mutual respect."[26(p457)] Examples of uncivil behaviors include putting others down, acting in a condescending manner, interrupting others, excluding individuals from meetings for which they should be included, and giving someone the "silent treatment."[27]

Incivility is more broadly defined than the concept of workplace bullying and encompasses behavior that also involves a power imbalance. Further, incivil behavior is behavior that occurs at least once per week lasting for at least 6 months.[28] Another important characteristic of incivility, distinguishing this behavior from bullying, is ambiguity regarding whether there is an intention to harm.[27] Individuals who are experiencing the impacts of workplace incivility behaviors, people observing the incivility behaviors, and even the perpetuators of incivility may not be clear that the intent of the behavior is harmful or malicious.[27] Therefore, for behavior to be qualified as incivility, "any harmful intent must be ambiguous to one or more of the parties involved."[20(p1580)] If there is clear intent to harm an individual through uncivil behavior, this rises to the level of workplace aggression, defined as "any form of behavior directed by one or more persons in a workplace toward the goal of harming one or more others in that workplace (or the entire organization) in ways the intended targets are motivated to avoid."[29(p27)]

A third distinguishing characteristic of workplace incivility is the low intensity of the behavior, as it is does not include physical assault. Further, this low intensity of behavior characteristic of incivility elicits a negative appraisal (eg, appraising the behavior as bothersome, annoying, frustrating, insensitive) by the target of such behavior.[27] Uncivil behavior in the workplace that does include physical assault is defined as workplace violence.[29] It is important to keep in mind that, though "incivility may be subtle, its impact is not—showing similar effects as more blatant and malicious forms of workplace hostility."[27(p285)]

Incivility as Workplace Discrimination

Women and racial and ethnic minorities may be subject to incivility at higher rates than White men.[1] As a result of the ambiguity inherent in incivility behavior (eg, using a condescending tone, belittling a coworker's contribution), those perpetuating this behavior may rationalize it as unbiased and as having nothing to do with gender or race.[1] Most troubling, this can result in individuals degrading women and racial and ethnic minorities while also maintaining that they are not sexist or racist. As noted by Cortina and colleagues,[20] this type of behavior is "highly consistent with the social-psychological notion of modern discrimination."[(p1581)] Research that has examined the experiences of incivility in non-sport workplaces (eg, the military, university faculty, police) indicates that women and minority men experience higher instances of incivility than White men.[20] Within the context of a sports organization, there has been limited research that has explored the incidence of incivility, yet limited findings do support that women and racial minorities experience greater levels of uncivil behavior.[30,31]

> Women and racial and ethnic minorities may be subject to incivility at higher rates than White men.

Workplace Mistreatment in Sports Organizations

Sports organizations in which athletic trainers work, including intercollegiate and professional sports medicine departments, are male dominated.[7,32a] As a result, within sports organizations, men hold greater power and access to leadership when compared to women.[33,34] This power imbalance and increased privilege can contribute to experiences of workplace mistreatment in the sport organization.[31] Though not examined directly in the athletic training context, the experiences of women officials in basketball demonstrated incidence of selective incivility behavior that was higher when compared to male basketball officials.[31]

In the context of intercollegiate sports medicine, young female athletic trainers reported experiencing incivility, most often by male head coaches or male athletes, though the female athletic trainers did not report this behavior as incivility specifically.[6] The participants described pervasive questioning of injury diagnoses, treatment protocols, and return-to-play guidelines by male coaches, something the participants did not witness for their male athletic training colleagues. Further work with regard to incivility within the context of sports medicine is warranted. This examination should include experiences of incivility of student athletic trainers working with college athletes and coaches, certified athletic trainers working with high-profile sports (revenue-producing sports), and those working in professional sports organizations. Given the noted differences in experiences of incivility, by women and minority men and women, their experiences of incivility may help uncover issues that contribute to their decreased representation in certain contexts (eg, high-profile intercollegiate sport, professional sports) in the field of sports medicine.

CONSEQUENCES OF DISCRIMINATION IN THE WORKPLACE

Access and Treatment Discrimination

An understanding of the outcomes associated with discrimination is necessary. There are not only negative effects on individuals, but also on organizations, and even more broadly the profession that supports this discrimination. One of the most obvious effects of access discrimination is the limitation on opportunities to obtain a job, enter an organization or pursue a career in a particular profession.[35] Access discrimination "influences not only those who experience it but also those who may consider that career path."[4(p59)] Considering the racial and ethnic diversity within athletic participation at the intercollegiate and professional level,[32a] and the underrepresentation of racial/ethnic minorities in athletic training within those areas (18.5% of intercollegiate athletic trainers are of minority status and only 2.3% of professional sports athletic trainers are of minority status), it is plausible to assume that access discrimination is a contributing factor.[32b] As noted by Cunningham,[33] there is a growing body of research that supports the notion that people who anticipate significant barriers in a profession are unlikely to choose that career path. Those working in the field of athletic training must consider how access discrimination is affecting perceptions of minorities and their decisions to enter or not enter the profession.

Individuals subjected to treatment discrimination experience both tangible and intangible outcomes. Tangible outcomes to treatment discrimination include job assignments, training and development opportunities, opportunities for promotions, and increases in salary.[4] Experiences reported by young female athletic trainers indicated outcomes associated with treatment discrimination, as they reported being denied opportunities to work with high-profile male sports because they were women.[6] Additional outcomes of treatment discrimination that are more difficult to detect include failing to integrate within the work group (eg, athletic training staff) and decreased support from supervisors. Though issues of treatment discrimination have not been directly examined in the athletic training workplace, scholars should consider this as a potential factor contributing to the attrition of female athletic trainers in some athletic training settings, such as intercollegiate athletics.

Consequences of Workplace Mistreatment

There is also a growing body of research that has examined the consequences of workplace aggression, bullying, and incivility for employees. Though there is only limited research to date that has explored the consequences of these behaviors within the athletic training workplace, it is likely that these outcomes would also be seen for those working in athletic training.

Workplace Aggression

As noted earlier in this chapter, supervisor aggression is one of the most troubling forms of workplace aggression; therefore, it is important to focus on some of the consequences associated with this form of aggression. One consequence of supervisor aggression is employee retaliation against the perceived aggressor. Further, displaced aggression is a consequence when direct retaliation against the perceived supervisor aggressor is not possible. This displaced aggression can be directed at peers or fellow co-workers.[36] When considered within the athletic training workplace, those victimized by supervisors could turn their aggression toward fellow athletic trainers, student athletic trainers, or athletes under their care and supervision. A more positive response to supervisor aggression has also been noted. Some victims have used this negative experience as an opportunity to use more constructive strategies, such as reconciliation and constructive resistance as responses.[36]

Bullying

Consequences associated with workplace bullying are associated with job-related, health- and well-being-related outcomes.[37] The most consistent findings with regard to outcomes associated with bullying include experiences of post-traumatic stress and mental health problems. Workplace bullying is also a major contributor to intentions to leave the workplace and decreased job satisfaction and commitment to the organization.[37]

Selective Incivility

As noted by Cortina and colleagues,[23] when compared to other more severe forms of harassment and workplace mistreatment (eg, workplace bullying, abusive supervisors), incivility may not appear to have as much of an impact on employees. However, workplace incivility has been a contributing factor in lower job satisfaction, burnout, and higher workplace turnover.[1,23] Incivility is also linked to employee depression, anxiety, and hostility.[23] Other outcomes to workplace incivility include decreased workplace creativity, cooperation, and organizational citizenship behaviors (eg, helping a co-worker with a job-related task).

These negative outcomes may also be experienced by those who witness incivility, but are not the targets of such behavior.[1] A troubling consequence that has also been noted in regard to workplace incivility is the potential for incivility to spiral, as those who are targets of uncivil behavior may then engage in uncivil acts toward other employees. An incivility spiral is also more likely to be perpetrated by men when the workplace tolerates rudeness or other uncivil behaviors (ie, supports an uncivil climate in the workplace).[38]

LEGAL CHALLENGES TO DISCRIMINATION

A full discussion of legal issues relevant to workplace discrimination is beyond the scope of this chapter. However, we must address some of the major laws that cover issues of workplace discrimination. You are encouraged to seek out additional resources to increase your knowledge of legal issues relative to workplace discrimination (see additional readings/resources for more information).

Employment Discrimination Claims

From the perspective of employees, discrimination can take the form of disparate treatment and disparate impact.[4] When an employer intentionally discriminates against individuals from groups (eg, minority men and women), that is considered disparate treatment. Disparate impact is the result of a neutral organizational policy (eg, employment test) that negatively affects one group (eg, men) relative to another (eg, women) though it is not the intent of the employer to discriminate.[4] If an individual believes that his or her employment rights have been violated, a charge of discrimination can be filed with the nearest Equal Employment Opportunity Commission (www.eeoc.org). All claims filed based on a violation of Title VII must be filed within 120 days of the discriminating event.[4]

Title IX

Most people involved in sports in the United States are familiar with Title IX, as it has provided significant opportunities for girls and women in sports since its passage in 1972.[7] However, Title IX was not passed merely to increase opportunities for girls and women in sports; it was passed to eliminate discrimination based on sex. Title IX states the following:

> *No person in the United States shall, on the basis of sex, be excluded from participation in, be denied the benefits of, or be subjected to discrimination under any educational program or activity receiving Federal financial assistance.*

Sexual harassment of any form can be considered a form of discrimination under Title IX. As noted on its website, the Department of Education states, "The Office for Civil Rights has long recognized that sexual harassment of students engaged in by school employees, other students, or third parties is covered by Title IX."[38] Of important note is the impact of Title IX on the context of the athletic training workplace, as athletic trainers working in the secondary school or intercollegiate context would be covered under Title IX as those institutions receive federal funding.

ADDRESSING ISSUES OF DISCRIMINATION IN THE ATHLETIC TRAINING WORKPLACE

To understand how to address issues of discrimination in the athletic training workplace, it is necessary to discuss factors that contribute to a discriminatory environment. In this section, organizational structures and processes that enable discrimination to occur and how masculine hegemony is perpetuated through sports can contribute to discrimination in the workplace will be discussed.

Masculine hegemony is a pattern of practices that subordinate women and other groups that do not represent dominant masculinity (eg, gay men).[40] Anderson[41] has argued that sports serve as a site of masculine hegemony because they reward traditional notions of masculinity and facilitate its reproduction. Further, competitive sports serve as a social institution principally organized around defining certain forms of masculinity as acceptable, while denigrating others. Sports operate as a space to define and reproduce hegemonic masculinity, in which one form of masculinity (ie, exclusively heterosexual and physically dominant) maintains dominance by suppressing all other forms of masculinity and subordinating women.[42] Within the social institution of sports, women are often situated as an "other" and the presence of women in sports, as athlete, coach, manager, athletic trainer or administrator, is under constant scrutiny.[6,43] Given the influence of masculine hegemony in sports, the athletic training workplace can also be affected by this influence. In addition, some athletic training workplaces have a male-dominated workforce, with men leading the sports medicine staff and men leading the athletic departments overseeing these sports medicine staffs.[7]

Organization Climate/Culture

Employees working in positive social climates and those that punish or discourage sexual harassing behaviors report lower incidents of harassment when compared to workplaces that show more tolerance of sexual harassment.[44] Workplace climate is also critical when considering incivility behavior, as the climate (ie, workplace culture, policies, procedures) can influence whether individuals will perpetuate uncivil behavior. Workplace climate appears to have a more significant impact on men, "as men who worked in an uncivil climate generally reported higher likelihood of perpetrating incivility than anyone else, even when they did not report being a target of incivility."[44(p150)] Climate does not appear to be as influential for women, as women are more likely to perpetuate incivility only when they are targets of incivility, regardless of the tolerance for incivility in the workplace. Again, given the male-dominated workforce of some athletic training workplaces, the importance of a positive social climate that does not tolerate uncivil behavior is critical.

> Workplace climate (ie, workplace culture, policies, procedures) can influence whether individuals will perpetuate uncivil behavior.

An additional issue to address is the perception of power imbalances within the athletic training workplace. With regard to bullying, one type of workplace mistreatment, if there is no power imbalance, no bullying can occur, as the "person toward whom the aggression is directed could withstand the direct or indirect attacks and retaliate, thus preventing the bullying from beginning."[25(p1219)] Also, bullying occurs more when employees perceive the costs associated with such behavior to be low (ie, low risk of punishment). If the risks of being caught bullying, being reprimanded, punished or socially isolated, or dismissed from the organization are perceived as low, a perpetrator is more likely to engage in bullying behavior. Further, "bullying seems to flourish when upper management abdicate responsibility and do not intervene in bullying."[25(p1220)]

Also, if employees are experiencing dissatisfaction, lack of control within the work environment, and frustration, workplace mistreatment behavior is more likely to occur.[25] Given the long hours and difficult work schedules many athletic trainers experience, as well as the lack of autonomy in setting their schedules, the athletic training workplace can be one that leads to dissatisfaction and frustration.[8] This may make the athletic training workplace one that is more likely to cultivate an uncivil work climate. Further, and important to consider within the athletic training workplace, a high degree of stress, high workload, and time pressures can also be contributing factors in workplace mistreatment.[25]

Strategies to Reduce Workplace Discrimination

As noted in the previous section, employment laws protect individuals who are victims of explicit forms of employment discrimination, including racial, ethnic, and sex discrimination.[45] However, as we have described, more implicit forms of workplace discrimination do occur and it is important to create a workplace that is free from explicit and implicit discrimination. Strategies that are supported to reduce implicit workplace discrimination begin with the attraction of employees into the workplace, continue with reducing discrimination in the selection of employees, reducing discrimination in the inclusion of employees into the workplace, and reducing discrimination in the retention of employees.[45] Also, leadership and establishing an organization climate and culture that promotes a civil and positive organizational culture also contributes to reductions in employee discrimination. Both individual and organizational approaches to reducing workplace discrimination will be discussed in this section.

In an effort to reduce workplace mistreatment, including harassment and incivility behavior, all senior level members of the organization (eg, head athletic trainer, head coach, athletic director, physician) must demonstrate respectful, appropriate workplace behavior, and also provide clearly stated expectations regarding a civil workplace that should be included in organizational policies and procedures.[20] Further, new athletic trainers employed in the workplace should undergo inter-personal skills training and receive education regarding civility expectations for the workplace.[20] Also of critical importance, if workplace mistreatment does occur, all perpetuators of that mis-treatment must be consistently, swiftly, and justly sanctioned.[20] To avoid a perceived power imbal-ance, clear organizational policies and procedures must be developed that allow athletes, coaches, athletic administrators, and site managers to recognize the role of the athletic trainer in making decisions regarding injury diagnosis, rehabilitation protocol decisions, and return-to-play criteria.

Discrimination reduction efforts begin with attracting diverse candidates for jobs within the workplace. The first step to attract diverse candidates is targeted recruitment in order to increase the diversity of the applicant pool. Efforts can include developing relationships with organizations representing the underrepresented groups such as educational institutions, professional organiza-tions, and minority organizations. In addition, having diverse representation of individuals in your organization can demonstrate to those applying that the organization has a commitment to diversity. Explicit discussion of the importance of diverse recruitment of applicants can also com-municate to those in the organization that diversity is valued and supported.

Strategies to reduce bias in the selection process can also reduce discrimination in the workplace. Within the context of athletic training, strategies that reduce subjectivity in the interview process can help to reduce selection bias. This would include training hiring managers (eg, head athletic trainers in the college setting) on nondiscrimination policies for hiring, following consistent and standardized procedures that minimize subjectivity throughout the hiring phase, using only struc-tured interview questions for all candidates, and finally selecting individuals with low implicit and explicit bias to be a part of the selection process. One test that can be employed to measure implicit bias is the Implicit Association Test. See, for example, https://implicit.harvard.edu/implicit.[46]

Inclusion of diverse groups in the workplace is also critical to reduce workplace discrimination. Examples of actions considered inclusionary would be diversity training for all members of the workplace and providing workplace benefits that assist diverse employees but that also benefit all employees (eg, flexible work hours for primary caregivers). When providing workplace benefits that support diverse employees, it is critical to emphasize that these benefits can and should be used by all members of the workplace.

Retention of diverse employees can also lead to decreased workplace discrimination. These efforts can include equitable compensation packages for all employees, training and development opportunities such as leadership or management training and mentorship programs, and career development programs that include clear pathways to career advancement. Further efforts should include monitoring programs to be sure that promotion, compensation, and development oppor-tunities are being used by diverse employees. If diverse employees choose to leave the athletic training workplace, exit interviews should be conducted to evaluate why retention efforts have failed and identify areas for improvement.

Summary

This chapter has focused on the concept of discrimination in the athletic training workplace. It is important to recognize the 2 types of discrimination, access discrimination and treatment dis-crimination, and that discrimination most often is directed toward individuals who are members of minority groups (eg, women, minority men and women, LGBT individuals). Within the athletic training workplace, discrimination can be either explicit or implicit. Victims of explicit forms of discrimination (eg, refusing to hire someone based on race) are covered by Title VII of the Civil Rights; and victims of sexual harassment in federally funded institutions (eg, public high schools, and colleges and universities) are protected by Title IX. However, as there has been a decline in explicit forms of discrimination in the workplace, there has been increased incidence of implicit forms of discrimination. Implicit discrimination can include workplace aggression, bullying, and incivility. It is important to recognize these more implicit forms of discrimination as the impact of these types of behavior can be detrimental to employees and others working within the athletic training workplace. Explicit and implicit discrimination can be reduced through programs to increase the number of underrepresented groups in the athletic training workplace and by establishing a culture and climate that support diversity and civility.

ACTIVITIES FOR REINFORCEMENT

Questions for Review

1. Describe the difference between explicit and implicit discrimination and provide an example of both.

2. What groups are most at risk of discrimination in the workplace?

3. What is meant by workplace mistreatment? How does this differ from discrimination?

Case Vignettes

Case #1

Steve has worked as the head athletic trainer at State University for almost 3 years. He is responsible for more than 20 varsity sports including a football bowl subdivision team. His staff includes 5 full-time athletic trainers and supports 15 clinical education students each academic year. Steve works closely with one of his staff members, Eric, who serves as the head athletic trainer for football; however, Steve does not directly oversee football.

During football preseason camp, Eric is the preceptor for 5 of the athletic training students. After the first full week of preseason camp, a few of the students start sharing stories of a weekend spent with some of the players at a party. Eric hears about the party and recognizes that players are not supposed to go out on weekends during camp. However, given that he does not hear that anything has happened (eg, excessive drinking) he does not report the incident to Steve. Camp concludes and the academic year begins. After the second week of the semester Steve calls Eric into his office to ask about a rumor he is hearing from the full-time staff members. Steve relays a rumor that one of the clinical students, Joshua, is helping provide players with answers to assignments in an accounting class. Eric confronts Joshua about this rumor but Joshua denies it. Over the course of the next 2 weeks, Eric notices that Joshua is being asked to do extra "work" for some of the players, including cleaning their lockers, gathering up laundry, and retrieving extra food for them from the training table. Eric again confronts Joshua and asks about the things he has observed. Joshua then breaks down and pleads with Eric to be removed from the football clinical assignment. With further questioning Eric discovers that 3 football players cornered Joshua after they discovered that Joshua had tweeted that they were present at a party during training camp. Joshua then tells Eric that the players are harassing him during practice, after practice, and during the accounting class they share. This has been happening since the week following the party.

1. How would you classify the behavior Joshua is describing?

2. What 3 steps should Eric take after learning what had taken place, based on Joshua's account?

3. What should Steve do based on what he knows of the situation?

Case #2

For the past 5 years, Susan has been working in a physical therapy clinic with 3 physical therapists, 2 athletic trainers, and 1 physical therapy assistant. She left a position as head athletic trainer for a small Division III college after 10 years leading a sports medicine staff of 3 athletic trainers covering 25 varsity sports (no football). During her time as a member of the physical therapy clinic staff, Susan has asked to be given more responsibilities as she has had experience leading a team, albeit a small team, and believes she has the managerial skills to help the busy clinic practice. Twice in the past 6 months she has requested meetings with her supervisor, David, the owner and managing director of the clinic. During these meetings she expressed her desire to take on more responsibility. David has agreed, yet, last week Susan learned that Joseph, the other athletic trainer in the clinic, was attending a leadership course that David recommended to him. Joseph told Susan he was getting 2 days' pay and travel reimbursement for attending the course. Susan decided to ask David why she was not offered that opportunity and David told her that given Susan's busy schedule with 2 young children, he did not think she had time to take the course so therefore he offered it to Joseph.

1. How would you describe what may be happening to Susan in her role within the physical therapy clinic?

2. Is there a better approach that David could use to help support both of the athletic trainer staff members?

3. What steps should Susan take to address this issue and be sure she is provided more opportunities for development in the future?

Discussion Questions

1. What is the difference between access and treatment discrimination? Provide examples of each that relate to athletic training.

2. How can workplace discrimination eventually be costly for an employer?

3. What is meant by the phrase "good old boy network" and how is it a form of discrimination?

4. What is the relationship between diversity and discrimination in the workplace?

Suggested Resources

- www.eeoc.gov
- www.ncaa.org/sites/default/files/S%2BHarassment%2BBrochure.pdf
- www.sportsmanagementresources.com/sexual-abuse-and-harassment
- www.sportsmanagementresources.com/coach-athlete-misconduct-sexual-harassment-legal-liability

REFERENCES

1. Cortina LM. Unseen injustice: incivility as modern discrimination in organizations. *Acad Manag Rev.* 2008;33(1):55.

2. Cunningham GB, Fink JS. Diversity issues in sport and leisure: introduction to a special issue. *J Sport Manag.* 2006;20:455-465.

3. Kabat-Farr D, Cortina LM. Selective incivility: gender, race and the discriminatory workplace. In: Fox S, Lituchy TR. *Gender and the Dysfunctional Workplace.* Cheltenham, UK: Edward Elgar Publishing; 2012:107-117.

4. Cunningham GB. *Diversity in Sport Organizations.* Scottsdale, AZ: Holcomb Hathaway; 2011.

5. Greenhaus JH, Parasuraman S, Wormley WM. Effects of race on organizational experiences, job performance evaluations, and career outcomes. *Acad Manag J.* 1990;33(1):64-86.

6. Burton LJ, Borland J, Mazerolle SM. "They cannot seem to get past the gender issue": Experiences of young female athletic trainers in NCAA Division I intercollegiate athletics. *Sport Manag Rev.* 2012;15(3):304-317.

7. Acosta RV, Carpenter LJ. Status of women in intercollegiate sport—37 Year Update—1977–2014; 2014. http://www.acostacarpenter.org/. Accessed July 27, 2014.
8. Mazerolle SM, Bruening JE, Casa DJ, Burton LJ. Work-family conflict, part II: Job and life satisfaction in National Collegiate Athletic Association Division I-A certified athletic trainers. *J Athl Train*. 2008;43(5):513-522.
9. Sharp LA, Moorman AM, Claussen CL. *Sport Law: A Managerial Approach*. Scottsdale, AZ: Holcomb-Hathaway; 2007.
10. Velasquez BJ. Sexual harassment: a concern for the athletic trainer. *J Athl Train*. 1998;33(2):171-176.
11a. Shingles RR, Smith Y. Perceptions of sexual harassment in athletic training. http://www.nataej.org/3.3/EJ53 SexualHarrassmentfinalsubmittedcopy.pdf. Accessed July 27, 2014.
11b. National Athletic Trainers' Association. Athletic Training Education Competencies, 5th Edition. 2011. http://www.nata.org/sites/default/files/5th_Edition_Competencies.pdf. Accessed August 11, 2015.
12. Mazerolle SM, Pitney WA, Casa DJ, Pagnotta KD. Assessing strategies to manage work and life balance of athletic trainers working in the National Collegiate Athletic Association Division I setting. *J Athl Train*. 2011;46(2):194-205.
13. Nussbaum E, Rogers MJ. Athletic training and mothering at the Division 1 level. *Coll Athl Train Soc Newsl*. 1999; 1-2.
14. Benson K. Comments on Crocker's "An analysis of university definitions of sexual harassment." *Signs*. 1984;9:516-519.
15. Rospenda KM, Richman JA, Nawyn SJ. Doing power: the confluence of gender, race, and class in contrapower sexual harassment. *Gender Soc*. 1998;12(1):40-60.
16. DeSouza E, Fansler AG. Contrapower sexual harassment: a survey of students and faculty members. *Sex Roles*. 2003; 48(11-12),529-542.
17. U.S. Equal Employment Opportunity Commission. Race/Color Discrimination. http://www.eeoc.gov/laws/types/race_color.cfm. Accessed July 27, 2014.
18. Human Rights Campaign. Maps of state laws and policies. http://www.hrc.org/state_maps. Accessed September 4, 2015.
19. Ensign KA, Yiamouyiannis A, White KM, Ridpath BD. Athletic trainers' attitudes toward lesbian, gay, and bisexual National Collegiate Athletic Association student-athletes. *J Athl Train*. 2011;46(1):69-75.
20. Cortina LM, Kabat-Farr D, Leskinen EA, Huerta M, Magley VJ. Selective incivility as modern discrimination in organizations: evidence and impact. *J Manag*. 2013;39(6):1579-1605.
21. Yang LQ, Caughlin DE, Gazica MW, Truxillo DM, Spector PE. Workplace mistreatment climate and potential employee and organizational outcomes: a meta-analytic review from the target's perspective. *J Occup Health Psychol*. 2014;99(1):310-321.
22. Neuman JH, Baron RA. Workplace violence and workplace aggression: Evidence concerning specific forms, potential causes, and preferred targets. *J Manag*. 1998;24(3):391-419.
23. Cortina LM, Magley VJ, Williams JH, Langhout RD. Incivility in the workplace: incidence and impact. *J Occup Health Psychol*. 2001;6(1):64-80.
24. Mitchell MS, Ambrose ML. Employees' behavioral reactions to supervisor aggression: an examination of individual and situational factors. *J Appl Psychol*. 2012;97(6):1148-1170.
25. Salin D. Ways of explaining workplace bullying: a review of enabling, motivating and precipitating structures and processes in the work environment. *Hum Relat*. 2013;56(10):1213-1232.
26. Andersson LM, Pearson CM. Tit for tat? The spiraling effect of incivility in the workplace. *Acad Manag Rev*. 1999;24(3):452-471.
27. Cortina LM, Magley VJ. Patterns and profiles of response to incivility in the workplace. *J Occup Health Psychol*. 2009;14(3):272-288.
28. Einarsen S, Hoel H, Zapf D, Cooper C. *Bullying and Harassment in the Workplace: Developments in Theory, Research, and Practice*. 2nd ed. Boca Raton, FL: CRC Press; 2010.
29. Baron RA. Workplace aggression and violence: insights from basic research. In: Griffin RW, O'Leary-Kelly A, eds. *The Dark Side of Organizational Behavior*. San Francisco, CA: John Wiley & Sons; 2004:23-46.
30. Cunningham GB, Miner K, McDonald J. Being different and suffering the consequences: the influence of head coach-player racial dissimilarity on experienced incivility. *Int Rev Sociol Sport*. 2013;48(6):689-705.
31. Tingle JK, Warner S, Sartore-Baldwin ML. The experience of former women officials and the impact on the sporting community. *Sex Roles*. 2014;71:7-20.
32a. Lapchick R. The racial and gender report card. http://www.tidesport.org/racialgenderreportcard.html. Accessed July 27, 2014.
32b. National Athletic Trainers' Association. May 2014 NATA Certified Membership by Job Setting. 2014. http://members.nata.org/members1/documents/membstats/2014-06.htm. Accessed August 12, 2015.
33. Cunningham GB. Creating and sustaining gender diversity in sport organizations. *Sex Roles*. 2008;58(1-2):136-145.
32. Fink JS, Pastore DL, Riemer H. Do differences make a difference? Managing diversity in Division IA intercollegiate athletics. *J Sport Manag*. 2001;15(1):10-50.
33. Button SB. Organizational efforts to affirm sexual diversity: a cross-level examination. *J Appl Psychol*. 2001;86(1):17-28.

34. Mitchell MS, Ambrose ML. Employees' behavioral reactions to supervisor aggression: an examination of individual and situational factors. *J Appl Psychol.* 2012;97(6):1148-1170.

35. Nielsen MB, Einarsen S. Outcomes of exposure to workplace bullying: a meta-analytic review. *Work Stress.* 2012;26(4):309-332.

36. Gallus JA, Bunk JA, Matthews RA, Barnes-Farrell JL, Magley VJ. An eye for an eye? Exploring the relationship between workplace incivility experiences and perpetration. *J Occup Health Psychol.* 2014;19(2):143-154.

37. U.S. Department of Education. Sexual harassment guidelines. http://www2.ed.gov/about/offices/list/ocr/docs/sexhar00.html. Accessed July 27, 2014.

38. Connell RW, Messerschmidt JW. Hegemonic masculinity rethinking the concept. *Gender Soc.* 2015;19(6):829-859.

39. Anderson ED. The maintenance of masculinity among the stakeholders of sport. *Sport Manag Rev.* 2009;12(1):3-14.

40. Connell RW. Masculinities and globalization. *Men Masc.* 1998;1(1):3-23.

41. Kane MJ. Resistance/transformation of the oppositional binary: exposing sport as a continuum. *J Sport Soc Issues.* 1995;19(2):191-218.

42. Bartlett KT. Making good on good intentions: the critical role of motivation in reducing implicit workplace discrimination. *Va Law Rev.* 2009;95(8):1893-1972.

43. Lindsey A, King E, McCausland T, Jones K, Dunleavy E. What we know and don't: eradicating employment discrimination 50 years after the Civil Rights Act. *Industr Organiz Psychol.* 2013;6(4):391-413.

44. Project Implicit. https://implicit.harvard.edu/implicit/. Accessed August 11, 2015.

7

Job Burnout in Athletic Training

Stephanie M. Mazerolle, PhD, ATC, LAT

OBJECTIVES

After reading this chapter, the reader will be able to do the following:

1. Define burnout.
2. Identify signs and symptoms of burnout.
3. Understand the impact burnout can have on the individual and workplace.
4. Identify effective strategies to help prevent or reduce the impact of burnout on the individual.
5. Recommend different ways supervisors can mitigate the occurrence of burnout for the employee.

INTRODUCTION

Burnout has become a central focus in the health professions, as there is growing concern that its impact reaches beyond just the affected person to include those who are in the care of the health care worker.[1] When burnout occurs, it is often coupled with compassion fatigue, meaning the person can no longer demonstrate the same level of effort and care, despite trying. This notion, which has been documented in nursing, has yet to be examined in athletic training; however, parallels can be drawn due to comparable job expectations and demands. Because burnout can affect not only professionals themselves but those in their care, increased attention has been seen in the literature.[2-5]

Burnout affects athletic training professionals in varying positions (eg, program directors, assistant athletic trainers) and practice settings (eg, high school, college). The condition, viewed as a negative response to stress, manifests when an individual is no longer able to cope and manage responsibilities associated with their professional roles. Burnout has been reported among many

Mazerolle SM, Pitney WA.
Workplace Concepts for Athletic Trainers (pp 107-121).
© 2016 Taylor & Francis Group.

professionals within various fields, but mostly among those working in service-related fields such as teaching, health care, and social work.[6]

In this chapter, we will define the concept of burnout, paying great attention to the signs and symptoms, causes, and the impact experiences with burnout can have on the athletic trainer. We will then identify ways to prevent burnout from happening. The aim of the chapter will be to help the athletic trainer recognize the early signs of burnout in the hopes to prevent its occurrence and allow for maintenance of personal and professional rejuvenation.

> Emotional and physical exhaustion are often the hallmark sign of burnout, which results when prolonged stressors go unaddressed or unrelieved.

DEFINING BURNOUT

Burnout is defined as a negative response to chronic stress in which a person often is exhausted emotionally and physically because of the demands placed on him or her.[7] Our first contemporary burnout definition came from a 1974 book, *Burnout: The High Cost of High Achievement*, by psychologist Herbert Freudenberger.[8] He defined burnout as "the extinction of motivation or incentive, especially where one's devotion to a cause or relationship fails to produce the desired results."[8] Since Freudenberger's work, burnout has been studied among a diverse group of working professionals, but largely with those who work in service or human-oriented positions such as nurses, doctors, psychologists, and athletic trainers. Moreover, burnout is often characterized on a spectrum ranging from mild to severe and acute to chronic.[9] Symptoms manifest progressively, and can range from emotional (apathy, guilt, anger) to physical (fatigue, insomnia). As the condition lingers, often an individual starts to disengage, particularly from roles that once brought pleasure and enjoyment.[10,11] The condition is often described by the symptoms that habitually manifest, including decreased motivation, ineffectiveness, and decreased productivity.

The most commonly accepted definition of burnout was developed by Maslach et al,[12,13] who characterized 3 subsets: emotional exhaustion, depersonalization, and reduced personal accomplishment. Emotional exhaustion measures feelings of being emotionally overstretched and exhausted by an individual's work-related responsibilities.[13] Depersonalization measures feelings, specifically the development of cynicism and impersonality to one's role as a worker. Reduced personal accomplishment measures people's feelings of competences and worth as it relates to their work goals and achievements.[13] After several decades of research, the 3 aforementioned concepts have become synonymous with operationalizing burnout. Other organizational or workplace factors have been discussed as possible influential facilitators for burnout, and researchers have therefore begun to investigate the potential for other subscales to describe burnout adequately.

In athletic training, Capel[14,15] was the first to suggest that role conflict, high time commitment, limited opportunities for career advancement, low salary, and inadequate working conditions are contributors to burnout. Using the Maslach Burnout Inventory (MBI) as the foundation, Clapper and Harris[16] developed an instrument designed to specifically measure burnout within athletic training, as it suggested that each profession offers its own set of unique environmental factors that can stimulate burnout. Four constructs emerged to operationalize burnout: *emotional exhaustion and depersonalization, administrative responsibility, time commitment,* and *organizational support.*[16]

Emotional exhaustion and depersonalization were largely based on the original subscale described by Maslach[11] and was descriptive of the athletic trainer's perceptions of relationships with athletes and coaches and the degree of "hardening" that occurred because of the role. Administrative responsibility as operationalized within athletic training represented the amount

TABLE 7-1		
CONTRIBUTORS TO BURNOUT		
WORK-RELATED	**LIFESTYLE**	**PERSONALITY**
• Locus of control issues • Role or job ambiguity • Dysfunctional workplace dynamics • Repetitive or monotonous job responsibilities • Employment in a high-pressure, chaotic environment • Lack of respect or reward for job responsibilities	• Lack of social support • Limited time for leisure or social activities • Lack of sleep or poor eating, exercise habits • Assuming too many roles with competing demands • Work and life imbalance	• Type A, high-achieving personalities • Negative affinity disposition • Control issues • Perfectionism tendencies • Self-sacrificing

of work-related responsibility that athletic trainers reported (eg, pressure to get work done, paperwork). The time commitment construct reflected feelings related to time spent away from personal life, mostly related to family issues. The final construct, organizational support, reflected the relationship an athletic trainer can have with his or her employer.

Together the Athletic Training Burnout Inventory (ATBI) and MBI provide the underpinnings for the construct of burnout. Conceptually, burnout is the result of role overload as the continued stress mounts and without relief triggers a host of emotional and physical symptoms.[11] A host of factors have been identified that contribute to burnout, including work environment, nature of one's work, personality, and coping strategies.

Emotional exhaustion references the depletion of an athletic trainer's emotional and internal resources.[13]
Depersonalization refers to athletic trainers' attempt to distance themselves from their role, as a cynical attitude begins to develop toward their job.
Reduced personal accomplishment is an outcome of exhaustion and cynicism, which manifests as feelings of insufficiency and evaluating one's work negatively, whereby an athletic trainer may fail to see value in his or her care of the student-athlete.[13]

CONTRIBUTORS TO BURNOUT

Experiences of burnout can be described as facilitated by 3 factors (Table 7-1). The first, work-related contributors, speak to those circumstances and stressors that are attributed to an individual's workplace. Job characteristics such as role overload, role ambiguity, and relationships between patients and the health care provider are often factors contributing to burnout. Also, some organizational pieces such as job performance and the link to consequences or reward can be contributors to work-related burnout factors. The second, lifestyle, reflects those aspects of one's life that encompass non-work items as well as personal habits and choices. The final piece, personality, speaks to the individuality of the person whereby individual traits and personal attributes can influence one's susceptibility to stress and burnout. Self-efficacy, coping, and social support are often characteristics associated with experiences of burnout. Each factor is discussed in greater detail next.

Work-Related Contributors

Those who endure greater job demands are more likely to experience burnout as they suffer from energy depletion and lack the resources to cope with undue stress.[17] Issues within the workplace that can stimulate burnout can include excessive workloads (too many roles, hours, etc), lack of administrative support or appreciation within workplace, budgetary constraints that affect work performance, lack of control, and other restricting or unfair workplace policies.[11]

Maslach and Leiter[11] describe 6 aspects within a workplace that contribute to burnout: *workload, control, reward, unfairness, community,* and *value conflict.* Workload encompasses an individual's work hours, job responsibilities, and understanding of the expectations and demands placed upon them. Control refers to the power in which a person has over their work scheduling, responsibilities placed upon them, and role they assume within their organization. Reward reflects the degree to which individuals are recognized for their accomplishments, hard work, and contributions to their job/organization. Unfairness includes compensation (paycheck vs expectations) or treatment within the workplace (unclear or inequity expectations). Community or, more specifically, breakdown of the workplace community, indicates a lack of cohesion between employers and employees whereby the environment is not conducive to productivity. Finally, value conflict suggests a disconnect between an organization's expectations and values and the individual's personal goals and beliefs.

Excessive workload, emotionally demanding interactions with patients, and lack of control over aspects of one's job can influence experiences of burnout,[6] circumstances that can be used to describe the athletic trainer's work environment, and why its prevalence has been found across all roles and settings in athletic training.[2,3,5] Fundamentally, the excessive work hours for the athletic trainer have been reported as the primary facilitator to burnout[2,5]; however, beyond hours worked, other workplace factors contribute to burnout for the athletic trainer. These include pressure from a coach to medically clear the student-athlete, high patient volumes coupled by multiple sport coverage assignments, high injury frequencies, and limited time for outside activities.[2,3,18] Role overload or strain can also contribute to experiences of burnout for athletic trainers, as those who assume multiple roles (program director and clinical athletic trainer; clinical athletic trainer and preceptor, etc) are at greater risk for burnout.[3,18] Workplace stressors play only a small role in the occurrence of burnout, as the construct is multifactorial.

Lifestyle Contributors

Daily exercise, diet, sleep, and alcohol consumption are often linked to lifestyle habits, and can be considered factors related to burnout. Individuals who fail to find work-life balance, have limited support networks, and demonstrate unhealthy behaviors (lack of sleep, no exercise, etc) are at greater risk for experiencing burnout.[2,19]

Exercise appears to have a positive influence on those experiencing burnout, as a recent study revealed that aerobic exercise reduced symptoms of burnout and improved the mood of working male professionals with documented levels of high burnout.[20] Athletic trainers report using exercise as a medium to help cope and manage stress as well as improve their work-life balance, thus findings from Gerber et al[20] support the need to include regular exercise as a burnout prevention strategy. Work-life balance has also been found to correlate with experiences in job burnout. Athletic trainers who experience greater levels of work-life conflict are also likely to experience job burnout. In fact, Mazerolle et al[21] found a positive relationship between the 2 constructs, and when compared to other working professionals demonstrated a strong, significant relationship.

Personal Contributors

Age is often linked to experiences of burnout, especially in health care, where those early in their careers (< 30 years of age) experience symptoms.[22] The concept of "reality shock" is often a reason cited as foundational to burnout among these young workers, as they are trying to gain role inductance while balancing a new role and expectations related to the position.[22] Burnout has been reported among graduate assistant athletic trainers,[2] the newest of the professionals illustrating that age can play a role in burnout. Burnout of young athletic training professionals has been mentioned as a contributing factor for departure,[23] although these have mostly been anecdotally based.

Beyond age, personality has also been discussed as playing a central role in the development of burnout. Personality variables include hardiness, locus of control, Type A vs B behavior, self-esteem, and achievement motivation.

Hardiness, otherwise known as personality or cognitive hardiness, is a personality construct that describes those individuals who can "weather" life stress and has been described as encompassing 3 general dispositions: commitment, control, and challenge.[24,25] The 3 attitudes influence how people view themselves, as well as how they interact with those in their life. An individual who is considered to be hardy is able to turn stressful circumstances into opportunities for personal growth.[26] Commitment refers to an individual's interests and curiosity (facing life with eagerness and a sense of purpose), control reflects the tendency to believe in one's power to influence his or her course of life, and challenge recognizes that change rather than stability is a normal aspect of life.[26,27] Individuals who are considered to have low levels of hardiness are at risk for experiencing burnout. In athletic training, for example, Hendrix et al[5] found that athletic trainers who scored lower on hardiness and social support and higher on athletic training issues reported higher levels of burnout.

Locus of control denotes the extent to which individuals believe they can control events that affect them and is intellectualized as internal (control over one's own life) or external (decision are affected and controlled by environmental factors, not the person).[28] Those who embody an internal locus of control are motivated and believe they control their own fate and the outcomes that result from their actions, attitudes, and behaviors are their own doing.[28] Those who embody an external locus of control, on the other hand, attribute outcomes to outside circumstances and therefore believe events are out of their control. Individuals who have an external locus of control tend to be more stressed and thus at greater risk for depression or other negative outcomes such as burnout.[29,30] Those with external control often have a negative affinity or outlook, and are quick to react negatively to stress. Nurses who had greater sense of control over work-related responsibilities and decision making reported experiencing less burnout.[31]

Type A and B personality behavior are 2 dichotomous constructs that describe a person's disposition, regular behaviors and patterns.[32,33] Type A personalities are often characterized as ambitious, organized, impatient, proactive, high-achieving, and deadline driven. Juxtaposed to the Type A are Type B personalities, who often live at a lower level of stress as they are often described as relaxed and easy going; they appear to adapt better to stressful situations, thus reducing their likeliness to suffer from stress-related syndromes. Type B personalities are creative, embrace differences, avoid competition, and enjoy being reflective and exploring new ideas and concepts. Professionals such as nurses and teachers who are identified as Type A personalities have demonstrated higher levels of stress, which then positively correlate to higher burnout scores.

| | TABLE 7-2 | |
| | SUMMARY OF RELATIONSHIP BETWEEN THE
BIG 5 AND BURNOUT SUBSCALES[39-41] | |
BIG 5 PERSONALITY CONSTRUCT	**BURNOUT SUBSCALE**	**RELATIONSHIP**
Extraversion	Emotional exhaustion	Negative
Agreeableness	Depersonalization	Negative
Agreeableness	Personal accomplishment	Positive
Conscientiousness	Personal accomplishment	Positive
Conscientiousness	Depersonalization	Positive
Neuroticism	Emotional exhaustion	Positive
Neuroticism	Depersonalization	Positive

"Internals" are those who perceive control over their own decisions and life choices. In contrast, an "external" is a person who perceives no control over his or her life course and happenings.
Individuals who have an internal locus of control are the people who are self-confident, find enjoyment in their jobs, and have successful strategies in place to help them adapt to their workplace stressors.
"Internals" have a greater chance of not experiencing occupational or emotional exhaustion as they have emotional adaptability and flexibility.

The use of the big 5 personality model has emerged recently as an integral model to evaluate the relationship to burnout. Using the acronym OCEAN (Table 7-2), the model has 5 broad dimensions of personality: *openness, conscientiousness, extraversion, agreeableness,* and *neuroticism.* Table 7-2 provides a brief summary of the relationships between burnout and personality as assessed using the big 5 model (Table 7-3). Associations with the model and other workplace issues, such as work-life balance,[34] have been reported previously, making personality a likely culprit with experiences of burnout.

Type A: aggressive, hard-working, impatient, time-urgent, competitive, achievement orientated. Type B: realistic self-expectations, realistic goals, unaware of time, less intense, calm, relaxed.

The findings are mixed in regards to openness and burnout, with most research suggesting a positive relationship between openness and personal accomplishment,[35] and negative relationships between emotional exhaustion and depersonalization.[36] Conscientiousness demonstrates a positive relationship with burnout, typically as those who demonstrate this trait are self-disciplined and goal-oriented, suggesting they complete tasks despite distractions or an increase in workload or demand.[36] Extraversion, in general, is associated with a negative relationship with

TABLE 7-3
BIG 5 MODEL[42]
Openness: Individual will demonstrate intellect, curiosity, and be open to new ideas and concepts. Viewed as your level of creativity and curiosity.
Conscientiousness: Individual is dutiful, high-achieving, and self-disciplined. Seen as your level of organization and work ethic.
Extraversion: Individuals who exhibit self-confidence, seek excitement, and want stimulation through social stimulation. Often are optimistic and reappraise problems in a positive manner. Your level of sociability and enthusiasm.
Agreeableness: Individual will be compassionate, cooperative, and trusting. One's level of friendliness and kindness.
Neuroticism: Individuals display irrational, unstable behaviors, and have a reduced impulse control. Your level of emotional stability and tranquility.

burnout as those who demonstrate this quality often use rational, problem-solving coping skills to manage their problems and issues. Moreover, they use social support and positive appraisal as means to manage their stress, both of which are effective practices for managing burnout.[37,38] Agreeableness has demonstrated a negative relationship with burnout, as those who are concerned with social harmony and getting along with others will exhibit or perceive less burnout in comparison to those who are selfish and self-centered.[39] Neuroticism demonstrates a positive relationship with burnout, as neurotics often respond irrationally to undue stress and under-use proven coping strategies for burnout.[39]

Neuroticism and conscientiousness are often linked to experiences of burnout, as those who are more likely to respond irrationally and negatively to stress are more likely to be unable to cope with those stressors.[41] Additionally, those who demonstrate extroversion and agreeableness characteristics are less likely to experience burnout, as their disposition appears to improve their work engagement and buffer issues that may lead to burnout.[41] Limited information is available regarding personality and experiences of burnout in athletic training. Personal factors have been reported to influence experiences of burnout in athletic training, as Kania et al[3] found that elevated stress levels and limited time for leisure were predictive of elevated levels of burnout.

CONSEQUENCES OF BURNOUT

The inability to cope with stressful situations will lead to experiences of burnout, which then begin to produce negative physical, behavioral, and emotional problems that vary from person to person (Table 7-4). The physical problems related to burnout are somatic in nature, often including feelings of chronic fatigue or exhaustion, sleeplessness, headaches, and respiratory issues.[8] Behavioral problems may include a shorter temper, verbally negative behavior, stubbornness, and inflexibility. Emotional problems associated with burnout include increased cynicism, decreased motivation, frustration and irritability, and a removal from social situations. In fact, a burned out person may exhibit symptoms of depression as they remove themselves from others.

On-the-job outcomes have also been found to occur in those who experience job burnout, which includes a reduction in productivity, increased absenteeism, decreased job satisfaction, and poor patient care outcomes. Compassion fatigue is also an issue related to burnout, as those who

TABLE 7-4 CONSEQUENCES OF BURNOUT		
PHYSICAL	**EMOTIONAL**	**BEHAVIOR**
• Exhaustion • Repeated illnesses • Headaches • Loss of sleep • Change in appetite • Unexplained back and neck pain	• Self-doubt • Loss of motivation • Reduction in satisfaction and accomplishments • Social isolation • Feelings of defeat and frustrations • Negative outlook and cynical thoughts	• Withdrawing from activities and involvement in normal activities • Isolation (social groups) • Procrastination • Increased emotional outbursts • Absenteeism or tardiness • Using unhealthy habits to cope (drinking, etc)

experience constant stress and are engaged in helping professions are likely to become cynical and withdraw from and disengage from their professional roles. Health care workers develop compassion fatigue, mostly due to the demands placed on them related to patient care and working conditions.[43,44] Experiences of burnout are also linked to career and job turnover, as constant experiences of stress lead to needing a change as the person can no longer stay committed or engaged in the role.[45,46] Although the link and understanding of the negative consequences of burnout is limited in athletic training, the condition has been linked to work-family conflict, another work-related issue, and it is well understood that work-family conflict leads to decreased job satisfaction and commitment to the profession.[21]

> Compassion fatigue is a gradual lessening of compassion over time. It is a common sequela of burnout, as those who work directly with patients are at risk for suffering from it as the constant stress can lead to self-doubt, withdrawing from their roles, and a lack of connection and commitment to their duties.

PREVENTING, REDUCING, AND MANAGING BURNOUT

Dealing with burnout can be simply summarized by the 3 Rs: recognize, reverse, and resilience. Simply, one must be aware of and recognize those factors that can contribute to experiences and feelings of burnout. Understanding the triggers and warning signs of burnout can help the athletic trainer avoid its occurrence. Next, it is important after recognizing the signs to slowly begin to manage that stress, often via stress-relieving techniques and practices, in order to reverse the burnout process. Once the reversal process has been initiated, the athletic trainer can then begin to develop resiliency by improving his or her overall health and mental disposition as the stresses are alleviated or removed. See Chapter 15 for more information on emotional resiliency.

Recognize: Be aware of the outward signs and causes of burnout.
Reverse: Establish a plan to help address concerns related to burnout.
Resilience: Use support, and other proven techniques to cope with feelings of burnout.

It is important to understand that there is a degree of individuality when it comes to managing and coping with stress. Everyone has different sets of stressors and triggers and, therefore, also has various ways to cope with those daily stresses. As discussed within the work-life chapter, self-reflection and evaluation of goals are critical in developing practices that can help reduce undue stress and prevent job burnout.

Circumvent the Stressors

Athletic trainers are going to work long hours, have some travel, and at times manage high patient loads, but it is still important to identify ways to reduce the number of stressors that affect them all at once. A simple method is to learn to say "no," a recommendation that has been reported as effective in establishing work-life balance for the athletic trainer.[47] Understanding your limits personally and professionally can help you assume or avoid additional roles that you can successfully balance. For example, an athletic trainer who is currently managing a high patient load and traveling extensively may say "no" to taking on an athletic training student to supervise as he or she may not have the time to do so, and the additional administrative load may not be manageable. Other means to avoid stress include a daily to-do list outlining the "musts" of the day vs the "shoulds," as well as establishing boundaries or expectations with coaches, administrators, patients, or student-athletes. This can include treatment hours and expectations and appropriate times for communication during the day.

Modify the Situation

Time management is a fundamental skill that allows individuals to manage their daily roles and responsibilities, thus planning ahead can allow for avoiding undue stress or at best altering the impact the stress can have on the person. Using time management skills can help athletic trainers take control over their time, which is a valuable resource. Planning for today and tomorrow can help reduce the "hold" job demands and expectations can have on the athletic trainer. For example, setting aside time weekly to address administrative loads (insurance, progress notes, etc) not only can increase the control assumed by the athletic trainer, it can allow for completion of monotonous, tedious tasks that are often a source of stress.

Altering the stressors is often about mindset, that is, how athletic trainers view those stressors that affect them. Job ambiguity is often a factor leading to burnout, thus it is important for an athletic trainer to communicate to a supervisor that expectations are unclear and a better job description is needed. Failure to express concerns or uncertainties can lead to frustration and burnout. Cohesion in the workplace, which is often facilitated by an effective supervisor, teamwork among co-workers, and a love of the job, has been shown to improve work-life balance and satisfaction in the workplace,[47-50] also key for a reduction in burnout.

Time Management

1. Organize: Draft a to-do list. This list should be exhaustive of all tasks for that day/ week.

2. Prioritize: Rewrite the to-do list to reflect order of importance. Priority should be given to only those that must be performed immediately.

3. Schedule: Establish the time that is necessary to complete the tasks. The time should be manageable and reasonable and set for each item of the list.

Adapting or Adjusting to the Stressor

Adjusting one's mindset can profoundly influence experiences of burnout, as it can reduce the negative affectivity that comes with seeing the undesirable aspects of the workplace and one's job responsibilities. It may be impossible to change the sources of stress (ie, hours worked, travel schedule), but the athletic trainer can adapt to the stressful situations by seeking support from co-workers who are sharing similar stresses, identifying the positives of the workplace (ie, remember why you took the position), or developing a plan or solution to address concerns that are creating the stressors in the first place.

Athletic trainers are attracted to the career because of a love of sports, an interest in health care, strong relationships forged with their co-workers and student-athletes, and the love of the workplace culture.[49-51] Adapting expectations, having reasonable expectations, and focusing on the positives can help athletic trainers manage their roles and responsibilities and thus reducing burnout.

Acknowledgment

As discussed previously, personality can play a factor in burnout; often those who have an optimistic outlook, react calmly to stress, and who are able to adapt to stress are likely to experience less burnout.[52] Embracing the workplace setting and its limitations is necessary to avoid undue stress and its negative impact. An athletic trainer must have a realistic impression of the workplace demands and expectations, and accept those benefits as well as the limitations. For example, many athletic trainers who have persisted in the Division I (D-I) setting have come to accept the "athletics lifestyle," which has allowed them to develop practices that enable them to manage the demands placed on them both at home and in the workplace.

Rejuvenation

Finding healthy ways to relax and recharge is critical not only for preventing burnout, but also for stimulating and maintaining professional commitment.[48] Adapting a positive attitude is important, and taking the time for fun and relaxation is also necessary to help the athletic trainer manage life- and work-related stressors. Often coined "me" time, this personal time has permeated the athletic training literature as a means to help the athletic trainer cope with the demands of the profession[19,47] and has direct applications to reducing job burnout. The concept of "me" time simply refers to the time athletic trainers take for themselves to engage in activities of leisure, fun, or relaxation that do not require their time or resources for the job-related responsibilities.

The use of exercise and sleep has surfaced as practices used by athletic training professionals[19,47] and athletic training students[53,54] as a means to cope with stress and prevent incidences of burnout. Beyond those 2 practices, other activities for creating rejuvenation include quiet time, having lunch with a friend, engaging in hobbies (gardening, reading, etc), and being active (hiking, biking, etc). Regardless of the act, creating time for disengagement from stressful roles can allow the athletic trainer to reinvest in the stressful role and likely prevent burnout while promoting commitment to the role.

Healthy Lifestyle Choices

Evidence suggests that at times, athletic trainers do not meet the recommendations set forth by the American College of Sports Medicine (ACSM) regarding living a healthy lifestyle.[55] Simply, they do not engage in regular exercise and fail to meet the daily reference for food intake. Engaging in unhealthy lifestyle habits can affect an athletic trainer's ability to cope and manage stress, but often athletic trainers place their own needs and interests aside to care or attend to their job-related responsibilities. Although exercise is a key piece to a healthy lifestyle and stress management, other strategies are necessary to prevent burnout, including eating a healthy diet, reducing caffeine intake, and getting enough sleep.

Getting enough sleep, however, is more than just about quantity (8 hours), the quality of sleep is important. Simple tips to improve overall sleep habits include having a regular bed time, consistent wake-up times, getting enough daytime light, maintaining room temperature that allows for comfort (~68°F), and avoiding overstimulation before bedtime.

American College of Sports Medicine (ACSM) Guidelines for Healthy Adults Under 65[56]

- Do moderately[a] intense cardio 30 minutes a day, 5 days a week, or
- Do vigorously intense cardio 20 minutes a day, 3 days a week, and
- Do 8 to 10 strength-training exercises, 8 to 12 repetitions of each exercise twice a week.

---

[a]Moderate-intensity physical activity means working hard enough to raise your heart rate and break a sweat, yet still being able to carry on a conversation.

SUMMARY

Within the profession of athletic training, the topic of burnout has become increasingly more popular because of the increase in attrition rates of athletic trainers. Capel[14] was the first to examine the construct of burnout in athletic training, finding that burnout was predicated by long working hours, insufficient salaries, and high patient volumes. Clapper and Harris[16] created the ATBI, an adaptation of the MBI that more specifically addressed issues faced by athletic trainers. The long hours, required travel, ever-changing schedules, and low pay have been found to cause burnout within the profession.[3] The research has continued to identify similar constructs as antecedents to burnout, along with coping strategies, hardiness, and perceived levels of stress.[3,5] Additionally, job-related duties such as pressures to medically clear a student-athlete have been found to mediate the occurrence of burnout.[3]

Kania el al[3] reported that 32% of athletic trainers experience moderate levels of burnout, and Giacobbi[4] found 17.2% of a random nationwide sample of athletic trainers were in advanced stages of burnout. Some argue that burnout occurs less frequently among athletic trainers than among other health care professionals, yet they still experience signs and symptoms of the condition. Thus burnout has been explored at all levels of athletic training from National Collegiate Athletic Association (NCAA) athletic trainers[3,5,16] to graduate assistant athletic trainers[2] to athletic training program directors.[57] While male and female athletic trainers experience burnout, Naugle et al[58] found that females report higher levels of burnout as compared to their male counterparts, a finding similar to Giacobbi.[4] The collegiate setting also appears to be the setting where burn-out manifests itself more strongly than in other practice settings.[4,58] While no one is immune to burnout in health care professions, there are ways to recognize it, see the effect it can have on an individual or a workplace, and find ways to reduce or prevent burnout from affecting a health care professional. Burnout has been identified as a concern in the profession as demonstrated by the increase in literature, empirically and anecdotally.[59]

Awareness of the signs and symptoms as well as the development of healthy lifestyle practices can help the athletic trainer reduce the prevalence of burnout. Working in health care can be emotionally and physically exhausting, but the rewards can often outweigh the demands. Athletic trainers are encouraged to balance their workloads and take time for themselves as a means to create rejuvenation and maintain professional commitment, without becoming burned out.

ACTIVITIES FOR REINFORCEMENT

Questions for Review

1. What are the signs and symptoms of burnout?

2. What are the causes of burnout?

3. How can an individual successfully deal with burnout?

Case Vignettes

Case #1

Payton is a 33-year-old assistant athletic trainer who has been employed for 7 years at a Division II college. Over the last month she has noted feeling exhausted after each day of work and has been suffering a migraine or tension headache once a week, an increase from her normal once every few months. Restless at night, she has been using the extra awake time to respond to emails and update treatment plans and subjective, objective, assessment, and planning (SOAP) notes.

Although she has been maintaining a normal 50-hour work week, Payton has been frustrated by the time she is away from her son and daughter (ages 6 and 8, respectively). Her frustrations have spilled over into her job, with her sometimes lashing out at her peers or dreading going in for the day. She has been limiting her running to only 3 days per week, but was regularly running 5 days a week 6 months ago.

1. What could be causing Payton's increase in headaches and exhaustion?

2. Would Payton's experiences of burnout be different if she were employed in a different practice setting?

3. What recommendations could you make to Payton to help her reduce her frustrations at work and improve her mood?

Case #2

Bobby is a 42-year-old high school athletic trainer who has been in his current position for 8 years. He is contracted through the local physical therapy clinic, where he is required to work 12 hours per week in addition to his 35 with the high school. He began the position with great enthusiasm as the position allowed for the integration of medical care, student-athlete interactions, and a job that was close to home.

A new supervisor has begun to micromanage his role, unlike the previous supervisor who allowed Bobby both flexibility with this clinic hours and autonomy to manage his high school responsibilities. Over time, his ability to create injury-prevention programs and seek out other opportunities to challenge his skills as a clinician has become a struggle. Despite his ability to have his wife and kids visit and be involved while he works, Bobby has become increasingly frustrated with his job. At times, he has appeared to be absent from the job and seems to go through the motions. He even called in sick twice in 2 weeks, something he hadn't done in 8 years on the job.

1. At this point, should Bobby be concerned about job burnout? Please explain.
2. What sources of stress appear to be the most problematic for Bobby?
3. What recommendations would you offer to Bobby to help address some of the issues that may be contributing to his burnout?

Discussion Questions

1. Based on your experience in athletic training, what do you believe is the most common sign and symptom of burnout?
2. What do you believe is the relationship between compassion fatigue and burnout?
3. Why is physical activity an effective way to deal with stress?

REFERENCES

1. Miller D. Stress and burnout among health-care staff working with people affected by HIV. *Br J Guid Couns.* 1995;23(1):19-32.
2. Mazerolle SM, Monsma E, Dixon C, Mensch J. An assessment of burnout in graduate assistant certified athletic trainers. *J Athl Train.* 2012;47(3):320.
3. Kania ML, Meyer BB, Ebersole KT. Personal and environmental characteristics predicting burnout among certified athletic trainers at National Collegiate Athletic Association institutions. *J Athl Train.* 2009;44(1):58.
4. Giacobbi PR Jr. Low burnout and high engagement levels in athletic trainers: results of a nationwide random sample. *J Athl Train.* 2009;44(4):370.
5. Hendrix AE, Acevedo EO, Hebert E. An examination of stress and burnout in certified athletic trainers at Division IA universities. *J Athl Train.* 2000;35(2):139-144.
6. Maslach C, Schaufeli WB, Leiter MP. Job burnout. *Annu Rev Psychol.* 2001;(52):397-422.
7. Gieck J, Brown R, Shank R. The burnout syndrome among athletic trainers. *J Athl Train.* 1982;17(1):36-40.
8. Freudenberger HJ, Richelson G. *Burn Out: The High Cost of High Achievement: What it Is and How to Survive it.* New York: Bantam Books; 1980.
9. Hamann DL, Gordon DG. Burnout: an occupational hazard. *Music Educ J.* 2000;87(3):34.
10. Maslach C, Goldberg J. Prevention of burnout: new perspectives. *Appl Prev Psychol.* 1999;7(1):63-74.
11. Maslach C, Leiter MP. *The Truth About Burnout.* San Francisco: Jossey-Bass; 1997.
12. Maslach C, Jackson SE. *Maslach Burnout Inventory Manual.* 2nd ed. Palo Alto, CA: Consulting Psychologists Press; 1986.
13. Schaufeli WB, Maslach C, Marek T. *Professional Burnout: Recent Developments in Theory and Research.* Washington, D.C.: Taylor & Francis; 1993.
14. Capel S. Attrition of athletic trainers. *J Athl Train.* 1990;25(1):34-39.
15. Capel SA. Psychological and organizational factors related to burnout in athletic trainers. *R Quarterly Exerc Sport.* 1986;57(4):321-328.
16. Clapper DC, Harris LL. Reliability and validity of an instrument to describe burnout among collegiate athletic trainers. *J Athl Train.* 2008;43(1):62-69.
17. Demerouti E, Bakker AB, Nachreiner F, Schaufeli WB. The job demands-resources model of burnout. *J Appl Psychol.* 2001;86(3):499-512.
18. Walter JM, Van Lunen BL, Walker SE, Ismaeli ZC, Oñate JA. An assessment of burnout in undergraduate athletic training education program directors. *J Athl Train.* 2009;44(2):190.
19. Mazerolle SM, Pitney WA, Casa DJ, Pagnotta KD. Assessing strategies to manage work and life balance of athletic trainers working in the National Collegiate Athletic Association Division I setting. *J Athl Train.* 2011;46(2):194.
20. Gerber M, Brand S, Elliot C, Holsboer-Trachsler E, Pühse U, Beck J. Aerobic exercise training and burnout: a pilot study with male participants suffering from burnout. *BMC Res Notes.* 2013;6(1):78.

21. Mazerolle SM, Bruening JE, Casa DJ, Burton LJ. Work-family conflict, part II: job and life satisfaction in National Collegiate Athletic Association Division IA certified athletic trainers. *J Athl Train.* 2008;43(5):513.

22. Van Dierendonck D, Schaufeli WB, Buunk BP. Burnout and inequity among human service professionals: a longitudinal study. *J Occup Health Psychol.* 2001;6(1):43.

23. Kahanov L, Eberman LE. Age, sex, and setting factors and labor force in athletic training. *J Athl Train.* 2011;46(4):424.

24. Kobasa SC, Maddi SR, Kahn S. Hardiness and health: a prospective study. *J Pers Soc Psychol.* 1982;42(1):168.

25. Kobasa SC. Stressful life events, personality, and health: an inquiry into hardiness. *J Pers Soc Psychol.* 1979;37(1):1.

26. Maddi SR. Hardiness: an operationalization of existential courage. *J Humanist Psychol.* 2004;44(3):279-298.

27. Smith R. Toward a cognitive-affective model of athletic burnout. *J Sport Psychol.* 1986;8:36-50.

28. Rotter JB. Generalized expectancies for internal versus external control of reinforcement. *Psychol Monogr Gen Appl.* 1966;80(1):1.

29. April KA, Dharani B, Peters K. Impact of locus of control expectancy on level of well-being. *Rev Eur Stud.* 2012;4(2).

30. Jacobs-Lawson JM, Waddell EL, Webb AK. Predictors of health locus of control in older adults. *Curr Psychol.* 2011;30(2):173-183.

31. Schmitz N, Neumann W, Oppermann R. Stress, burnout and locus of control in German nurses. *Int J Nurs Stud.* 2000;37(2):95-99.

32. Furnham A. Response bias, social desirability and dissimulation. *Personal Individ Differ.* 1986;7(3):385-400.

33. Schmied LA, Lawler KA. Hardiness, Type A behavior, and the stress-illness relation in working women. *J Pers Soc Psychol.* 1986;51(6):1218-1223.

34. Bruck CS, Allen TD. The relationship between big five personality traits, negative affectivity, type A behavior, and work-family conflict. *J Vocat Behav.* 2003;63(3):457-472.

35. Zellars KL, Perrewé PL, Hochwarter WA. Burnout in health care: the role of the five factors of personality. *J Appl Soc Psychol.* 2000;30(8):1570-1598.

36. Deary I, Watson R, Hogston R. A longitudinal cohort study of burnout and attrition in nursing students. *J Adv Nurs.* 2003;43(1):71-81.

37. Watson D, Hubbard B. Adaptational style and dispositional structure: coping in the context of the five-factor model. *J Pers.* 1996;64(4):737-774.

38. Eastburg MC, Williamson M, Gorsuch R, Ridley C. Social support, personality, and burnout in nurses. *J Appl Soc Psychol.* 1994;24(14):1233-1250.

39. Bakker AB, Van Der Zee KI, Lewig KA, Dollard MF. The relationship between the Big Five personality factors and burnout: a study among volunteers. *J Soc Psychol.* 2006;146(1):31-50.

40. Kim HJ, Shin KH, Umbreit WT. Hotel job burnout: the role of personality characteristics. *Spec Issue Self-Cater Accommod.* 2007;26(2):421-434.

41. Kim HJ, Shin KH, Swanger N. Burnout and engagement: a comparative analysis using the Big Five personality dimensions. *Int J Hosp Manag.* 2009;28(1):96-104.

42. Costa PT Jr, McCrae RR. *Revised NEO Personality Inventory (NEO-PI R) and NEO Five Factor Inventory (NEO-FFI) Manual.* Odessa, FL: Psychological Assessment Resources; 1992.

43. Beck CT. Secondary traumatic stress in nurses: a systematic review. *Arch Psychiatr Nurs.* 2011;25(1):1-10.

44. Hooper C, Craig J, Janvrin DR, Wetsel MA, Reimels E. Compassion satisfaction, burnout, and compassion fatigue among emergency nurses compared with nurses in other selected inpatient specialties. *J Emerg Nurs.* 2010;36(5):420-427.

45. Landon B, Aseltine R, Shaul J, Miller Y, Auerbach B, Cleary P. The evolving dissatisfaction among primary care physicians. *Am J Manag Care* 2002;8(10):890-901.

46. Zhang Y, Feng X. The relationship between job satisfaction, burnout, and turnover intention among physicians from urban state-owned medical institutions in Hubei, China: a cross-sectional study. *BMC Health Serv Res.* 2011;11(1):235.

47. Mazerolle SM, Pitney WA, Goodman A, Eason CM. NATA Position Statement on Work-Life Balance for the Athletic Trainer. Paper presented at:66th National Athletic Trainers' Association Annual Meeting and Clinical Symposia; June, 2015; St. Louis, MO.

48. Pitney WA. A qualitative examination of professional role commitment among athletic trainers working in the secondary school setting. *J Athl Train.* 2010;45(2):198.

49. Goodman A, Mensch JM, Jay M, French KE, Mitchell MF, Fritz SL. Retention and attrition factors for female certified athletic trainers in the National Collegiate Athletic Association Division I Football Bowl Subdivision setting. *J Athl Train.* 2010;45(3):287.

50. Mazerolle SM, Goodman A, Pitney WA. Factors influencing retention of male athletic trainers in the NCAA Division I setting. *Int J Athl Ther Train.* 2013;18(5):6-9.

51. Mensch JM, Ennis CD. Pedagogic strategies perceived to enhance student learning in athletic training education. *J Athl Train.* 2002;37(4 Suppl):S-199-S-207.

52. Zellars KL, Hochwarter WA, Perrewé PL, Hoffman N, Ford EW. Experiencing job burnout: the roles of positive and negative traits and states. *J Appl Soc Psychol.* 2004;34(5):887-911.

53. Mazerolle SM, Pagnotta KD. Student perspectives on burnout. *Athl Train Educ J.* 2011;6(2):60-68.

54. Mazerolle SM, Bowman T, Fister C. Coping strategies utilized by athletic training majors to manage clinical and academic responsibilities. *Int J Athl Ther Train.* 2015;20(3):4-12.

55. Gorant J. *Female head athletic trainers in NCAA Division I (IA football) athletics: How they made it to the top.* [doctoral dissertation]. Kalamazoo: Western Michigan University; 2012.

56. Garber CE, Blissmer B, Deschenes MR, et al. Quantity and quality of exercise for developing and maintaining cardiorespiratory, musculoskeletal, and neuromotor fitness in apparently healthy adults: guidance for prescribing exercise. *Med Sci Sports Exerc.* 2011;43(7):1334-1359.

57. Judd MR, Perkins SA. Athletic training education program directors' perceptions on job selection, satisfaction, and attrition. *J Athl Train.* 2004;39(2):185.

58. Naugle KE, Behar-Horenstein LS, Dodd VJ, Tillman MD, Borsa PA. Perceptions of wellness and burnout among certified athletic trainers: sex differences. *J Athl Train.* 2013;48(3):424-430.

59. Hunt V. Dangerous dedication: burnout a risk in profession. *NATA News.* 2000:8-10.

Job Satisfaction in Athletic Training

Stephanie M. Mazerolle, PhD, ATC, LAT and
Ashley Goodman, PhD, LAT, ATC

OBJECTIVES

After reading this chapter, the reader will be able to do the following:

1. Define job satisfaction.

2. Discuss models of job satisfaction.

3. Share valid methods used to evaluate job satisfaction.

4. Review the literature on job satisfaction in health care and athletic training.

5. Identify the causes of dissatisfaction and outcomes related to reduced job satisfaction.

6. Present strategies to improve job satisfaction in the workplace.

INTRODUCTION

Over the last few years there has been growing concern about the declining National Athletic Trainers' Association (NATA) membership, which has been loosely linked to the level of satisfaction athletic trainers may or may not have with their job. The association is based on the knowledge that job satisfaction is a predictor to a person's intention to leave a job or profession.[1] Issues surrounding job satisfaction surface within every profession, but owing to the continued discourse regarding departure of young professionals from athletic training,[2,3] the topic is of acute importance.

Job satisfaction is expressed as the degree to which a person likes his or her job.[4] Multifaceted, the construct can be greatly influenced by one's level of work-related stress, pay, professional recognition, work-life balance, and overall nature of their job.[5-7] The greatest consequence of low job satisfaction is intention to leave a position or the profession entirely. Other consequences include

Mazerolle SM, Pitney WA.
Workplace Concepts for Athletic Trainers (pp 123-135).
© 2016 Taylor & Francis Group.

reduction in productivity, work withdrawal, and reduced commitment to the organization, which have also been identified as precursors to departure.[8]

Organizationally, job satisfaction can be improved through positive work environments, rewards and recognitions, and support networks. Individuals are encouraged to develop strong relationships with co-workers, use effective communication skills to share expectations and needs related to one's job, and develop short- and long-term goals to maintain commitment and engagement in their role. This chapter will focus on defining job satisfaction, discussing those factors that lead to an improved level of satisfaction, and methods to help promote satisfaction within the workplace.

DEFINING JOB SATISFACTION

Job satisfaction is a complex concept that has been conceptualized differently, but pragmatically it is how content people are regarding their job and the tasks that comprise that position. Most refer to this assessment of one's job as "job satisfaction" but it can also be referred to as employee satisfaction. Spector[4,9] describes the construct as "the extent to which people like (satisfaction) or dislike (dissatisfaction) their jobs." Within organizational research, Locke's widely used definition is, "a pleasurable or positive emotional state resulting from the appraisal of one's job or experiences."[10(p1304)] Lawler[11] suggests that job satisfaction is the actualization between an employee's needs and feelings that should encompass a job and what actually is provided to him or her. In the end, job satisfaction is a blend of an employee's expectations, values, and attitudes.

Although it is believed that the term is simplistic, many facets comprise the construct of job satisfaction, and often the individuality of each employee can greatly influence the assessment of job satisfaction. This construct can be viewed globally, which indicates an overall assessment of and reaction to one's job. It also can be measured by varying facets or dimensions that traditionally include pay, rewards, co-workers, nature of the job, and job conditions.[4,9] A facet can be articulated as a portion of the job that can produce feelings of satisfaction or dissatisfaction.[4] Debate exists as to whether job satisfaction is evaluated globally or at the facet level. Spector[4] suggests there are 9 components whereby an employee evaluates their job (Table 8-1).

Job satisfaction (Figure 8-1) is also viewed as an attitude an employee has toward his or her organization. Hulin and Judge[12] suggest that job satisfaction is multidimensional and is the psychological response to a person's job. The response can be viewed as cognitive (evaluative), affective (emotional), and behavioral. The evaluative component of their theory addresses an individual's overall employee satisfaction and is often viewed as "How satisfied are you with your job?" The affective component is the emotional response evoked by one's job such as pleasure, stress, anger, or joy. The behavioral component relates to one's goals and aspirations and how they can align with one's current position.

MODELS OF SATISFACTION

Several theories or models have emerged to explain how one evaluates the level of satisfaction with their job. The most popular is *Locke's Range of Affect Theory*, which articulates that a discrepancy can manifest between an individual's wants and what one actually has in a job.[10] The value one places of the facets of the job, as described by Spector,[4] can positively or negatively affect that person's assessment. For example, if athletic trainers value autonomy in the workplace, and are provided that in their position, they will be more likely to be satisfied with their job.

The *dispositional approach*, detailed by Staw and peers,[13] illustrates individuality in desires and wants in a job. That is, satisfaction is a product of a person's personality traits. The theory has

TABLE 8-1	
JOB SATISFACTION FACETS[4]	
FACET	**DESCRIPTION**
Pay	The financial compensation associated with the job. It can include salary and pay raises.
Promotion	The chance for personal growth, more responsibilities, and increased social status.
Supervision	An employee's direct supervisor and the communication and relationship between the 2.
Fringe benefits	Non-monetary and monetary benefits associated with the job such as health insurance and time off.
Contingent rewards	Include recognition, appreciation, and rewards for good work.
Operating conditions	The policies and procedures associated with the organization, structural hierarchy, and other aspects of the workplace.
Co-Workers	Individuals whom the employee works with and the relationship and culture created within the workplace.
Nature of the work	The responsibilities and expectations related to the person's role/job in the organization.
Communication	Includes formation of goals, feedback on goal achievement, and performance within the role.

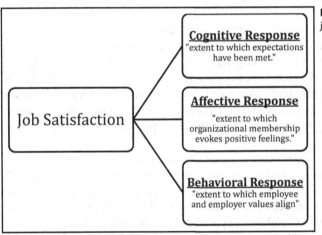

Figure 8-1. The multidimensional aspects of job satisfaction.

gained much support as a means to explain varying levels of satisfaction among different employees, as links have been documented between trait taxonomies (neuroticism, extroversion) and job satisfaction. Specifically, those who demonstrate a negative affectivity (negative emotions—anger, nervousness, etc, or a predisposition to be predominately negative or unhappy)[14] are more likely to experience more job-related stress and will be dissatisfied[15] quickly and more often. Neuroticism, a personality trait that is associated with anger and other irrational responses, has been negatively related to job satisfaction. Conversely, those who display a positive affectivity (positive emotions—energetic, confident, active, etc, or a predisposition to be predominately positive or happy) will

TABLE 8-2

CORE JOB CHARACTERISTICS[20]

CORE CHARACTERISTICS	DESCRIPTOR
Skill variety	The degree to which a job requires various skills and allows the employee to become multi-faceted within his or her role.
Task identity	The degree to which the job allows the worker to become a stakeholder in the job. The tasks that are meaningful to the employees help them develop an identity.
Task significance	The degree to which the job can affect others' lives. It is the reach that the role can have beyond the individual and the organization.
Autonomy	The degree to which the job allows for independence, critical thinking, and discretion to plan and carry out job responsibilities.
Feedback	The degree to which the employee is provided with consistent, clear, detailed, and effective feedback on job performance.

have a greater level of satisfaction with their jobs;[16] mostly due to a positive outlook on life and greater coping resources.[17] Extroversion, similar to positive affectivity,[14] is a trait quantified as energetic and outgoing and can be viewed as how one gains energy or is recharged from being social and assertive.[15] The idea of locus of control, another personality factor, has also tentatively been linked to job satisfaction; that is, those who have a greater internal locus of control are likely to be more satisfied.[16]

The *2-factor theory* depicts job satisfaction as a dichotomous construct that is driven by motivation and hygiene, or simply intrinsic motivation of a person and the aspects of the workplace that define it.[18] Individuals can be seen as inherently motivated, but beyond that they have factors that can influence drive and motivation to achieve personal and professional goals.[19] On-the-job motivators can include professional goals, recognition, and promotion opportunities, and they are thought to be internally motivating. Hygiene factors are related to working conditions and other job facets such as pay, policies and procedures outlined by the employer, and supervisory practices within the organization.[19]

The *job characteristics model* focuses on 5 core job characteristics that can affect one's view of his or her job.[19] Skill variety, task identity, task significance, autonomy, and feedback (Table 8-2) are the characteristics that affect work outcomes such as satisfaction and motivation in the workplace. These core job characteristics as developed by Hackman and Oldham should then stimulate 3 psychological states: experienced meaningfulness, experienced responsibility, and knowledge of results (Table 8-3). The relationship forged between characteristics and psychological states creates contextual satisfaction for one's job.

MEASUREMENTS OF JOB SATISFACTION

Measurements of job satisfaction are self-reporting scales by which an individual assesses their own affective and cognitive levels of satisfaction.[20] Much speculation exists on the instrument that provides the most reliable or valid tool, thus a "gold-standard" instrument has not been used

TABLE 8-3	
CRITICAL PSYCHOLOGICAL STATES	
PSYCHOLOGICAL STATES	**DESCRIPTOR**
Experienced meaningfulness	The intrinsical meaningfulness of the job as perceived by the employee and how the value transcends to the organization.
Experienced responsibility for outcome of the work	The accountability and responsibility held by the employees as it pertains to their work.
Knowledge of the results of the work activities	The understanding the employee has regarding job performance and task completion.

across all disciplines and by researchers. Instruments used in previous literature have included global measurements, single-item scales, and specific tools that are trade or profession dependent (ie, the nursing satisfaction scale or emergency physician job satisfaction scale). Several scales do exist to measure job satisfaction; however, within athletic training only 3 scales have been used to measure the construct. Each is presented next.

The *Job Satisfaction Survey (JSS)* is one of the most widely used tools. First developed for the social service sector, the instrument has been modified across professions including athletic training. The multidimensional scale included 9 subscales based on Spector's[21] work: salary (pay), promotion, supervision, fringe benefits, contingent rewards, operating procedures, nature of work, co-workers, and communication. Responses are on a 6-point Likert scale from "disagree very much" (1) to "agree very much." In total, the JSS is a 36-question instrument that demonstrates strong reliability and validity (α.91).[20] The scale has been used in several athletic training research studies examining job satisfaction.[6,21]

The *Job Descriptive Index (JDI)*[22] measures cognitive job satisfaction specific to 5 facets: *pay, promotions and promotion opportunities, coworkers, supervisor,* and *the job itself.* The questions are scaled by "yes" or "no" responses regarding one's job. Respondents are provided various short-term phrases or words that describe the aforementioned facets (ie, co-workers—stimulating, boring, slow, helpful). The responses are tallied and an overall score is derived. The scale has been modified and modernized twice since its initial development in 1969 by Smith and colleagues. The JDI, like the JSS, has been shown to be valid and reliable ($\alpha = .88$ to .91).

The *Minnesota Satisfaction Questionnaire (MSQ)*[9] is a robust measurement of an employee satisfaction with their job. The instrument measures satisfaction across 20 different dimensions using both a long and short version of the instrument. The 100-item, self-report instrument has 5 questions per each dimension, where the 20-item survey has 1 question per dimension. The dimensions include: *ability utilization* (ability to use skill sets), *achievement* (feelings of accomplishment), *activity* (ability to stay busy), *advancement* (chance to move up), *authority* (direct others), *company* (company policies), *compensation* (pay), *coworkers* (relationships with peers), *creativity* (chance to try out own ideas), *independence* (work alone), *moral values* (not having to violate conscience), *recognition* (praise received), *responsibility* (freedom to use judgment), *security* (stability of job), *social service* (to do things for others), *social status* (chance to be 'somebody'), *supervision* (human resources), *supervision* (supervisor managerial style), *variety* (change to do different things), *and working conditions* (work environment).

JOB SATISFACTION AND VOLUNTARY TURNOVER

Conventional belief has been that job satisfaction is a driving force in employee voluntary turn-over (henceforth "turnover"), that leaving a dissatisfying job is the most traditional path to depar-ture. Early turnover models supported this; however, recent turnover research has challenged this belief. In the late 1970s, the job satisfaction determinant of Price's[23] causal model of turnover contained several job-structure variables, including pay, promotional chances, distributive justice, social support, job stress (role ambiguity, overload, and conflict), autonomy, and routinization. In 2000, meta-analytic research on this model found all these variables were directly related to job satisfaction, except for pay.[24] Also in 2000, Griffeth and colleagues[25] published the most recent meta-analysis on turnover predictors and found that overall job satisfaction is one of the most con-sistent predictors of individual turnover decisions. However, this study and other recent research have shown that quit intentions, job search, weighted application blanks, organizational commit-ment, supervisor relationships, role clarity, and tenure are stronger predictors of turnover than job satisfaction. In fact, recent retention research[26] suggests that job satisfaction explains less than half of the variation in individual departure decisions.

The consensus in turnover research is there are multiple paths to departure from a job or a profession.[26,27] The decision to quit may or may not involve job satisfaction, because many dis-satisfied employees stay, and many satisfied employees leave. New turnover research by Maertz and colleagues[28] even suggests the actual motives that cause employees to leave a job may be different from the reason(s) they provide, both to themselves and to others; the real reason emerges after the decision to quit has been made. Some newer turnover models still include job satisfaction, but also introduce other important variables. According to Lee and Mitchell's[29] unfolding model of turnover, which has a job satisfaction component, many individuals who are very satisfied in their current position will quit if they are offered a more attractive alternative, if their spouse's job requires that the family relocate, or if they experience a negative "shock" (eg, an immediate family member becomes very ill).

Turnover research involving job satisfaction is trending toward investigations of "overall job attitude" (a combination of job satisfaction and organizational commitment) and changes in job satisfaction over time.[27] Although overall job satisfaction has been a consistent predictor of turn-over, one should consider multiple predictors when evaluating retention, turnover and attrition of employees. For a more robust discussion on retention, turnover, and attrition in athletic training, refer to Chapter 9.

JOB SATISFACTION AND HEALTH CARE

Job satisfaction has become a central focus within health care organizations, simply because job satisfaction has direct implications on the care provided to a patient and documented patient outcomes. Job satisfaction concerns can affect all professionals working in the health care industry, including physicians and nurses. In a 2011 study, McHugh[30] reported that patient satisfaction was correlated to nurses' satisfaction with their jobs and working conditions. Beyond patient care, it is well understood that when health care workers are satisfied with their job, they are more vested, committed, and less likely to consider leaving their position.[31] Productivity in the workplace, how-ever, is likely the most important factor stimulating continuous investigations of job satisfaction among health care workers.

Nursing literature is robust regarding job satisfaction. Factors influencing nursing satisfaction can be multifactorial and often includes working relationships with supervisors, coworkers, and physicians.[32,33] Cohesion is often a positive mediating factor for satisfaction in the workplace for the nurse along with collaboration and professionalism between the medical staff.[33] Other

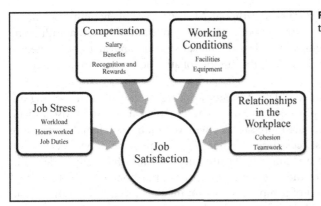

Figure 8-2. Factors influencing job satisfaction.

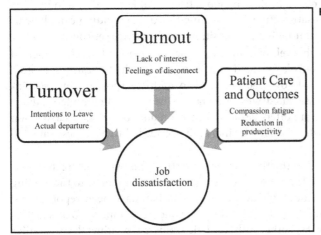

Figure 8-3. Impact of job dissatisfaction.

contributing factors in nursing satisfaction include working conditions,[33] the work itself (workload, requirements, etc), salary, promotion, and job security[34-36] (Figure 8-2).

Within the nursing profession, the greatest impact of job dissatisfaction can be found with intentions to stay, and as previously mentioned the level of care provided to the nurses' patients (Figure 8-3).[37] Burnout has also been found to be present as the experience of job dissatisfaction grows.[38,39] Outcomes of job dissatisfaction have also been reported and often include those previously mentioned, such as turnover, absenteeism, low morale, increased stress, and in some cases work-family conflict. The impact of job dissatisfaction is often comparable to other consequences of the workplace including burnout, work-life conflict, and professional commitment.

Whereas job satisfaction seems to be concerning within the nursing field, some evidence suggests that physicians are overall satisfied with their careers in medicine. In fact Leigh and peers[40] report that 70% of all physicians are happy or satisfied with their positions. One plausible explanation for this is the relationship between job autonomy and decision making, whereby increased levels of control increases overall assessments of job satisfaction; thus for physicians who are often in control of patient loads and decision making, they view their positions favorably.[33]

JOB SATISFACTION AND ATHLETIC TRAINING

Studies investigating job satisfaction within athletic training have grown over the last decade. The growth has been stimulated with growing concern about membership statistics and the decline of athletic trainers over the last few years. Although the causes are likely multifaceted, job satisfaction has often been a primary discussion point. It is also important to note that unlike the nursing literature, which is robust, studies investigating job satisfaction appear to be limited to the collegiate practice setting. The culprit is likely the number of athletic trainers employed in the setting as compared to others.

Brumels and Beach[41] found that most athletic trainers working in the collegiate setting are satisfied with their positions. Demographically speaking, male athletic trainers and those athletic trainers with a greater level of experience are more satisfied with their jobs than females and those with less experience[42] Mixed data exist regarding whether job type mediates experiences of job satisfaction; some report that program directors and faculty members may have greater levels in comparison to assistant athletic trainers and others in more clinical positions.[6,42] Terranova and Henning[6] suggest that job type and level of competition do not mediate levels of job satisfaction. Deficient from the literature, and a possible explanation to the conflicting data, is the idea of personality and one's mindset when it comes to evaluating job satisfaction. Personality and outlook can play a role in the assessment of job satisfaction, thus having this understanding can allow us to understand why individuals select certain job types, positions, and practice settings.

Athletic trainers are susceptible to high levels of job stress; in fact Brumels and Beach[41] reported that 38% report high levels of stress from role overload. Role overload in athletic training is often stimulated by long hours, travel, medical coverage provided to multiple sports/teams, administrative tasks, and supervisory roles associated with graduate assistants and/or undergraduate students.[6,43,44] Increased levels of stress are often associated with a reduction in one's satisfaction with the job, thus it makes sense that when athletic trainers are overloaded they are less satisfied with their job.[41]

The impact of job dissatisfaction within athletic training is mostly unknown. The greatest connection has been made with intentions to leave the profession,[6] which is comparable to the nursing field. Although job satisfaction, like burnout and work-family conflict, have been reported and linked to intention to leave in athletic training,[3] little is known beyond what impact job dissatisfaction has on patient care or productivity. Hypothetically, athletic trainers are vulnerable to similar outcomes such as compassion fatigue and turnover like nurses because of job dissatisfaction, but direct connections have yet to be made, empirically.

IMPROVING JOB SATISFACTION

Working can be stressful, and when the job grows due to a myriad of factors, job satisfaction can be negatively affected. It is important to recognize that job satisfaction can be improved at both the individual and organizational level. As previously discussed within the chapter, personality plays a critical role in how one perceives one's own level of job satisfaction. So, the approach in which an individual takes toward his or her job can help change their evaluation of it. For example, if you value pay and benefits, it is important to find a job that allows for adequate compensation for the work performed. If one perceives a job as a life-long career, he or she will want the chance to grow within the organization, having a chance to "climb" the ranks of hierarchy. Or, if one believes the job is a calling, then he or she may be more concerned with work tasks, and less on the financial rewards or benefits. Individuals should be aware of what aspects they value most when searching for a job and organization that shares similar values and expectations. A positive attitude can also help improve assessment of one's job. Positive affectivity can allow an employee to manage and cope with stress and work expectations without adverse effect. Goal setting can also help employees remain satisfied with their jobs and careers, as they can reflect on their achievements and stay challenged while reaching those goals.

Creating job enrichment is one way supervisors and organizations can improve job satisfaction for their employees. Job enrichment can be simply created, as it is founded on allowing more control over decision making and work completion as well as being provided with feedback on job performance. In athletic training, supervising athletic trainers can rotate jobs, such as morning treatments, weekend coverage for off-season sport practices or competitions, and more monotonous or tedious tasks (ie, inventory and cleaning). Frequency of feedback and communication can also help create job enrichment. Take the chance to acknowledge hard work informally during staff meetings, but also take the time to formally provide constructive and positive feedback for role growth and increased productivity. Allowing for autonomy and participative management can improve job morale and enrich an athletic trainer's satisfaction with his or her job. For example, allowing trainers to manage certain aspects of their role (treatment schedules, injury managements, work schedules, etc) can improve their commitment and satisfaction, as they feel like they are a part of the process and invested in the mission and goals of the sports medicine team. Reflecting back on Hackman and Oldham's 5 factors of job design that promote job satisfaction, supervisors should try to provide *skill variety* (promote growth and use of skills—creativity and skill growth), *task identity* (allow for job completion and full understanding role and expectations), *tasks significance* (provide opportunity for meaningful work), *autonomy* (increase chances for decision making), and *feedback* (increase the frequency of formal feedback). We provide athletic training-specific examples in Table 8-4. Many workplace strategies exists; we present more examples in Table 8-5. It is important to remember employee needs, such as having clear objectives and job descriptions, allowing them to be a part of the team and being valued, as well as being allowed to grow within their position.

SUMMARY

Job satisfaction is an important aspect to helping promote career commitment and professional enthusiasm. The topic is well understood in health care, but is still in its infancy in terms of full consideration in athletic training. The concept is multidimensional, whereby many factors appear to influence a person's assessment of his or her job. Many parallels can be drawn from the literature within other professions that suggest satisfaction is cultivated when individuals can work independently, make decisions that affect the well-being of their patients as well as their schedules, and are provided feedback related to their performance.

ACTIVITIES FOR REINFORCEMENT

Questions for Review

1. How is job satisfaction defined?
2. What factors affect job satisfaction?
3. What are the primary causes of job dissatisfaction?
4. What are examples of cognitive, affective and behavioral responses to job satisfaction?
5. What are the core job characteristics that lead to job satisfaction?

TABLE 8-4		
HACKMAN AND OLDHAM'S[18] TIPS FOR IMPROVED JOB SATISFACTION		
JOB FACTOR	**DESCRIPTOR**	**EXAMPLE**
Skill variety	Increase number of skills used while working	Support attendance of a workshop designed to increase knowledge and skill for use of kinesio-taping.
Task identity	Enabling people to perform a job from start to finish. Providing clear expectations and job details.	Provide initial, realistic job previews and socialization tactics for new employees. Evaluate and update/clarify job descriptions with employees annually.
Task significance	Providing work that has a direct impact on the organization or stakeholders of the organization.	Use patient outcomes to highlight to administrators the impact the athletic trainer has on the success of the organization.
Autonomy	Increasing the degree of decision making, the freedom and independence to choose how and when work is done.	Advocate to administrators that athletic trainers be considered and consulted when events that need medical coverage are scheduled. Allow athletic trainers to create a schedule that satisfies personal goals and gets the job done.
Feedback	Increasing the amount of recognition for doing a job well. Communication of constructive and positive feedback for role development and growth.	Announce accomplishments, positive patient outcomes, and milestone years of service in administrative meetings, newsletters and alumni pages. Provide clear, constructive, and *consistent* feedback to athletic training staff members.

Case Vignettes

Case #1

Ben is in his third year of his assistant athletic training position at a mid-major university. During his first year, Ben was working with the women's soccer team, crew, and tennis. He continued working with all 3 teams until the return of his third season, in which he was switched to men's ice hockey and track and field. His head athletic trainer made the change without his input, and he was given very little information on the change in sport assignments. Although his hours worked are unchanged, the nature of his work and coaching staff interactions are much different. He has noticed over the last 2 months since the change that he is less positive in the workplace, and often is quick to be upset; something that was not like him last year. His relationships with the previous teams were upbeat and energetic. The team dynamics this year with his new teams are different, and the coaching staff for hockey is more demanding and at times more abrasive.

1. What factors seem to have led to Ben's reduction in job satisfaction?

2. If you were Ben's supervisor, how would you have approached the change in sport coverage?

TABLE 8-5	
STRATEGIES TO IMPROVE JOB SATISFACTION	
STRATEGY	**DESCRIPTION**
Recognize and reward employees	Achievement and recognition are high motivators for employees. It can be the small things, such as an afternoon off, saying "thank you," or providing them a free lunch.
Autonomy and decision making	Allow employees to make decisions regarding work schedules or management of their responsibilities. Supervisors should minimize micro-management tendencies, as this can suppress creativity and "flexing" of the brain and skills.
Stakeholder mentality	Ask employees for their opinions and input, regarding policy development, staffing decisions, or other important aspects related to working conditions. Key is listening and respecting input.
Career development and continuing education	Offer and provide employees the chance for skill development and advancement of skills. This can be done with support for continuing education and attendance of workshops, etc. An employee who feels supported will be more productive and feel vested.
Communication	This includes feedback on performance and expectations of their role. Be transparent with expectations. Clearly communicate feedback and expectations, and feedback should be timely.
Mentoring	Can help provide support networks within the workplace, which allows for greater dialogue and rapport among peers and coworkers, a necessary facet of job satisfaction.
Cohesion and teamwork	Supervisors and employees should embrace teamwork and collegiality in the workplace. Supervisors should be creative and tolerant of employees' needs and requests, but also provide structure and consistency with policy development and adherence to them.

3. What recommendations can you give Ben to help improve his overall job satisfaction?

4. Based on the information provided, what factors does Ben value in his job?

Case #2

Kennedy worked for the last 5 years at the collegiate practice setting, working with the women's basketball team. She loved her job, but when her husband's job was relocated to a new region, she decided to take a new position with a local clinic with outreach to a high school. Although she had previous experience in the setting as a graduate student, she hasn't worked in the setting in 7 years. The high school setting is rewarding for Kennedy as she loves the interactions with the student-athletes, but she rarely sees any other athletic trainers or health care professionals, something she loved about her previous job. She has been in her job for 6 months now and was supposed to have a 3-month review, but that didn't happen because of schedule conflicts and the hustle and bustle of the fall season and the holidays. She feels as though she is making good inroads with her position and developing strong relationships with the athletic director, coaching staff, and parents when she interacts with them. Kennedy, however, feels as though she isn't as happy with her position, despite a pay raise and working on average 5 to 8 hours less per week. Over the last few weeks, she has been feeling slightly unmotivated, but still goes to work with a positive outlook.

1. What factors appear to influence Kennedy's assessment of her job satisfaction?
2. What, if any signs, of dissatisfaction does Kennedy display?
3. If you were Kennedy, what changes could you make to improve your level of job satisfaction?
4. What aspects of the job does Kennedy value, and based on that could she make a full commitment to her new job?

Discussion Questions

1. If you were an employer of athletic trainers, what steps would you take to create a work environment that promoted job satisfaction?
2. Consider a time when you were not satisfied with your employment. What steps did you take as an employee to cope and make your work more satisfying?
3. Think of the roles of an athletic trainer. How might a supervisor attempt to develop specific job skills to promote job satisfaction? Give a specific example.

REFERENCES

1. Mobley WH, Horner SO, Hollingsworth AT. An evaluation of precursors of hospital employee turnover. *J Appl Psychol.* 1978 63(4):408-14.
2. Kahnov L, Eberman LE. Age, sex, and setting factors and labor force in athletic training. *J Athl Train.* 2011;46(4):424-430.
3. Mazerolle SM, Bruening JE, Casa DJ, Burton LJ. Work-family conflict, part II: job and life satisfaction in National Collegiate Athletic Association Division I-A certified athletic trainers. *J Athl Train.* 2008;43(5):513-522.
4. Spector PE. *Job Satisfaction: Application, Assessment, Causes, and Consequences.* United Kingdom: Sage Publications; 1997.
5. Weiss HM. Deconstructing job satisfaction: separating evaluations, believes and affective experiences. *Human Res Manag Rev.* 2002;12:173-194.
6. Terranova AB, Henning JM. National Collegiate Athletic Association Division and primary job titled of athletic trainers and their job satisfaction or intention to leave athletic training. *J Athl Train.* 2011;46(3):312-318.
7. Mensch JM, Wham G. It's a quality-of-life issue. *Athl Ther Today.* 2005;10(1):34-35.
8. Coomber B, Barriball KL. Impact of job satisfaction components on intent to leave and turnover for hospital-based nurses: a review of the research literature. *Int J Nurs Stud.* 2007;44(2):297-314.
9. Spector PE. Measurement of human service staff satisfaction: development of the job satisfaction survey. *Am J Community Psych.* 1985;13(6), 693-713.
10. Locke EA. The nature and causes of job satisfaction. In: Dunnette MD, ed. *Handbook of Industrial and Organizational Psychology.* Chicago, IL: Rand McNally; 1976:1297-1349.
11. Lawler EE. *Motivation in Work Organizations.* Monterey: CA, Brooks/Cole; 1973.
12. Hulin CL, Judge TA. Job attitudes. In: WC Borman, Ligen DR, Klimoski RJ, eds. *Handbook of Psychology: Industrial and Organizational Psychology.* Hoboken, NJ: Wiley; 2003:255-276.
13. Staw, BM, Bell NE, Clausen JA. The dispositional approach to job attitudes: A lifetime longitudinal test. *Admin Science Q.* 1986;31, 56-77.
14. Heller D, Judge TA, Watson D. The confounding role of personality and trait affectivity in the relationship between job and life satisfaction. *J Organiz Behav.* 2002;23:815-835.
15. Judge TA, Heller D, Mount MK. Five-factor model of personality and job satisfaction: a meta-analysis. *J Applied Psych.* 2002;87(3):530-541.
16. Bruk-Lee V, Khoury HA, Nixon AE, Goh A, Spector PE. Replicating and extending past personality/job satisfaction meta-analyses. *Hum Perform.* 2009;22(2):156-189.
17. Brief AP, Weiss HM. Organizational behavior: affect in the workplace. *Annual Rev Psych.* 2002;53:279-307.
18. Hackman JR, Oldham GR. Motivation through design of work. *Organiz Behav Human Perform.* 1976;16(2):250-279.
19. Aristovnik A, Jaklic K. Job satisfaction of older workers as a factor of promoting labour market participation in the EU: the case of Slovenia. *Rev So Polit.* 2013;20(2):123-148.
20. van Saane V, Sluiter JK, Verbeek JH, Frings-Dresen MH. Reliability and validity of instruments measuring job satisfaction: a systematic review. *Occup Med (Lond).* 2003;53(3):191-200.

21. Spector PE. Measurement of human service staff satisfaction: development of the job satisfaction survey. *Am J Community Psychol.* 1985;13(6):693-713.

22. Smith PC, Kendall LM, Hulin CL. *The Measurement of Satisfaction in Work and Retirement.* Chicago: Rand McNally; 1969.

23. Price JL. *The Study of Turnover.* Ames, IA: Iowa State University Press; 1977.

24. Gaertner S. Structural determinants of job satisfaction and organizational commitment in turnover models. *Human Res Manag Rev.* 2000;9(4):479-493.

25. Griffeth RW, Hom PW, Gaertner S. A meta-analysis of antecedents and correlates of employee turnover: update, moderator tests, and research implications for the next millennium. *J Manag.* 2000;26:463-488.

26. Allen DG, Bryant P. *Managing Employee Turnover: Dispelling Myths and Fostering Evidence-Based Retention Strategies.* New York: Business Expert Press; 2012.

27. Holtom BC, Mitchell TR, Lee TW, Eberly MB. Turnover and retention research. *Acad Manag Ann.* 2008;2(1):231-274.

28. Maertz CP, Griffeth RW. Eight motivational forces and voluntary turnover: a theoretical synthesis with implications for research. *J Manag.* 2004;30:667-683.

29. Lee TW, Mitchell TR. An alternative approach: the unfolding model of voluntary employee turnover. *Acad Manag Rev.* 1994;19:51-89.

30. McHugh MD, Kutney-Lee A, Cimiotti JP, Sloane DM, Aiken LH. Nurses' widespread job dissatisfaction, burnout, and frustration with health benefits signal problems for patient care. *Health Aff.* 2011;30(2):202-210.

31. Ramoo V, Abdullah KL, Piaw CY. The relationship between job satisfaction and intention to leave current employment among registered nurses in a teaching hospital. *J Clin Nurs.* 2013;22(21-22):3141-3152.

32. Adams A, Bond S. Hospital nurses' job satisfaction, individual and organizational characteristics. *J Adv Nurs.* 2000;32(3):536-543.

33. Tovey E, Adams A., The changing nature of nurses' job satisfaction: an exploration of sources of satisfaction in the 1990s. *J Adv Nurs.* 1999;30(1):150-158.

34. Price M. Job satisfaction of registered nurses working in an acute hospital. *Br J Nurs.* 2002;11(4):275-280.

35. Nolan M, Nolan J, Grant G. Maintaining nurses' job satisfaction and morale. *Br J Nurs.* 1995;4(19):1148-1154.

36. Nolan M, Brown J, Naughton M, Nolan J. Developing nursing's future role 2: nurses' job satisfaction and morale. *Br J Nurs.* 1998;7(17):1044-1048.

37. Lee H, Song R, Cho YS, Lee GZ, Daly B. A comprehensive model for predicting burnout in Korean nurses. *J Adv Nurs.* 2003;44(5):534-545.

38. Tzeng HM. The influence of nurses' working motivation and job satisfaction on intention to quit: an empirical investigation in Taiwan. *Int J Nurs Stud.* 2002;39(8):867-878.

39. Tzeng HM. Satisfying nurses on job factors they care about: a Taiwanese perspective. *J Nurs Admin.* 2002;32(6):306-309.

40. Leigh JP, Kravitz RL, Schembri M, Samuels SJ, Mobley S. Physician career satisfaction across specialties. *Arch Intern Med.* 2002;162:1577-1584.

41. Brumels K, Beach A. Professional role complexity and job satisfaction of collegiate certified athletic trainers. *J Athl Train.* 2008;43(4):373-378.

42. Herrera R, Lim JY. Job satisfaction among athletic trainers in NCAA Division I-AA institutions. *Sport J.* 2003;6(1).

43. Henning JM, Weidner TG. Role strain in collegiate athletic training approved clinical instructors. *J Athl Train.* 2008;43(3):275-283.

44. Mazerolle SM, Bruening JE, Casa DJ. Work family conflict, part I: antecedents of work family conflict in National Collegiate Athletic Association Division I-A certified athletic trainers. *J Athl Train.* 2008;43(5):505-512.

9

Retention, Turnover, and Attrition in Athletic Training

Ashley Goodman, PhD, LAT, ATC

OBJECTIVES

After reading this chapter, the reader will be able to do the following:
1. Define retention, turnover, and attrition in the workplace.
2. Explain why retention, turnover, and attrition matter in the workplace.
3. Understand the advancement of retention and turnover research, and process models.
4. Identify evidence-based antecedents and consequences of employee turnover.
5. Compare retention, turnover, and attrition within the healthcare industry and the athletic training profession.
6. Develop an effective retention management plan.
7. Identify evidence-based retention strategies and best practices to reduce avoidable and undesirable turnover and attrition.

INTRODUCTION

Athletic trainer retention, turnover, and attrition issues have received increased attention in recent years. These issues have been discussed and researched at many levels, including organizational, setting, employer, and individual levels. The retention of high-quality athletic trainers is an important employment issue for organizations. Understanding why athletic trainers stay in and why they leave certain positions, settings or the profession has important implications for athletic training organizations, as well as the growth of the profession. The purpose of this chapter is to bridge research with evidence-based employee retention strategies to assist athletic trainers and employers with managing retention, turnover, and attrition in the workplace.

Mazerolle SM, Pitney WA.
Workplace Concepts for Athletic Trainers (pp 137-163).
© 2016 Taylor & Francis Group.

DEFINING RETENTION, TURNOVER, AND ATTRITION IN THE WORKPLACE

Retention in the workplace, simply, refers to an organization's ability to keep its employees. Retention rate is the percentage of employees who remain with an organization during a period of time. Terms such as retention, persistence, and perseverance have been used interchangeably in athletic training literature; however, this chapter will use the organizational term *retention* to discuss why athletic trainers stay. The retention rate is used to track particular employees over a particular period of time and is not affected by subsequent employee hires. Although calculating retention rate is useful, it does not track employees who joined and subsequently left during this period of time. Retention research in the workplace examines why employees stay with a particular organization, setting or profession, which can be quite useful to an organization's retention and turnover management strategies.

The terms *turnover* and *attrition* have been interchanged within the literature. Although these terms are similar, they are, in fact, different. The difference involves employee replacement. Turnover is the movement of employees across an organization or organizational setting.[1] Departure is other term that has been used to describe this movement, although turnover has been the preferred term in organizational and socioeconomic research. Another way to view turnover is the rate at which an employer gains and loses employees (eg, an employee resigns and a new employee is hired to replace him or her). Refer to Figure 9-1 for how to calculate retention and turnover rates.

Attrition is a reduction in the number of employees due to voluntary or involuntary reasons; however, the employee is not replaced. These positions remain unfilled or are eliminated. In the professional athletic training context, the term *setting-changer* has been used to describe turnover in professional settings (eg, an athletic trainer who leaves the collegiate setting for a more "family-friendly" work environment in the hospital/clinic setting). Attrition has been used to describe employees who leave the athletic training profession entirely.[2] Their departure may or may not include a lapse or expiration of their certification and/or state licensure.

DEFINING TERMS

Retention is referred to as an organization's ability keep its employees. *Turnover* is the movement of employees across an organization or setting. *Attrition* is the reduction or removal of employees within an organization, and the employee is not replaced.

Employees leave positions, organizations, settings, and entire professions for many reasons. Hence, there are several types of employee turnover highlighted in the literature[3-5] (refer to Figure 9-2).

One of the most important distinctions is that turnover can be *voluntary* or *involuntary*. Voluntary turnover (eg, quits, leaving for another job) is initiated by the employee. Involuntary turnover (eg, firings for poor performance, layoffs, organizational restructuring) is initiated by the organization. Voluntary and involuntary turnover have different organizational outcomes and require very different management techniques.[3,4] The majority of turnover research has focused on voluntary turnover, and this chapter also focuses on voluntary turnover.

Voluntary turnover, henceforth, called *turnover*, is divided into *functional* and *dysfunctional*.[5] Dysfunctional turnover can take on many forms and is detrimental to an organization. Examples include 1) departure of high-performing employees, 2) departure of minority employees, affecting workforce diversity, and 3) high turnover rates that lead to high replacement costs. Functional

$$Retention\ Rate\ =\ \frac{Number\ of\ employees\ at\ the\ beginning\ of\ a\ period}{Number\ of\ employees\ who\ remain\ during\ that\ period} \times 100$$

$$Turnover\ Rate\ =\ \frac{Average\ number\ of\ employees}{Number\ of\ employees\ leaving} \times 100$$

Figure 9-1. How to calculate retention and turnover rates.

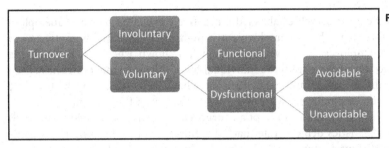

Figure 9-2. Types of turnover.[5]

turnover, by contrast, is not detrimental to an organization and may even be helpful. For instance, the departure of employees whose skills or talents are easily replaceable may not be detrimental to an organization. The departure of poor-performing employees who are replaced with better-performing employees may improve organizational performance and efficiency. Allen[3] makes an important point about this division of turnover: "This distinction between functional and dysfunctional turnover is relative. What makes an employee valuable and difficult to replace will vary by job, organization, industry, and other factors."(p3)

Dysfunctional turnover is divided into *avoidable* or *unavoidable*.[5] Avoidable turnover is created from causes an organization may be able to influence (eg, employee departures due to low job satisfaction or low wages/benefits). Unavoidable turnover is created from causes over which an organization has little or no control. Examples include employees leaving because 1) their spouse's job causes the family to relocate, 2) unforeseen health problems, either personal or familial, arise, or 3) they desire to return to school or become a stay-at-home parent. It is important for an organization to attempt to distinguish between avoidable and unavoidable turnover, although this can be a difficult, blurred line. It is likely fruitless for an organization to invest huge efforts in reducing turnover that stems from unavoidable reasons. However, departure situations that may be seen as unavoidable to some could be seen as avoidable to others. For instance, an organization has no control over whether an employee decides to start a family, or if an employee's immediate family member falls ill. However, administration can choose to offer paid maternity/paternity leave, on-site child care, or paid family leave to assist the employee and entice him or her to stay.[3] Understanding the definitions of retention, turnover, and attrition is important to understanding why these terms matter in the athletic training workplace.

WHY DO RETENTION, TURNOVER, AND ATTRITION MATTER IN THE WORKPLACE?

Recruiting and retaining high-quality employees, while effectively managing voluntary turnover, is a critical component of an organization's performance and success. Emerging trends such as globalization, the increase in work knowledge, and the accelerating rate of advanced technology, among others, have made it vital for employers to acquire and retain quality human capital.[4] Holtom and colleagues[4] may have said it best in their recent review of retention and voluntary turnover research by stating, "... the topic of voluntary turnover is a vital bridge between macro strategies and micro behavior in organizations. It is the one variable that conceptually connects the experiences of individuals in organizations to critical measures of success for those organizations."[(p232)] Human resource organizations and sound research have shown that retention and turnover management does matter for 3 key reasons: 1) high turnover is costly, 2) high turnover affects organizational performance, and 3) retention and turnover may become increasingly difficult to manage.[3-5] These key reasons will be discussed later in further detail in the "Consequences of Turnover" section.

Traditional thought and early research established a negative correlation between unemployment rates and turnover rates (eg, when unemployment is high, people are highly motivated to remain with their current employer).[3,4] However, research has shown when you examine the decision-making process to stay or leave from the individual-level, unemployment rates have little to no effect on turnover, and even high unemployment rates have little impact on the turnover of top-performing employees, or employees with in-demand talents.[6] In the previous section we learned there are several types of turnover and not all turnover is equal. The United States (US) Bureau of Labor's turnover statistics demonstrate that different types of professions and organizations face very different turnover rates.[7] For instance, the 2013 annual quit rate (ie, voluntary separations by employees, excluding retirement) for the health care and social assistance industry was 18%, compared to 11.9% for educational services, and 28.5% for professional and business services. Turnover is a complex process that involves much more than just labor market conditions. For example, in a 2003 study, researchers found that 30% to 40% of market value can be attributed to intangible factors (execution of strategies, managerial credibility and experience, attracting and retaining the best talent, compensation strategies, etc).[8] Furthermore, one must consider the implications on the individual leaving a job, such as the energy used to find a new job, and to adjust, both personally and professionally. Therefore, understanding retention and turnover is important not only to researchers, managers and organizations, and professional associations, but also to individuals as well.

From a research standpoint, retention research is much easier to conduct than turnover and attrition research, the primary reason being participants are difficult to find or track once they leave a position, setting, or the profession. In light of this dilemma, new approaches to research methodology and technology, labor market dynamism and human resource practices have allowed retention and turnover research to remain vibrant with more than 1500 academic studies on the topic.[3-5,9]

THE EVOLUTION OF RETENTION AND TURNOVER RESEARCH: UNDERSTANDING WHY EMPLOYEES LEAVE AND WHY THEY STAY

Early Turnover Models

Since the 1950s, many research models on retention and turnover have emerged. The inception of this scientific research was mainly focused on turnover at the individual level, with the intent of explaining the process one goes through when leaving a job.[4] In 1958, March and Simon[10] introduced a theory of organizational equilibrium, emphasizing the importance of balanced employee and organization contributions and incentives. Their research introduced and focused on the concepts we know today as job satisfaction and perceived alternatives.[4]

In the 1970s, several turnover models were introduced that focused on met expectations and the withdrawal process.[4] Price and Mueller[1] developed the Causal Model of Turnover, a comprehensive, structural, socioeconomic model. Several environmental (eg, job opportunities, kinship responsibility), individual (eg, personality affects), and job structural (eg, autonomy, job stressors, pay) variables were shown to positively or negatively affect job satisfaction, organizational commitment, search behavior, and intent to leave. Price and Mueller's model was one of the first to include organizational commitment as a mediating variable between job satisfaction and intent to leave. Their work began a major shift in focus, horizontally and vertically, toward the causes of job satisfaction.[4]

Several other turnover models emerged in the 1980s, and all of these early models introduced and significantly advanced turnover research. Recent turnover models are grounded in one or more of these traditional theories.[4] Many other studies examined antecedents or predictors of turnover during this time, which will be discussed later in the "Antecedents of Turnover" section. Refer to the article by Holtom et al article[4] for a comprehensive review of early turnover research.

Modern Retention and Turnover Models

Early turnover models primarily focused on traditional determinants of job satisfaction, commitment, search behavior, and distal antecedents of turnover. Research on retention and turnover during the mid-1980s to mid-1990s shifted toward complex organizational/macro-level variables (eg, organizational culture) and personal/micro-level variables (eg, perceived supervisor or administrative support).[4] Two popular models used in today's research were also developed during this period: The 3-component model of organizational commitment[11] and the unfolding model of turnover.[12] Furthermore, research by Hulin[13] produced an integrative adaptation-withdrawal model that redefined the withdrawal process. Hulin argued "withdrawal" incorporates many behaviors, including lateness, absenteeism, reduced performance and retirement, and intent to leave; that subsequent turnover behavior is only one subset of the withdrawal construct. Maertz and Campion[14] introduced an interesting model in 2004 that combined process and content turnover models to demonstrate that turnover motive forces (affective, calculative, contractual, behavioral, alternative, normative, moral and constituent) are systematically related to 4 turnover decision types—impulsive, comparison, preplanned, and condition quitters. In other words, different forces motivate different groups of quitters. An interesting finding of their empirical research was those who quit with no job alternative actually had more negative affect than employees with other decision types, suggesting affect-driven, impulsive quitting.

Holtom and colleagues[4] recognized several major trends in the research over the past 15 years: 1) a focus on individual (personality and motivational) difference predictions of turnover, 2) an emphasis on interpersonal relationships (eg, supervisor-employee exchanges), 3) enhanced focus on strong intent-to-stay factors, and 4) dynamic modeling of the turnover process considering changes over time. The following sub-sections present the major models introduced during this period, while the next section, Antecedents of Turnover, discusses the individual and interpersonal relationship predictors of turnover.

THE WITHDRAWAL PROCESS

Turnover is a complex process that involves much more than just the actual act of leaving a job. Research by Hulin[13] redefined the behavioral process of withdrawal to include lateness, absenteeism, reduced performance, and retirement. Intent to quit and subsequent turnover is only one part of the withdrawal process.

The 3-Component Model of Organizational Commitment

In the late 1980s to early 1990s, organizational commitment was a major focus of research.[15] Meyer and Allen[11] developed the 3-component model of organizational commitment backed by years of extensive empirical research. The 3 distinct components of this model are 1) affective commitment; the emotional attachment, identification and involvement in an organization, 2) continuance commitment, one's perceived costs of leaving an organization; and 3) normative commitment, one's perceived obligation to remain with an organization. Research, including a 2002 meta-analysis of the construct,[15] showed that each of the 3 components had a negative relationship to turnover. Furthermore, each component related differently to work-related withdrawal cognition (eg, reduced attendance, employee performance, or organizational citizenship behavior). Affective commitment demonstrated the strongest positive correlation with these outcomes, followed by normative commitment. Continuance commitment has shown to be either neutral or negatively related. Subsequent research found links between commitment and other employee-related outcomes, such as stress and work-life conflict.[15]

ORGANIZATIONAL COMMITMENT

Organizational commitment, or an individual's psychological attachment to an organization, has 3 components of commitment: affective (identification with the organization), continuance (sacrifice of leaving the organization), and normative (obligation to the organization).[11]

The Unfolding Model of Turnover

In 1994, Lee and Mitchell[12] developed a new, alternative theory for understanding and describing turnover: the unfolding model of turnover. The researchers proposed that an individual's decision to leave is not always induced by a negative effect (eg, job dissatisfaction, organizational commitment), but because of a variety of precipitating events).[16] Sometimes leaving may even occur impulsively. The model has 5 key components: shocks, scripts, job search, image violations, and job dissatisfaction. "A *shock* is a particular, jarring event that initiates the psychological analyses involved in quitting a job."[17(p51)] Shocks can be an expected or unexpected event and can be perceived as positive, negative, or neutral. A *script* is a pre-existing plan of action an employee may prepare and carry out if a shock occurs—a plan for leaving. The script may be based on prior experience, observation or information gathering. An *image violation* occurs when an employee's values, goals, and strategies for goal attainment do not fit with either those of the organization or those implied by the shock. Low levels of job satisfaction occur, over time, when the job no longer provides the benefits desired. Finally, the *job search* component includes activities involved with looking for and evaluating alternatives. The model is one of the first to include alternatives that are work and non-work related.[12,16]

Lee and Mitchell[12,17,18] found these components unfold over time and most employees follow 1 of 4 psychological and behavioral decision paths prior to actual turnover. Paths 1, 2, and 3 are initiated by shocks, while paths 4a and 4b are initiated by job dissatisfaction. Path 1, *following a plan*, involves leaving a job in response to a shock or a script (plan) already in place. This decision to quit has little or nothing to do with job satisfaction and contains no active job search. Path 2, *leaving without a plan*, is an impulsive action, usually in response to a negative shock. The decision to quit may or may not be associated with job dissatisfaction, but does not include an active job search. Path 3, *leaving for something better*, entails a shock that is usually positive, producing image violations that, in turn, initiate a comparison of job opportunities (current and alternative). Ultimately, the employee leaves for the more attractive alternative (work or non-work related). This path may or may not involve job dissatisfaction. Path 4 contains 2 sub-paths. The first sub-path, 4a, *leaving*

TABLE 9-1	
THE UNFOLDING MODEL[16]: DECISION PATHS AND EXAMPLES	
DECISION PATH	**EXAMPLES**
Path 1: Following a plan Involves a shock and a script.	You planned to enroll in physician's assistant school in 3 years; you quit your athletic training job when successfully enrolled.
Path 2: Leaving without a plan Involves a shock and possibly image violations.	You were passed over on a promotion, or experienced sexual harassment or the death of a patient, or a family member becomes ill.
Path 3: Leaving for something better Involves a shock, image violations, and an active job search.	You receive an unsolicited, irresistible job offer that appears much better than your current job; or the opportunity arises to stay home with your children.
Path 4a: Leaving without a plan Involves job dissatisfaction and image violations.	You encounter escalating dissatisfaction with the job or athletic training setting climate that causes you to quit without searching for another job.
Path 4b: Leaving for something better Involves job dissatisfaction, image violations, and an active job search.	Accumulating job dissatisfaction results in an active and successful job search. You quit your current job for another job in the same athletic training setting, another setting, or another profession.

without a plan, is fueled by mounting job dissatisfaction. The employee quits without searching for another job. The second sub-path, 4b, *leaving for something better*, involves accumulating job dissatisfaction that encourages the employee to actively search for better alternatives. When a new job is found and accepted, the employee quits.[3,4,12,16-18] Table 9-1 provides a summary of the unfolding model decision paths and examples related to athletic training.

Empirical studies have continued to support the unfolding model and the shock component as a way to better understand turnover.[19-21] For example, a large, recent study[20] reported that in more than 60% of turnover cases examined across multiple professions (1200 "leavers"), the antecedent to quitting was a shock rather than accumulating job dissatisfaction. Fifty-nine percent of the shock-induced quits were expected, 41% were unexpected, 60% were organizational-related shocks (40% of these were personal), 64% were positive, 27% were negative, and 8% were neutral. Donnelly and Quinn[19] successfully classified 86% of their sample and, interestingly, reported women experience more shocks than men, and follow paths 1, 2, and 3 more than men. Morrell et al[21] found in their study of more than 300 nurse leavers the role of shocks significantly correlated with nurse turnover. Furthermore, shocks that were expected were more likely to be positive, personal shocks that result in unavoidable turnover. Shocks that were negative were more likely to be work related and associated with job dissatisfaction, more likely to affect others, and result in avoidable turnover.

The Job Embeddedness Model: Understanding Why Employees Stay

In 2001, Mitchell and colleagues,[22] who had previously developed the unfolding model, introduced job embeddedness, a construct that is focused on a broad cluster of factors or ideas that influence an employee's choice to remain in a job. The construct operates like a web in which the employee becomes enmeshed or embedded in a variety of ways, both work and non-work related. There are 3 dimensions of the job embeddedness model and each dimension has an organizational and a community component. First, *fit* involves how an employee's personal values, career goals, and future plans fit with the larger organizational culture, the demands of the job, as well as the community. As an example, a single, ambitious athletic trainer who has a strong love of all sports and a career goal to become a head athletic trainer in the college setting would likely be a good fit to work in an intercollegiate athletics position that has long hours, interactions with many different patient populations, and some added administrative responsibilities. Second, *links* are the threads that connect employees and/or their family to professional, social, psychological, and financial aspects of their lives (including work and non-work friends, social groups, immediate and extended family, the community, and the local physical environment. An athletic trainer who is married with children, and has immediate family in the local area to not only spend time and holidays with, but who can also help with day care/school drop-off/pick-up and sick days, may display high levels of job embeddedness. An athletic trainer, who, despite being dissatisfied with the job, has strong connections with work and/or non-work social and community groups and is able to spend time doing the outdoor hobbies in the local area, may likely remain at the job, despite professional dissatisfaction. Third, *sacrifice* represents the perceived cost of psychological benefits and/or materials that are forfeited by leaving. Examples include sacrificing the perks that come with a high-profile collegiate or professional sports athletic training position, or forfeiting the relationships formed with patients, colleagues and community members.

JOB EMBEDDEDNESS

Job embeddedness centers on the factors that influence an employee's choice to remain at a particular job. Like a web of connection, an employee becomes embedded in the organization and/or the community. Athletic trainers' fit within the organization, setting, and/or community, their links to the work and non-work aspects of their lives and the sacrifices they would have to make if they left a particular job affect their decision to stay or leave.

The critical focus of the job embeddedness model is the overall level of connectedness, not the influence of one specific connection. The construct encompasses the extent to which a job fits with the other aspects of an individual's life, the extent to which the individual has links to people, activities, and environment, and the ease with which those connections can be broken—what the individual would sacrifice if he or she left.[16,22] The more employees will have to give up when they depart, the more difficult it is to leave the organization.[20] Empirical studies on employees in several industries, including health care, have demonstrated aggregated job embeddedness is negatively correlated with turnover and predicts variance in turnover after controlled for job satisfaction, organizational commitment, job search, perceived alternatives, and gender.[22]

Holtom and Inderrieden[16] recently conducted a large-scale, national study on nearly 2000 stayers and leavers that integrated the job embeddedness and unfolding models. Results indicated job stayers had the highest levels of job embeddedness, shock-induced leavers had the next highest levels, and non-shock-induced leavers had the lowest levels. This implies that job embeddedness has a buffering role when employees experience shocks.[4,16]

The Comprehensive Voluntary Turnover Model

Allen and colleagues[3,23] recently presented a "comprehensive voluntary turnover model" that attempts to capture the complex process of turnover through an evidence-based approach. The model displays turnover drivers that affect key job attitudes. Low satisfaction and commitment initiates the withdrawal process, leading to turnover, if the organization fails to manage it effectively, or other withdrawal behaviors (absenteeism, reduced performance, etc). A new aspect includes "target populations" (eg, high performers, minorities) an organization may choose to focus on rather than trying to retain every employee. The model also includes on-boarding (realistic previews and socialization) and other aspects of previously discussed models including the organizational equilibrium theory[10] in the process of evaluating attractive alternatives, the unfolding model (shocks/scripts)[12] and job embeddedness.[22]

Researchers have significantly advanced the field of retention and turnover over the years. Understanding and describing why employees stay and why they leave has evolved from simpler models of job satisfaction and organizational commitment, into a complex, dynamic, temporal process with multiple pathways, indicators, and outcomes. Holtom and colleagues[4] suggest future research on retention and turnover should include studies on the influence of social networks (eg, interpersonal, relational, community, social/team dynamics and ties), cultural differences, temporal aspects (eg, the turnover process over time, early vs late turnover and longitudinal, mixed-methods studies), consequences of turnover, the impact of managerial practice, other types of withdrawal (eg, retirement), and multi-level investigations of turnover (eg, individual, department, organization, profession).

ANTECEDENTS OF EMPLOYEE TURNOVER

In the context of turnover, an antecedent is a mechanism or event that precedes or predicts the decision to depart; a precursor or a factor responsible for the decision to leave. An antecedent can have a positive or negative relationship or correlation to turnover. A positive antecedent is positively correlated to turnover, and a negative antecedent is negatively correlated to turnover. In other words, as a positive antecedent increases, so does turnover. As a negative antecedent increases, turnover decreases. Over the past 5 decades, researchers have identified many antecedents of turnover. Griffeth and colleagues[9] performed the latest and most comprehensive meta-analysis on the antecedents and correlates of employee turnover. Some of the strongest, positive antecedents of general employee turnover are related to the withdrawal process (eg, turnover intentions [0.45], job search intentions [0.34] and behavior [0.31], thoughts of quitting [0.29]). Other strong, positive antecedents include weighted application blanks (0.31) (eg, a standardized job application form used to predict an employee's success in the organization) and role conflict (0.22).[9] Becton et al[24] used biodata (application blanks, questionnaires, multiple choice items, structured interview questions, etc) to predict turnover, job performance, and organizational commitment in hospital employees. The authors found their instrument correlated well with these outcomes, and that collecting and using biodata to select health care employees could result in more committed employees, better performers, and less turnover.

Strong but negative antecedents of turnover are organizational commitment (−0.27), leader-member exchange (−0.25), role clarity (−0.24), job and work satisfaction (−0.22), and tenure (−0.23). Interestingly, pay (−0.11) and pay satisfaction (−0.08) are relatively weak antecedents of turnover.[9] Therefore, offering raises or bonuses in order to retain an employee may not be the best way to address retention. Recent research has consistently showed demographics (gender, race, marital status, education) are also weak antecedents of turnover.[9] For instance, the quit rate of women is very similar to that of men, and educated women resemble men in turnover rate and pattern (ie, leaving for another job rather than leaving the workforce entirely). However, it is important to keep in mind that the strength of these antecedents varies across job types, organizations, professions, and individual situations.[3] Many of these antecedents have been identified in research on retention, turnover, and attrition in athletic training. A comparison of general labor market and athletic training turnover antecedents are discussed in a later section.

ANTECEDENTS/PREDICTORS OF TURNOVER

Strong, positive antecedents of turnover include turnover intentions, job search intentions, job search behavior, thoughts of quitting, weighted application blanks and biodata, and role conflict. Strong, negative antecedents of turnover include organizational commitment, leader-member exchange, role clarity, job and work satisfaction, and tenure.

CONSEQUENCES OF TURNOVER

Before the consequences of employee turnover are discussed, it is important to remember that not all turnover is harmful or avoidable. A certain amount of turnover is not only necessary and helpful (ie, functional turnover), but also inevitable (eg, unavoidable turnover) in organizations.[1,3,4] An organization will not be able to retain every employer it hires—people leave for unavoidable reasons (pregnancy, family illness, better job alternatives, etc) and the vast majority of people who stay eventually age into retirement. On the other hand, functional turnover can generate important benefits for an organization. Therefore, organizational members should understand and consider both the costs and benefits associated with turnover (refer to Table 9-2).[3]

Managing dysfunctional turnover in the workplace matters to individuals, managers/supervisors, and organizations, because 1) turnover is costly, 2) turnover affects organizational performance and effectiveness, and 3) retention and turnover may become difficult to manage over time.[1,3,4,16,25] These consequences of turnover are discussed in detail below.

Turnover Is Costly

The total cost of an employee's departure includes not only aspects of the employee's entire withdrawal process (ie, absence, lateness, the withholding of effort, actual departure) but also the costs of an organization's time (eg, new hire recruiting, selecting, and training), money, and other resources.[16] Research on the cost of turnover suggests direct replacement costs can reach 50% to 60% of an employee's annual salary, with total costs ranging from 90% to 200% of an employee's annual salary.[26] In the health care industry, studies have demonstrated remarkable costs associated with turnover among nurses[27] and respiratory therapists.[28] Cortese et al[29] found that workers subjected to stressor agents incur increased costs for their organization associated with inefficiency, absenteeism, reduced job satisfaction, and productivity. Clearly, the direct and indirect costs of turnover can have an alarming impact on an organization.

Turnover Adversely Affects Organizational Performance, Workplace Morale, and the Efficiency and Quality of Patient Care

A number of studies have linked high turnover rates to shortfalls in organizational performance, workplace morale, value, efficiency, and quality of patient care.[3,25] A nationwide study[30] of nurses at more than 300 hospitals demonstrated turnover among registered nurses accounted for 68% of the variability in per-bed operating costs. Batt and Valcour[31] found good human resource practices (eg, strategies to reduce dysfunctional turnover rates) improve sales growth, workforce morale, and organizational profitability and market value. Shaw and colleagues[32] demonstrate the importance of understanding who, in particular, is leaving, because high turnover among employees with high social capital can dramatically erode organizational performance.

TABLE 9-2 **TURNOVER COSTS AND BENEFITS[5]**	
Separation costs	*Tangible*
	• Human resource time (exit interview, payroll, benefits)
	• Supervisor's time (retention attempts, exit interview)
	• Temporary medical coverage and administrative duties
	Intangible
	• Diminished quality/coverage while the position is unfilled
	• Loss of clients/patients
	• Contagion (other athletic trainers decide to leave)
	• Disruptions to team-based work
	• Loss of seasoned mentors
Replacement costs	*General Costs*
	• Human resource/staff time (benefits, enrollment, orientation)
	• Supervisor's time (search committee, orientation, training)
	Recruitment
	• Advertising
	• Hiring inducements (bonus, relocation expenses, perks)
	Orientation and Training
	• Orientation and socialization time and resources
	• Formal and informal training (time, materials, equipment, mentoring)
	• Productivity loss (until the replacement is proficient)
Turnover/ attrition benefits	• Financially better not to replace the leaver, or hire a less experienced employee
	• New skills, creativity, teamwork is infused into the organization
	• Vacancy creates promotion opportunities for others
	• Replacement is a better performer and citizen
	• Departure may offer the opportunity to reorganize the work unit

In the health care industry, quality of patient care, including patient outcomes and safety outcomes, is an important aspect of an organization's performance and efficiency. Research shows this quality declines and malpractice claims increase with high dysfunctional turnover.[33] This type of turnover has been negatively correlated with patient satisfaction with their care[34] and positively correlated with patient complication rates.[35] Studies show high nurse turnover can negatively affect an organization's capacity to meet patient needs and provide quality care.[27] At the unit level, high turnover affects nurse morale and the productivity of those who remain to provide care while new members are hired, oriented, and trained.[36] Clearly, high turnover can adversely affect health care organizations' capacity to respond to today's demands for health care.

Today's Challenge of Managing Retention and Turnover

A white paper by Manpower Incorporated[37] reported in its ninth annual Talent Shortage Survey that, globally, 36% of employers reported talent shortages in 2014, the highest percentage in 7 years. The United States reported a 40% talent shortage rate. Although the actual cause is unknown, the shortage has been attributed to demographics shifts (eg, aging populations, declining birthrates, economic migration) along with social evolution, globalization, inadequate educational programs, and entrepreneurial practices. Specifically, these shortages are not just about availability of talent, but also about employees with the specific skills required for certain industries. If an organization does not effectively manage employee turnover, it may make finding and retaining high-quality employees increasingly challenging.[3]

EMPLOYMENT OUTLOOK FOR THE HEALTH CARE INDUSTRY

Health care is the largest industry in the United States. It is also an industry that is changing rapidly with health care reform, demographic shifts, and globalization.[24,38] The US Bureau of Labor Statistics'[7] 6-year aggregate annual hires and quits rate for the "health care and social assistance" industry is just under the national rates for all industries, and health care was the only sector that experienced growth during the economic downturn of 2008. Eleven of the 20 occupations listed with the highest percentage change of employment between 2012 and 2022 are health care occupations. However, a shortage of health care's clinical workforce, especially in certain professions, is well documented.[38-40] The aging health care workforce and aging population, combined with health care reform, is expected to increase demand for many health care professionals and expand the roles and necessary skill sets for existing professionals.[39] A recent 25-year retrospective study by Hillard and Burton[38] on US public health workforce research suggests the workforce is facing several urgent priorities that should be addressed, including, ". . . recruiting and retaining highly trained, well-prepared employees, and succession planning to replace retirees . . . and ensuring competitive salaries, opportunities for career advancement, standards for workplace performance, and fostering organizational cultures which generate high levels of job satisfaction for effective delivery of services."[(pS17)] Because of these findings and the consequences of turnover discussed above, management of retention and turnover in the health care industry is and should be a primary concern.

RETENTION AND TURNOVER OF HEALTH CARE PROFESSIONALS IN NURSING AND REHABILITATION SCIENCES

Nursing, by far, has been the health care profession most studied in regards to retention and turnover. In a global study, commonly stated reasons for nurses leaving included emotional exhaustion and problems in work design.[41] Haynes and colleagues[25] published a review of nursing turnover research in 2006. In light of methodological challenges noted when comparing turnover studies, the authors concluded that strong, consistent factors associated with nurse turnover include job dissatisfaction and expressed intent to leave, which can be moderated by organizational commitment and personal disposition.[25] Several studies demonstrated that organizational characteristics (eg, workload, management style, empowerment and autonomy, promotional opportunities, and work schedules) contribute to nurse turnover as well. Socio-demographic characteristics (eg, age, inexperience, education level, and kinship responsibilities) show inconsistent findings and are not usually considered explanatory in nurse turnover behavior.[25]

Currently, few studies have examined retention, turnover, and attrition in the rehabilitation professions. The current lack of attention within these fields is only speculative, but does warrant further investigation. One possible reason can be drawn from the structure that some rehabilitation professionals are allowed to have in regards to their work schedules, which allows for a more normal (8 am to 5 pm) workday. In the limited literature, McGuire et al[40] reported that respect, recognition, and organizational commitment, not pay and benefits, were found to be primary reasons for job satisfaction and subsequent retention of physical therapists, medical technicians, and rural hospital employees. Tran et al[42] found the recruitment and retention strategies that rehabilitation therapists in Ontario, Canada, considered most important and feasible were employer-worker communication, compensation packages, access to research, and professional development in budget planning. McLaughlin et al[43] studied turnover and attrition among Australian speech pathologists who had entered the withdrawal process in their current job. Those searching for a new job or profession were more likely to be less than 35 years of age, and perceive low levels of job security and benefits of the profession. Those employees who were intending to leave the profession entirely were more likely to spend more than half their work time on administrative duties, have a higher negative affect score, not have children under 18 years of age, and perceive speech pathology did not offer benefits that met their needs. Noh and Beggs[44] examined retention, turnover, and regional attrition factors among physiotherapists in Northern Ontario via a longitudinal study. Initial results indicated the most significant factor affecting retention was perceived opportunity for career development. In the follow-up part of the study, researchers found a 12% regional attrition rate (participants who left their job and left Northern Ontario). Turnover/attrition factors included professional experience, practice location, and community size. However, job satisfaction, the perceived lack of opportunity for career development, and the intention to leave Northern Ontario were the strongest predictors of turnover. Turnover was significantly more prevalent among young therapists and those with less professional experience.

EMPLOYMENT OUTLOOK FOR THE ATHLETIC TRAINING PROFESSION

In light of the growing need for health care services, and specifically the growing need and demand for athletic trainers in certain settings/environments (eg, the secondary school, occupational settings, and youth leagues), retention of quality athletic trainers is certainly desirable. The US Bureau of Labor Statistics predicts the employment of athletic trainers will grow 21% from 2012 to 2022.[7] This growth is larger than registered nurses (19%) but smaller than occupational therapists (29%) and physical therapists (36%). There are a few other avenues of employment data on the athletic training profession. For instance, the National Athletic Trainers' Association (NATA) conducts periodic member salary surveys and graduate placement reports. The NATA has reported studies with positive employment trends and outcomes in the occupational[45] and hospital settings.[46] However, more data and national data comparison outlets are needed for our profession's retention and turnover rates, and employment outlook. For instance, the Health Resources and Services Administration, National Center for Health Workforce Analysis, of the US Department of Health and Human Services publishes an annual US Health Workforce Chartbook[47] that provides valuable data on the size and characteristics of 35 health occupations. Yet, the athletic training profession is not among the data.

According to the Board of Certification (BOC),[48] the number of certified athletic trainers averaged an 8% growth from the years 2011 to 2013. The NATA membership has steadily grown over the years, including a 6.9% growth in members from 2012 to 2013.[49] However, a recent study by

Kahanov and Eberman[50] showed the NATA has a general decline in membership at the age of 30, with a marked decline in female membership at age 28. Interestingly, male NATA member representation in the secondary school setting increased, suggesting a setting shift. Although this was a cross-sectional study of NATA membership and not of certification or state licensure status, these results suggest an early exit from certain athletic training settings and/or the profession entirely. Therefore, understanding retention, turnover, and attrition in athletic training, especially *who* is staying and *who* is leaving, is important to the profession's growth and goal achievement.

RETENTION, ATTRITION, AND TURNOVER IN ATHLETIC TRAINING: WHY DO ATHLETIC TRAINERS STAY AND WHY DO THEY LEAVE?

There are few empirical data available on actual athletic training turnover and attrition rates from a NATA membership, a certification, or a state licensure perspective. However, there are studies in progress examining attrition rates via actual BOC certification inception and expiration rates. Capel[51] was the first to examine athletic trainer attrition nearly 25 years ago, and surveyed persons who were no longer employed as an athletic trainer asking why they had left the profession. Although there was a low response rate ($n = 82$, 37%), results showed the primary reasons for leaving were as follows:

1. Entering private practice as a physical therapist (28%)
2. Returning to school (14%)
3. Moved, no job available (12%)
4. Salary too low (9%)
5. Limited opportunities (9%)
6. Enjoyed another job more (6%)
7. Teach/direct athletic training programs (4%)
8. Long hours (3%)
9. Other (15%)

Recently, the National Collegiate Athletics Association Division-I (NCAA D-I) setting has been the most-studied setting in regards to retention, attrition, and turnover.[2,52-59] According to NATA membership statistics, the college/university setting contained the largest amount of members, and this is often why it is the focus of many of the investigations.[49] Moreover, the unique nature of work demands in this setting, combined with the dwindling "off-season" in college sports, has prompted researchers to investigate the professional and personal lives of collegiate athletic trainers, especially female collegiate athletic trainers. Female athletic trainers comprise approximately 28% of full-time collegiate positions.[49] Mazerolle and colleagues[53,54] found that only 22 females with children were employed at the NCAA D-I collegiate setting. In several studies examining retention and work-life balance, female athletic trainers have identified the time commitment of the profession, particularly in the collegiate setting, as problematic, especially when trying to balance motherhood and athletic training.[2,52,53,55] Time demands appear to permeate several of the employment settings as major challenges to work-life balance, a common thread to turnover in athletic training.

Goodman and colleagues[2] performed a qualitative inquiry, interviewing one current and one former female athletic trainer from each university in the Southeastern Conference. The Price Muller Causal Model of Turnover[1] guided their inquiry. Through a grounded theory analysis, the researchers found the factors affecting the decision to persist in the NCAA D-I setting were increased autonomy, increased social support (eg, supervisor, co-worker, and family), enjoyment of the NCAA D-I job and atmosphere, and kinship responsibility (eg, spouse or immediate family in the local area). Factors affecting the decision to leave the NCAA D-I setting or the profession entirely were work-life conflict, role strain (ie, primarily role conflict with supervisors and/or coaches and role overload), and decreased autonomy and kinship responsibility (eg, spouse accepts another job requiring a move). In 2 similar studies, Mazerolle and colleagues examined the retention[59] and turnover/attrition[58] of male NCAA D-I athletic trainers. Factors affecting the decision to persist in the NCAA D-I setting were enjoyment of the high-profile atmosphere and workplace environment (eg, the positive connections and experiences with their supervisor and co-workers). Factors affecting the decision to depart the setting were: role strain (role conflict with administration/coaches and role overload), work-family conflict, role transition (eg, phased retirement) and a lack of opportunities for career advancement (eg, promotional chances and raises).

Enjoyment of NCAA D-I setting, including the competitive atmosphere and positive dynamics with student-athletes, has emerged as a main athletic trainer retention factor in the collegiate setting. A recent study[60] on the retention of head athletic trainers at the NCAA D-I setting reported the decision to remain in their jobs and the setting was because of the rewarding relationships they had with staff members and student-athletes. Furthermore, a commitment to lifelong learning for professional development also exerted a positive influence for retention.

The most recent published study of athletic trainer attrition was conducted by Bowman and peers.[61] The authors performed a qualitative inquiry of graduates of post-professional athletic training programs who subsequently decided to leave the athletic training profession. The 2 primary reasons for departure were decreased recognition of value and work-life conflict. Low salaries and long work hours primarily fueled departure due to decreased recognition of value.

In general, the characteristics of athletic training turnover are similar to nursing turnover (eg, job dissatisfaction, workload, management style, value, autonomy, promotional opportunities, and work schedules). Continued research is needed in athletic training regarding turnover, mostly because it appears to be problematic, yet the data is from a small sample from the field. Table 9-3 provides a summary of retention, turnover, and attrition factors in athletic training and other health care professions.

RELATING ANTECEDENTS OF TURNOVER TO THE ATHLETIC TRAINING LITERATURE

Many antecedents or predictors of turnover have been identified in workplace research. Although many of the studies have been qualitative (ie, not quantitative studies examining the significance and strength of relationships), several of these antecedents have been examined in the literature on turnover and professional issues in athletic training:

1. *Socialization* of the athletic trainer has been studied in different settings and found to be an important facet affecting the professional lives of athletic trainers.[62,63]

2. Moderate to high levels of role strain were found in collegiate athletic trainers who were also preceptors.[64] Furthermore, organizational socialization and *role clarity* influenced the role strain of these preceptors. As discussed in the previous section, *role conflict* and *role overload* are primary factors for leaving an athletic training position, setting or the entire profession.

3. A lack of *promotional opportunities* at the NCAA D-I level emerged as a main departure factor for male athletic trainers.[58]

TABLE 9-3
RETENTION, ATTRITION, AND TURNOVER IN ATHLETIC TRAINING AND OTHER HEALTH CARE PROFESSIONS[2,51,58-61]

RETENTION—WHY ATHLETIC TRAINERS STAY	**TURNOVER/ATTRITION— WHY ATHLETIC TRAINERS LEAVE**	**TURNOVER/ATTRITION FACTORS IN OTHER HEALTH CARE PROFESSIONS***

• Workplace environment
• Social support
  ○ Administration
  ○ Supervisor
  ○ Co-workers
  ○ Non-work
• Enjoyment of the setting
  ○ Competitive environment
  ○ Positive patient dynamics
• Increased autonomy
• Kinship responsibility
• Lifelong learning
	• Work-life conflict
	  ○ Work-family conflict
	• Role strain
	  ○ Role overload
	  ○ Role conflict
	• Decreased recognition of value
	• Low salaries
	• Workload (long work hours)
	• Decreased autonomy
	• Limited career advancement
	• Role transition
	• Kinship responsibility
	• Entering another profession
	• Returning to school
	• Moving away, no job available
	• Low pay
	• Enjoyed another job more
	• Teach/direct athletic training programs
		• Job dissatisfaction
		• Intent to leave
		• Emotional exhaustion
		• Work design issues
		• Low organizational commitment
		• Workload
		• Management style
		• Lack of empowerment
		• Decreased autonomy
		• Limited promotional opportunities
		• Lack of career development
		• Work schedules
		• Value
		• Professional experience

*Research from nursing, physical therapy, occupational therapy, and speech pathology.[25,42-44]

4. *Pay* and *pay satisfaction* is generally a weak predictor of turnover/attrition.[9] However, it has long been discussed anecdotally that athletic trainer salaries are not commensurate with the number of hours worked or the level of responsibility. Goodman and colleagues[2] found pay did not influence the decision of female athletic trainers to leave the NCAA D-I setting. However, low salaries have been identified as a contributing departure factor from the NCAA D-I athletic training setting for males,[58] and from the profession entirely for both sexes.[61] According

to the 2014 NATA Salary Survey,[65] the mean, annual athletic trainer salary was $52,837; up from $48,317 in 2012. Yet, the median was $45,690, and 25% of athletic trainers surveyed made less than $38,000. Although athletic training salaries are increasing, salary data comparing peer health care professions highlight the sharp differences in pay. According to 2014 data from the US Bureau of Labor,[7] the mean annual salary for an athletic trainer is $44,720, which is 36% lower than registered nurses ($68,910), 40% lower than speech-language pathologists ($74,900), 43% lower than occupational therapists ($77,890), and 46% lower than physical therapists ($82,180). A recent white paper[66] examining the professional degree level for athletic training also provided data that highlighted the sharp differences in pay between athletic trainers, compared to physical therapists, occupational therapists, and physician assistants. Furthermore, the papers revealed a startling fact that, ". . . growth in [athletic trainer] salaries has barely kept pace with inflation since the 2008–09 period."[(p17)] Lack of engagement in third-party reimbursement and the profession's connection to public sector jobs have been hypothesized as reasons for this salary disparity and the slower recovery of athletic training pay after the 2008 economic recession.[66]

5. *Leader-member exchange, supervisor satisfaction,* and *co-worker satisfaction* have been consistent factors found in studies of athletic trainer retention and turnover,[2,59] work-life conflict,[53,54,67] and organizational structure.[56] The quality of the relationships between employees and their immediate supervisor and between employees and their co-workers set the work climate and influence the decision to stay or leave.

6. *Work group cohesion* has been discussed in studies involving athletic training organizational structure,[56] head athletic trainers,[67] and retention-turnover.[2,58,59]

7. *Kinship responsibilities* were found to be a major factor in both the decision to stay and leave the NCAA D-I setting for female athletic trainers.[2] The decision to stay was influenced by the fact their spouse/partner had a good job in the local area. The decision to leave was highly influenced by their spouse/partner taking another job, which required a substantial move. Other studies have referred to these responsibilities (eg, to a spouse, children or other immediate family) through work-family conflict[2,53,54,58] and how the struggle to maintain a balance between work and kinship responsibilities influenced the intent to leave or the decision to leave.

8. Winterstein[68] examined *organizational commitment* among collegiate head athletic trainers and found the positive attachment to the student-athletes and obligation toward athletic training students were the primary focus of their commitment. Across the sample, continuance commitment scores were significantly lower than affective and normative scores. Pitney[69] studied professional commitment of secondary school athletic trainers and found similar results. A central feature of their professional commitment was the strong sense of responsibility to their patients. Commitment was influenced by both intrinsic and extrinsic rewards, and respect from others. Co-worker support and the ability to rejuvenate away from the job have also been found to facilitate professional commitment of collegiate athletic trainers,[70] while stage of life, work overload, organizational climate, and human resources have been found to be barriers to this commitment.[71]

9. Athletic trainer *job satisfaction* has been predominately studied in the collegiate setting.[54,72,73] The studies have contrasted, somewhat, in terms of who and what type of collegiate athletic trainer is more or less satisfied. In regards to job satisfaction's influence on turnover of collegiate athletic trainers, Terranova and Henning[73] found the job satisfaction subscale, nature of work, was the best predictor of intent to leave, and Mazerolle and colleagues[54] found work-family conflict had a direct negative relationship to job satisfaction and a direct positive relationship to intent to leave.

Based on the available research, studies support traditional thought and show that athletic trainers stay in and leave positions, settings, and the profession for all kinds of reasons. Some of the most common retention factors were workplace environment, social support, and enjoyment of the athletic training setting. The most common turnover/attrition factors were work-life conflict, role strain, and decreased recognition of value.

Future research on athletic training retention, turnover, and attrition should focus on: 1) actual retention and attrition/turnover rates based on certification and licensure data, 2) longitudinal, mixed-method studies using modern retention and turnover models (eg, the unfolding model, the job embeddedness model) and 3) multi-departmental, -organizational and -setting investigations. A better, global representation of athletic training retention, attrition, and turnover can assist organizational members in developing effective retention strategies and foster sustainable growth in the athletic training profession.

DEVELOPING AN EFFECTIVE RETENTION MANAGEMENT PLAN TO ACTIVELY REDUCE AVOIDABLE AND UNDESIRABLE TURNOVER: DIAGNOSE, IMPLEMENT, AND ADAPT

In the previous sections of this chapter, we defined retention, turnover, and attrition; discussed why turnover matters and the process involved when employees decide to stay or leave; and examined the professional issues involved in athletic trainer retention, turnover, and attrition. This knowledge is helpful in creating retention management strategies, and in order to effectively manage retention, "... you need to engage in an ongoing diagnosis of the nature and causes of turnover, as well as develop (and constantly hone) the right mix of retention initiatives. That calls for thinking about retention before employees are hired, while they're working at your company and after they leave."[3(p11)] However, we must keep in mind that every organization is unique and will have its own human capital strategies and challenges that may differ across departments, divisions, programs, settings, geographic locations, and individuals.[3] Therefore, you must develop a plan that works best for your organization. Allen and colleagues[3,5,23] provide practical steps and evidenced-based strategies for developing an effective retention management plan and this process is discussed in the following paragraphs.

Step 1: Performing an Effective Turnover Analysis

The development of an effective plan involves a process that begins with answering this question: Is turnover a problem for our organization? Remember, not all turnover is bad, and you cannot possibly prevent every employee from leaving. However, turnover becomes dysfunctional when the wrong people leave, or when high turnover creates instability and high costs that outweigh the benefits. An effective turnover analysis tries to answer 3 questions: 1) What is our turnover rate (ie, how many people are leaving)? 2) Who is actually leaving? and 3) What are the relative costs and benefits of this turnover?[3] First, calculate your turnover rate (eg, monthly or yearly); using Figure 9-1, track bulleted types of turnover, actual reasons for departure, and other useful demographic data (gender, race, job type, job level, performance, etc). Second, use these data to create a clearer picture of who is actually leaving (eg, women are leaving more than men; more higher-skilled, higher-performing employees are leaving). These data will help determine your organization-specific turnover drivers. Third, develop a cost-benefit formula that works best for your unique organization.[3,23] Examples of formulas, metrics, and other resources are available at websites like www.shrm.org and www.retensa.com.

In the organizational context, benchmarking and needs assessment can provide you additional information while determining whether turnover is a problem.[3,23] Through internal benchmarking, you track your organization's turnover rates and characteristics longitudinally to find red flags. Through external benchmarking you compare your turnover rates with other similar organizations and/or professions using data from government,[7] regional, state, BOC, state licensure board resources, etc. Performing an external needs assessment will help you evaluate turnover implications for your organization in the context of future labor market trends, demand, and availability. Performing an internal needs assessment will assist you in evaluating your organization's strategic plan and its implications for your staff's labor requirements.

Overall, this step will enable you to determine if turnover in your organization is problematic. If turnover does not appear to be a problem, you may likely maintain the status quo, yet continually monitor turnover.[3,5] If turnover is a problem, this analysis provides a view through an organizational context lens, enabling organizational members to create data-based retention goals.[23]

Step 2: Developing an Effective Retention Management Plan

An effective plan will include systemic or targeted retention strategies, or a combination of both. Systemic, or broad-based, strategies are based on general principles intended to reduce overall turnover. These general strategies can come from sources such as retention research, published best-practices, and benchmarking surveys conducted by professional associations (eg, salary surveys).[23] Evidence-based retention strategies and best practices are discussed in the next section.

Targeted strategies are based on organization-specific turnover drivers, intended to address organization-specific issues and address turnover among specific employee populations.[23] Systemic and targeted strategies are not mutually exclusive. For example, a systemic strategy can help retain specific employees, while a targeted strategy can help reduce overall turnover. However, an effective retention plan uses data and strategies that have been personalized to your organization's particular turnover problem(s).[23] Data from several sources can be used to create a targeted strategy, including qualitative research via current employee interviews, focus groups and follow-ups, linkage research, predictive surveys, exit interviews, and post-exit surveys. Qualitative research on current employees is valuable because the in-depth data can shed light on reason(s) employees have considered leaving and why they chose to stay. Linkage research usually involves measuring employee attitudes/opinions through an anonymous survey to look for connections between trends at the unit-level and overall turnover rates. Predictive turnover studies examine direct relationships between individual survey responses and turnover decisions—employees are surveyed on their attitudes and opinions and then followed over time to see who stays and who leaves. This type of study provides important data on the strength of relationships between turnover antecedents and actual turnover, which can help you develop specific, targeted retention strategies. Exit interviews and post-exit surveys are the least reliable target strategies often because of the employees' reluctant behavior to report negative facets of the job or organization that caused them to depart. This may be due to a fear they may end the professional relationship on a negative note, which burns bridges needed for future employment.[3] Most important, in order to receive valuable data, interviewers should be neutral, interviews should be structured, quantitative and qualitative data should be cross-checked, and confidentiality should be ensured to the extent possible.[3,5]

Steps 3 and 4: Implement and Evaluate

Steps 3 and 4 involve implementing the retention management plan and evaluating the results. This plan can be implemented organization wide, at the unit level or in specific employee groups (women, minorities, high-performers, etc). As with any organizational change, having top administrative support of your plan is important. Continuous evaluation of the plan's results allows you to examine the impact of the retention investment and relative cost, and the realistic and practical nature of implemented strategies and objectify the plan's success. These results are important data that will assist you with modifying and adapting the plan, if needed, to meet the organization's retention goals, and align with the organization's strategic plan.[3,5]

DEVELOPING AN EFFECTIVE RETENTION PLAN

In order to develop a plan that proactively reduces undesirable turnover and retains quality athletic trainers, organizational members must 1) perform a turnover analysis, 2) develop and implement a quality retention plan, and 3) consistently evaluate and adapt the retention plan.

EVIDENCE-BASED RETENTION STRATEGIES AND BEST PRACTICES

Retention strategies involve many aspects of the employer-employee relationship, and they can begin before the employee is even hired. Research demonstrates that certain human resource practices can be a powerful enabler to achieving organizational retention goals.[3,9,74,75] The following sections discuss evidence-based retention strategies/practices, and Table 9-4 provides a summary of these best practices.

RECRUITMENT

The recruitment process is the first formal opportunity supervisors and administration have to manage turnover. A "realistic job preview" (RJP) is "the presentation by an organization of both favorable and unfavorable job-related information to job candidates."[76(p41)] RJPs can come in many formats (verbal, booklets, etc) and should be delivered through multiple credible sources. Research has shown RJPs can have an important role in attracting "good fit" employees and improve retention. However, an honest, accurate RJP may reduce your applicant pool. Therefore, they are most appropriate when you have enough qualified applicants.[3] RJPs for positions in athletic training with the potential for role ambiguity (eg, the collegiate and secondary school settings) may be helpful with the socialization and retention of quality athletic trainers. Allen[3] provides useful information on how to create an RJP. Another recruitment practice is employee referrals, which is common in the athletic training employment sector. Employees recruited and hired through employee referrals, not through recruitment sources, may be less likely to leave.

Selection

The use of biodata and weighted application blanks (discussed in previous sections) can be used during the selection process to predict retention.[24,74] Weighted-application blanks (WABs) have been used since the 1950s and are among the strongest antecedents to turnover.[9] Many organizations assess person-job and person-organization *fit*, or the compatibility of an individual within the work environment, during the selection process to influence retention. Researchers suggest using WABs and structured rather than traditional interviews in the selection process. Also, structured questionnaires such as the Organizational Culture Profile, the Job Compatibility Questionnaire, or values/personality profile matching[74] can assist employers with measuring the fit of a potential athletic trainer, which can often be challenging and subjective.

TABLE 9-4 EVIDENCED-BASED HUMAN RESOURCE RETENTION MANAGEMENT STRATEGIES[23]	
Recruitment	• Provide realistic job previews. • Use employee referrals.
Selection	• Use biodata (biographical data) and weighted application blanks to predict who is most likely to leave. • Assess fit with the organization and job.
Socialization	• Involve experienced organization members as role models and mentors. • Provide new hires with positive feedback as they adapt. • Group structured orientation activities. • Provide clear information about socialization stages.
Training and development	• Offer training and development opportunities. • Link developmental opportunities to tenure.
Compensation and rewards	• Lead the market in rewards tailored to individual needs and preferences. • Promote justice and fairness in pay and reward decisions. • Link rewards to retention.
Supervision	• Train supervisors on retention management (eg, how to lead, how to develop effective relationships with subordinates) • Evaluate supervisors on retention. • Identify and remove abusive supervisors.
Engagement	• Increase meaningfulness, autonomy, variety, and co-worker support. • Provide orientation that communicates how jobs contribute to the organizational mission. • Offer ongoing skills development and provide challenging goals. • Consider competency-based and pay-for-performance systems. • Provide positive feedback and recognition of all types of contributions.

Socialization

Turnover rates are often high among new employees.[77] Often in athletic training, the first few weeks or even months are highly stressful. A lack of socialization, or on-boarding, can have adverse effects on an athletic trainer's professional and personal lives.[62,63] Allen[77] found that socialization practices can reduce turnover, mainly through job embeddedness. Socialization best practices are 1) formal and clearly defined, 2) collective using cohort-centered learning experiences, 3) sequential rather than random, 4) fixed with clear and set learning activities, 5) serial with experienced members as role models and mentors, and 6) investitive with positive feedback and social support.[5]

Training and Development

Making investments in training and development can often be perceived as a double-edged sword, with the fear these investments might make employees more marketable, attractive, and mobile, leading to increased turnover.[5] However, employees who receive more training and development opportunities are less likely to quit,[75] likely because employees' perceptions of organizational support increase. This increases job satisfaction and organizational commitment, decreases the intent to leave, and produces more internal mobility and less external mobility. Furthermore, the training of supervisors/managers may reduce turnover at all levels.[5] Continuing education is mandatory for athletic trainers to maintain their certification and licensure. Therefore, employers should provide funding and opportunities for continuing education, as well as training and career development programs, especially for athletic trainers who are supervisors. Other best practices include offering job-specific training rather than generalized training and linking developmental opportunities to tenure.[3,75] These training and development opportunities should be coupled with corresponding internal career advancement opportunities, which can be difficult in organizations with limited promotional opportunities (eg, collegiate and secondary school athletic training settings).

Compensation and Rewards

Although pay and pay satisfaction are weak turnover antecedents,[9] we have seen in athletic training turnover research that sometimes pay does matter. There are several best practices in this area to consider. Compensation and rewards program managers should consider "leading the market" for some types of pay and rewards and some types of positions, yet in ways that fit the organization and strategic plan (this is practiced heavily in the college and professional coaching job market). Cash is not always the driving force in low pay and benefits satisfaction. Therefore, programs should try to tailor rewards to meet employee needs and values (with pay, benefits, work-family arrangements, etc). Also, linking compensation and rewards to "tenure milestones" (eg, retention bonuses) can have a positive effect on retention.[3,5]

Perceptions of fairness and equity in pay and rewards are also important in managing turnover. In order to manage these perceptions you should know what similar organizations are paying their athletic trainers, pay similar positions comparatively, use objective criteria to determine pay differences (eg, education, experience, performance), understand how employees are "calculating" equity to arrive at these perceptions, and practice transparency about procedures used to make pay and rewards decisions.[5]

Supervision

A common statement in the labor market is "... people leave supervisors, not companies."[5] Research does support this statement. As noted earlier, the quality of the employee-immediate supervisor relationship, employee-supervisor satisfaction, fair treatment from supervisors, and perceived organizational support are all strong turnover antecedents[9] and have been consistent factors of retention and turnover in athletic training research.[2,58,59] In order to have good leadership, supervisors must be *prepared* and often *trained* to lead and develop effective employee relationships. Too often employees are promoted to supervisory positions based on performance and not on managerial abilities. Organizations should provide training for supervisors that not only helps them be a good "boss," but also helps them understand how to retain talent.[3] Other best practices include holding supervisors accountable for retention, and identifying, addressing, and/

or removing abusive, bullying supervisors. Effective supervisors who support their employees are 1) physically present and available to their employees, 2) provide positive, constructive feedback, mentoring, and appropriate recognition, 3) provide fair and flexible work schedules and appropriate job autonomy, and 4) reward employee accomplishments sufficiently and fairly. Perceived organizational support is also important in employee retention and interacts with perceived supervisor support. High levels of organizational support may compensate for low levels of supervisor support and vice versa.[5] Employees want to know their administrators care and respect them as important organizational members, that they will listen to them and assist with continuing education, development and internal career advancement and that they are fair and equitable in terms of pay and rewards.[3,5]

Engagement and Embeddedness

Engaged employees are less likely to leave than those who not engaged.[5] Providing employees with mentors, proper rewards and recognition, fair procedures, clear communication, guidance and support, specific and challenging goals, and enriched job experiences (autonomy, feedback, etc) can foster engagement and job embeddedness. Community engagement and embeddedness can be strengthened through links to service organizations and recreational leagues (eg, the company's softball team). Fit within the community can be built and strengthened by recruiting locally when feasible, and by providing extensive community information (eg, housing and day care assistance) to new employees who are relocating. Fit can also be established when the organization sponsors local events (eg, a 5K walk/run for charity) and builds ties within the community.[22]

SUMMARY

Employee retention and turnover are complex processes with multiple indicators and outcomes. High, dysfunctional employee turnover can be expensive, disruptive, and damaging to organizational success and patient care.[5] This chapter provides evidenced-based perspectives on retention, turnover, and attrition: 1) not all turnover is the same, nor is all turnover bad, 2) causes of turnover and attrition go beyond pay and job dissatisfaction, 3) supervisors and administrators can greatly affect retention and turnover, and 4) retention management is multifaceted and attainable.[23] Understanding what drives turnover can help organizational members move beyond the common misconceptions of turnover and attrition in athletic training, and make evidence-based decisions on retention management in athletic training organizations and the entire profession. Retaining quality and committed athletic trainers is in the best interest of the profession, the organizations, and the patients we serve.

ACTIVITIES FOR REINFORCEMENT

Questions for Review

1. What is the difference between retention, turnover, and attrition in the workplace?
2. How does turnover and attrition affect organizations?
3. Why do some employees leave and others stay in their employment organization?
4. What is organizational commitment and how can it be promoted?
5. How can organizational leaders improve employee retention?

Case Vignettes

Case #1

Marcus and Kayla are good friends and both are assistant athletic trainers at a large NCAA D-I university, entering their seventh year of employment. Marcus provides medical care for the men's basketball team, and Kayla for the women's basketball team. They have both received excellent performance evaluations and are considered high-quality employees. Both athletic trainers are married. Marcus and his wife have 2 children, and Kayla and her husband have 1 child. Marcus and Kayla enjoy the perks of the D-I atmosphere, and being a D-I athletic trainer was a lifelong professional dream for both. However, they now speak often about the high demands of the job, and the effects on their career mobility and personal life. Even though they love the university and the community they live in, they are considering either a setting-change or leaving the athletic training profession entirely.

1. Discuss any differences between these 2 athletic trainers from a societal lens. Based on the research, what can affect their decision to stay or leave their jobs?

2. What can the organization do in their attempt to retain these high-quality employees?

3. What can Marcus and Kayla do to improve their situations?

Case #2

Kelley is an athletic training coordinator who supervises other athletic trainers at an organization in the clinic-outreach setting. She discovers that previous employees and new hires were/are routinely reporting high stress levels and being unpleasantly surprised at certain facets of their work environment, and the organization is experiencing moderate levels of undesirable turnover. She obtained these data through exit interviews, post-exit surveys, and current employee interviews. She recognizes these findings as a shock.

1. How can Kelley develop and implement an effective retention management plan?

2. What evidenced-based strategies should she consider?

3. What can Kelley do, as a supervisor, to improve retention at her organization?

Discussion Questions

1. What do you believe is a primary reason that athletic trainers leave a job setting?

2. What employee retention strategies do you believe are most appropriate and applicable to athletic training practice settings?

3. What are some avoidable and unavoidable causes of turnover in athletic training practice settings?

REFERENCES

1. Price JL. Reflections on the determinants of voluntary turnover. *Int J Manpower.* 2001;22:600-624.
2. Goodman A, Mensch JM, Jay M, French KE, Mitchell MF, Fritz SL. Retention and attrition factors for female certified athletic trainers in the National Collegiate Athletic Association Division I football bowl subdivision setting. *J Athl Train.* 2010;45(3):287-298.
3. Allen DG. Retaining talent: a guide to analyzing and managing employee turnover. http://www.shrm.org/TemplatesTools/hrqa/Pages/CalculatingRetentionandTurnover.aspx. Accessed July 11, 2014.
4. Holtom BC, Mitchell TR, Lee TW, Eberly MB. Turnover and retention research. *Acad Manag Annals.* 2008;2(1):231-274.

5. Allen DG, Bryant P. *Managing Employee Turnover: Dispelling Myths and Fostering Evidence-Based Retention Strategies.* New York: Business Expert Press; 2012.

6. Trevor CO. Interactions among actual ease-of-movement determinants and job satisfaction in the prediction of voluntary turnover. *Acad Manag J.* 2001;44:621-638.

7. United States Bureau of Labor Statistics. Employment situation summary. http://www.bls.gov. Accessed July 20, 2014.

8. Beatty RW, Huselid MA, Schneier CE. Scoring on the balanced scorecard. *Organiz Dynamics.* 2003;32:107-121.

9. Griffeth RW, Hom PW, Gaertner S. A meta-analysis of antecedents and correlates of employee turnover: update, moderator tests, and research implications for the next millennium. *J Manage* 2000;26:463-488.

10. March JG, Simon HA. *Organizations.* New York: John Wiley; 1958.

11. Meyer JP, Allen NJ. A three-component conceptualization of organizational commitment. *Hum Res Manag Rev.* 1991;1:61-89.

12. Lee TW, Mitchell TR. An alternative approach: the unfolding model of voluntary employee turnover. *Acad Manag Rev.* 1994;19:51-89.

13. Hulin CL. Adaptation, persistence and commitment in organizations. In: Dunnette MD, Hough LM, eds. *Handbook of Industrial and Organizational Psychology.* 2nd ed. Palo Alto, CA: Consulting Psychologists Press; 1991:445-507.

14. Maertz CP, Campion MA. Profiles in quitting: integrating process and content turnover theory. *Acad Manag J.* 2004;47:566-582.

15. Meyer JP, Stanley DJ, Herscovitch L, Topolnytsky L. Affective, continuance, and normative commitment to the organization: a meta-analysis of antecedents, correlates, and consequences. *J Voc Beh.* 2002;61:20-52.

16. Holtom BC, Inderrieden EJ. Integrating the unfolding model and job embeddedness model in better understand voluntary turnover. *J Manag Iss.* 2006;18(4):435-452.

17. Lee TW, Maurer SD. The effects of family structure on organizational intention to leave and turnover commitment. *J Manag Iss.* 1999;11(4):493-514.

18. Lee TW, Mitchell TR, Wise L, Fireman S. An unfolding model of voluntary employee turnover. *Acad Manag J.* 1996;39:5-36.

19. Donnelly DP, Quinn JJ. An extension of Lee and Mitchell's unfolding model of voluntary turnover. *J Org Behav.* 2006;27:59-77.

20. Holtom BC, Mitchell TR, Lee TW, Inderrieden EJ. Shocks as causes of turnover: what they are and how organizations can manage them. *Hum Res Manag.* 2005;44:337-352.

21. Morrell K, Loan-Clarke J, Wilkinson A. The role of shocks in employee turnover. *Br J Manag.* 2004;15(4):335-349.

22. Mitchell TR, Holtom BC, Lee TW, Sablynski C, Erez M. Why people stay: using job embeddedness to predict voluntary turnover. *Acad Manag J.* 2001;44:1102-1121.

23. Allen DG, Bryant PC, Vardaman JM. Retaining talent: replacing misconceptions with evidence-based strategies. *Acad Manag Persp.* 2010;24(2):48-64.

24. Becton JB, Matthews MC, Hartley DL, Whitaker DH. Using biodata to predict turnover, organizational commitment, and job performance in healthcare. *Int J Select Assess.* 2009;17(2):189-202.

25. Hayes LJ, Brien-Pallas LO, Duffield C, et al. Nurse turnover: a literature review. *Int J Nurs Stud.* 2006;43:237-263.

26. Mitchell TR, Holtom BC, Lee TW. How to keep your best employees: developing an effective retention policy. *Acad Manag Exec.* 2001;15:96-108.

27. Gray AM, Phillips VL, Normand C. The costs of nursing turnover: evidence from the British National Health Service. *Health Policy.* 1996;38:117-128.

28. Stoller JK, Orens DK, Kester L. The impact of turnover among respiratory care practitioners in a healthcare system: frequency and associated costs. *Respir Care.* 2001;46:238-242.

29. Cortese CG, Colombo L, Ghislieri C. Determinants of nurses' job satisfaction: the role of work-family conflict, job demand, emotional charge and social support. *J Nurs Manag.* 2010;18(1):35-43.

30. Alexander JA, Bloom JR, Nuchols BA. Nursing turnover and hospital efficiency: an organization-level analysis. *Indus Rel J Econ Soc.* 1994;33(4):505-520.

31. Batt R, Valcour PM. Human resource practices as predictors of work-family outcomes and employee turnover. *Indus Rel.* 2003;42(2):189-220.

32. Shaw JD, Duffy MK, Johnson JJ, Lockhart D. Turnover, social capital losses and performance. *Acad Manag J.* 2005;48:594-606.

33. Aiken LH, Clarke SP, Sloane DM, Sochalski J, Silber JH. Hospital nurse staffing and patient mortality, nurse burnout, and job dissatisfaction. *JAMA.* 2002;286:1987-1993.

34. Leiter M, Harvie P, Frizzell C. The correspondence of patient satisfaction and nurse burnout. *Soc Sci Med.* 1998;47:1611-1617.

35. Blegen MA, Goode CJ, Reed L. Nursing staffing and patient outcomes. *Nurs Res.* 1998;47:43-50.

36. Sofer S. Determinants of nursing turnover. *Diss Abstr Inter.* 1995;Section B: The Sciences and Engineering(55):9-B.

37. Manpower. The talent shortage continues: how the ever changing role of HR can bridge the gap. http://www.manpowergroup.com/wps/wcm/connect/manpowergroup-en/home/thought-leadership/research-insights/Talent+Shortage/ - .U-IJCla1_wJ. Accessed July 20, 2014.

38. Hilliard TM, Biulton ML. Public health workforce research in review: a 25-year retrospective. *J Prev Med.* 2012;42(5 Suppl 1):S17-S28.

39. Healthcare Association of New York State. 2013 Health care professionals workforce survey. http://www.hanys.org/workforce/survey/reports/2013_nursing_allied_workforce_survey_report.pdf. Accessed July 17, 2014.

40. McGuire M, Houser J, Jarrar T, Moy W, Wall M. Retention: it's all about respect. *Health Care Man.* 2003;22(1):38-44.

41. Aiken LH, Clarke SP, Sloane DM, et al. Nurses' reports on hospital care in five countries. *Health Affairs.* 2001;20(3):43-53.

42. Tran D, Davis A, McGillis-Hall L, Jaglal SB. Comparing recruitment and retention strategies for rehabilitation professionals among hospital and home care employers. *Physiother Canada.* 2012;64(1):31-41.

43. McLaughlin EG, Adamson BJ, Lincoln MA, Pallant JF, Cooper CL. Turnover and intent to leave among speech pathologists. *Australian Health Rev.* 2010;34(2):227-233.

44. Noh S, Beggs CE. Job turnover and regional attrition among physiotherapists in northern Ontario. *Physiother Canada.* 1993;45(4):239-244.

45. National Athletic Trainers' Association. Executive summary: certified athletic trainers deliver ROI in occupational work settings. http://www.nata.org/ATCsROIinOccupationalSettings. Accessed July 17, 2014.

46. National Athletic Trainers' Association. Growing number of ATCs find hospitals offer increased job & career opportunities, higher salaries and fewer work hours. http://www.nata.org/NR11032003. Accessed July 17, 2014.

47. US Department of Health and Human Services, Health Resources and Services Administration. The US Health Workforce Chartbook. http://bhpr.hrsa.gov/healthworkforce/supplydemand/usworkforce/chartbook/. Accessed July 17, 2014.

48. Board of Certification. 2013 BOC annual report. http://www.bocatc.org/images/stories/multiple_references/boc_annual_report_1402bf.pdf. Accessed July 17, 2014.

49. National Athletic Trainers' Association. NATA 2013 certified membership statistics. http://members.nata.org/members1/documents/membstats/2013EOY-stats.htm. Accessed July 14, 2014.

50. Kahanov L, Eberman LE. Age, sex, and setting factors and labor force in athletic training. *J Athl Train.* 2011;46(4):424-430.

51. Capel SA. Attrition of athletic trainers. *J Athl Train.* 1990;25(1):34-39.

52. Kahanov L, Loebsack AR, Masucci MA, Roberts J. Perspectives on parenthood and working of female athletic trainers in the secondary school and collegiate settings. *J Athl Train.* 2010;45(5):459-466.

53. Mazerolle SM, Bruening JE, Casa DJ. Work-family conflict, part I: antecedents of work-family conflict in National Collegiate Athletic Association Division I-A certified athletic trainers. *J Athl Train.* 2008;43(5):505-512.

54. Mazerolle SM, Bruening JE, Casa DJ, Burton LJ. Work-family conflict, part II: job and life satisfaction in National Collegiate Athletic Association Division I-A certified athletic trainers. *J Athl Train.* 2008;43(5):513-522.

55. Mazerolle SM, Goodman A. Athletic trainers with children: finding a balance in the collegiate practice setting. *Int J Athl Ther Train.* 2011;16(3):9-12.

56. Mazerolle SM, Goodman A. Fulfillment of work-life balance from the organizational perspective: a case study. *J Athl Train.* 2013;48(5):668-677.

57. Mazerolle SM, Pitney WA, Casa DJ, Pagnotta KD. Assessing strategies to manage work and life balance of certified athletic trainers working in the Division I setting. *J Athl Train.* 2011;46(2):194-205.

58. Mazerolle SM, Pitney WA, Goodman A. Factors influencing departure of male athletic trainers in the NCAA Division I setting. *Int J Athl Ther Train.* 2013;18(6):7-12.

59. Mazerolle SM, Goodman A, Pitney WA. Factors influencing retention of male athletic trainers in the NCAA Division I setting. *Int J Athl Ther Train.* 2013;18(5):6-9.

60. Mazerolle SM, Pitney WA, Goodman A. Retention factors for head athletic trainers in the NCAA Division I collegiate setting. *Int J Athl Ther Train.* 2013;18(4):10-13.

61. Bowman T, Mazerolle SM, Goodman A. Career commitment of post-professional athletic training program graduates. *J Athl Train.* In press.

62. Pitney WA. Organizational influences and quality-of-life issues during the professional socialization of certified athletic trainers working in the National Collegiate Athletic Association Division I setting. *J Athl Train.* 2006;41:189-195.

63. Pitney WA. The professional socialization of certified athletic trainers in high school settings: a grounded theory investigation. *J Athl Train.* 2002;37(3):286-292.

64. Henning JM, Weidner TG. Role strain in collegiate athletic training approved clinical instructors. *J Athl Train.* 2008;43(3):275-283.

65. National Athletic Trainers' Association. NATA 2014 salary survey. http://members.nata.org/members1/salary survey2014/results2.cfm. Accessed February 12, 2015.

66. National Athletic Trainers' Association. Professional education in athletic training: an examination of the professional degree level. http://www.nata.org/sites/default/files/The_Professional_Degree_in_Athletic_Training.pdf. Accessed February 12, 2015.

67. Goodman A, Mazerolle S, Pitney W. Achieving work-life balance in the NCAA division I setting part 2: perspectives from head athletic trainers. *J Athl Train.* In press.

68. Winterstein AP. Organizational commitment among intercollegiate head athletic trainers: examining our work environment. *J Athl Train.* 1998;33:54-61.

69. Pitney WA. A qualitative examination of professional role commitment among athletic trainers working in the secondary school setting. *J Athl Train.* 2010;45(2):198-204.

70. Eason CM, Mazerolle SM, Pitney WA. Facilitators of professional commitment for the Athletic Trainer in the college setting. *J Athl Train.* In press; accepted June 3, 2014.

71. Mazerolle SM, Eason CM, Pitney WA. Athletic trainers' barriers to maintaining professional commitment in the collegiate setting. *J Athl Train.* 2015;50(5):524-531.

72. Barrett JJ, Gillentine A, Lamberth J, Daughtrey CL. Job satisfaction of NATABOC certified athletic trainers at Division One National Collegiate Athletic Association institutions in the Southeastern Conference. *Int Sports J.* 2002;6(2):1-13.

73. Terranova AB, Henning JM. National Collegiate Athletic Association division and primary job title of athletic trainers and their job satisfaction or intention to leave athletic training. *J Athl Train.* 2011;46(3):312-318.

74. Griffeth RW, Hom PW. *Retaining Valued Employees.* Thousand Oaks, CA: Sage; 2001.

75. Hom PW, Griffeth RW. *Employee Turnover.* Cincinnati: Southwestern; 1995.

76. Phillips JM. Effects of realistic job previews on multiple organizational outcomes: a meta-analysis. *Acad Manag J.* 1998;41:673-690.

77. Allen DG. Do organizational socialization tactics influence newcomer embeddedness and turnover? *J Manag.* 2006;32:237-256.

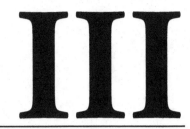

Personal Skills to
Foster Success and
Commitment in the Workplace

10

Role Modeling and Mentoring

Christianne M. Eason, MS, ATC

Objectives

After reading this chapter, the reader will be able to do the following:
1. Define mentor and role model.
2. Distinguish the difference between a role model and a mentor.
3. Understand the personal and career benefits of role models and mentors.
4. Help predict the success of mentoring relationships.
5. Recognize important steps in establishing a mentoring program within your own organization.

Introduction

Mentoring can be best described as a professional relationship in which a seasoned individual assists another, typically referred to as the mentee or protégé, in developing specific knowledge and skills that will enhance the mentee's professional and personal growth. The functions of a mentor include teaching, coaching, facilitation, and challenging. The purpose of this chapter is to highlight the personal and professional advantages of being mentored, to help guide an establishment of a formal mentoring program, and to specifically show the benefit of role modeling and mentoring within athletic training.

> "Mentoring is a brain to pick, an ear to listen, and a push in the right direction."
> —John C. Crosby

- 167 -

Mazerolle SM, Pitney WA.
Workplace Concepts for Athletic Trainers (pp 167-177).
© 2016 Taylor & Francis Group.

TABLE 10-1
COMPARISON OF A ROLE MODEL AND MENTOR

ROLE MODEL	MENTOR
• Teaches primarily through example • Facilitates professional identity by way of promoting observation and comparison • Less intentional, more informal	• Hierarchical relationship—typically senior members of an organization • Intentionally supports younger colleagues in their career • Developmental relationship that is implanted within the context of careers

MENTORS AND ROLE MODELS

Working within an organization does have many pros, one of which is the possible exposure to mentors and role models. The benefits of mentoring relationships have been publicized for several decades. The notion of mentoring was described by Levinson[1] in the late 1970s, exposing the mentoring relationship to be one of the most significant factors an individual can have in early adulthood. The literature is saturated with the benefits of mentoring, though much is anecdotal. Kram's[2] work in 1985 provided the first true foothold for empirical evidence. The majority of the research focuses on the benefits for the protégé and comes from various occupations with a large content focus from nursing and education.[3-7] The term *mentor* dates back to Greek mythology and describes a relationship between a younger adult and an older, more experienced adult who is able to help the younger individual navigate the adult world.[2]

Role models and mentors have the faculty to impart life-altering experiences that can inspire erudition, maturity, and reciprocal growth.[8] There is a difference between mentors and role models, however. Mentors are senior members of a group who intentionally encourage and support younger colleagues in their careers.[9] Mentors serve as career guides and serve as critical figures in times of transition by fostering their protégé's personal growth and professional development by conveying vision and simultaneously facilitating the development of their protégé's own vision.[10] Though the characterization of mentoring has been cultivated over the years, a fundamental feature that defines the mentoring relationships and separates it from other types of personal relationships is that mentoring is a developmental relationship that is implanted within the context of careers.[8] What makes mentoring relationships unique is that the primary focus of the relationship is on career development and growth. It is also important to remember that there is significant variation within the range and degree of functioning mentoring relationships and that these relationships are not static.[8]

Conversely, a role model teaches primarily by example and facilitates the formation of professional identity and commitment by way of promoting observation and comparison.[9,10] Role modeling is less intentional, more informal, and more episodic than mentoring. Mentoring does often include role modeling. A role model teaches predominantly by example and helps to form professional identity and commitment by way of promoting observation and comparison.[9] Table 10-1 compares and contrasts role modeling and mentoring.

WHAT IS A MENTOR RELATIONSHIP?

Within the mentoring literature there are 3 distinct areas of mentoring scholarship: youth mentoring, academic mentoring, and workplace mentoring. While these areas of research have developed relatively independently, they do share a common belief that through sustained interactions, mentoring has positive, significant, and enduring effects on protégés.

Youth mentoring consists of a supportive relationship between a non-parental adult and a young individual and promotes positive youth development. A youth mentor may serve as a protective factor against a wide range of negative things including drug use, poor academic performance, and psychological distress.[4] Academic mentoring is mentoring that occurs in academic programs and university settings. This is based on the apprenticeship education model and involves a faculty member providing academic and nonacademic issues. Academic mentoring may lead to improvements in academic achievement, professional and identity development, scholarly production, academic persistence, and psychological health.[11]

Mentoring relationships that exist in organizational settings are referred to as workplace mentoring. This type of mentoring relationship is geared toward helping the protégé develop personally and professionally within his or her career.[2] Workplace mentors are able to offer assistance by helping the protégé become oriented to the organization and socialized into the profession, while simultaneously preparing the protégé for career advancement.[3] Workplace mentoring is associated with more positive career attitudes, greater career success, and lower intentions to depart from the organization.[7] A workplace mentoring relationship is defined as one that is 1) time bound, 2) is sometimes role prescribed (meaning the protégé may or may not be assigned to a mentor), and 3) has a moderate to high level of reciprocity (benefits for both the mentor and protégé).

Workplace mentors serve the career-related ends of protégés by helping them learn the ropes of organizational life and gain exposure. The career-related support that workplace mentoring offers provides the protégé with enhanced opportunity for advancement within his or her organization. This mentor function is possible owing to mentors' more senior position, experience, and organizational influence. Workplace mentoring also provides psychosocial support to protégés by enhancing their sense of competence, identity, and effectiveness in a professional role.[2] The psychosocial functions of the workplace mentor include role modeling, acceptance, confirmation, counseling, and friendship.

The career impacts can be hard to measure because of limited long-term data. While a 2013 meta-analysis[3] found many small reciprocal relationships, the combined benefits should not be ignored. In fact, small effects may matter. Tables 10-2 and 10-3 highlight the results of the meta-analysis[3] showing the relationship between mentoring and career outcomes. It is important to note that the quality of mentoring relationships varies. An effective mentoring relationship should be graded based on the overall satisfaction of the relationship. When looking at what can predict mentoring relationship quality, the following are considered important:[3]

- **Deep-level similarity:** Similar shared attitudes, values, beliefs, and personality between the mentor and protégé
- **Experiential similarity:** Similar academic discipline, geographic location, and department affiliation between the mentor and the protégé
- **Interaction frequency:** Amount of time spent with mentor; there needs to be an opportunity for interaction between the mentor and the protégé (moderately correlated with all 3 aspects of mentoring)
- **Relationship length:** Tenure between the protégé and mentor; the relationship needs time to develop (though this is more apparent in academic mentoring relationships compared to workplace mentoring relationships)

TABLE 10-2

2004 META-ANALYSIS OF THE RELATIONSHIP BETWEEN CAREER OUTCOMES AND CAREER MENTORING[7]

DEPENDENT VARIABLE	WEIGHTED MEAN	95% CONFIDENCE INTERVAL
Objective		
Compensation	$r = 0.08$	.04, .11
Salary growth	$r = 0.19$	.11, .27
Promotions	$r = 0.10$	.05, .14
Subjective		
Career satisfaction	$r = 0.29$	.22, .36
Job satisfaction	$r = 0.30$	.25, .35
Satisfaction with mentor	$r = 0.37$	.26, .49

TABLE 10-3

OUTCOMES ASSOCIATED WITH MENTOR RELATIONSHIPS FOR PROTÉGÉS[3]

OUTCOMES	RELATIONSHIPS
Attitudinal -Satisfaction, commitment, positive attitudes	Small to medium effect
Behavioral -Performance, retention, intention to stay	Near zero to medium effect
Health related -Stress, strain	Near zero
Interpersonal -Positive relationships with others	Small effect
Motivational -Work/school/career involvement	Small effect
Career -Career success, skill development	Near zero to small effect

- **Social capital:** A perception that the relationship is supported by others, the extent to which a protégé's social network contacts create value for him or her (co-workers, supervisors, family, access to female role models) will enhance the relationship between the mentor and protégé

- **Institutional support:** The perception of institutional support is also important

When assessing the quality of the relationship, mentor or protégé, demographics do not seem to affect the relationship. The race and/or gender of the protégé and mentor do not need to be similar in order to establish a quality relationship.[3] It is important to look beyond surface characteristics to make good matches between the mentor and protégé. What does seem to be key is frequent interaction. A mentor needs to be available for the mentee. While there are possibilities for athletic trainers to interact with numerous people throughout their days working within an organization, it is recommended that athletic trainers seek out a mentor (or a supervisor assign them a mentor) within their own department as experiential and deep-level similarities will help enhance the relationship. For those athletic trainers who may not have exposure to a career mentor within their current organization, it is recommended that they rely on academic mentor relationships that developed during their education. Additionally, the athletic training profession has a wonderful network of professionals that are easily accessed through the National Athletic Trainers' Association (NATA). While a mentor in close proximity is ideal and will create a more high-quality relationship, athletic trainers are encouraged to ask questions of their peers and learn from the experiences of others within the profession.

MENTORING AND ROLE MODELING RESEARCH IN ATHLETIC TRAINING

Currently there is limited research on mentoring and role modeling within the context of athletic training, though it is a topic of growing interest. Pitney has examined the athletic training students' perception of effective mentoring.[12,13] Other studies have looked at the key attributes of preceptors, individuals who fill the role of mentor and role model to athletic training students during their clinical education.[14,15] Two studies[16,17] examined the effects of professional socialization among athletic trainers employed at the collegiate and secondary school settings. Comparable to mentoring, professional socialization is a method by which individuals learn the knowledge, skills, values, roles, and attitudes associated with their professional responsibilities.[18] The mentoring roles of athletic trainers evolve over their careers. At the outset of their careers, athletic trainers make network connections in order to learn, but as they become more experienced, they take on more of a mentoring role. This occurs as a result of being contacted by less-experienced colleagues for advice about how to deal with issues in their clinical settings.

Importance of Mentors and Role Models for Athletic Training Students

Mentorship has been identified as a significant factor that can affect the personal and professional development of a young adult,[5] while also being recognized as a strong socializing agent for athletic training students and young professionals.[16] In the context of athletic training, the presence of positive mentorship has been associated with increased student engagement and retention within the profession.[3] A recent study[19] questioning female athletic training students' perceptions on motherhood in the athletic training profession illustrated that female athletic training students felt strongly that a female mentor who had children would greatly benefit them personally as well as the profession. Remarkably, these athletic training students were already considering what clinical settings would permit career persistence in athletic training based on the setting's conduciveness to being a mother. These athletic training students, who themselves are still in their education process, are already contemplating limiting their clinical opportunities based on fears that they cannot be both a successful athletic trainer and a dedicated mother. Though the students named mentorship as an important retention factor, they themselves had very limited direct mentorship from a female athletic trainer with children employed in the collegiate setting. This parallels research in the medical literature[20] underlining a lack of role models or mentors being identified by females in respective professions.

Although case studies have been suggested as a way to encourage athletic training students, they lack the realism of a true mentoring relationship. Because of the lack of reality, case studies do not make managing motherhood seem authentic or believable to athletic training students. Rather, athletic training education programs should seek out female preceptors who have established a solid work-life balance strategy to mentor female athletic training students in order to help them develop the necessary skills to be successful in the profession while maintaining a solid work-life balance.

Importance of Mentors and Role Models for Female Athletic Trainers

A recent study by Eason et al[21] investigated experiences of female athletic trainers employed in the Division I (D-I) collegiate setting representing the 3 life stage groups (single, married, married with children) regarding work-life balance and the impact of role models and mentors. The female participants were able to identify mentors throughout their career and noted how those mentors shaped the views of professionalism among female athletic trainers in this study.[21] Identification of career impacts including clinical skills, professional interaction tips, and traveling advice occurred. Consistent with the literature from other health care fields,[6,22] the value of mentors' impact on career development and advancement is evident among female athletic trainers working in the D-I collegiate setting.

It is especially important to examine the potential benefits of mentors and role models on female athletic trainers owing to reports that there is a trend for females to leave the profession at the age of 28.[23] Additionally, the 35-year update on a longitudinal examination of women in sports reported that 92.2% of all National Collegiate Athletic Association (NCAA) member institutions that have athletic training services available, approximately 1 out of 3 have a female head athletic trainer.[24] Only 17.5% of D-I head athletic trainers are female despite the fact that the duties and skills of an athletic trainer are independent of their gender.[24] This paucity of females in leadership positions limits the exposure to and availability of female role models and mentors.

While the Acosta and Carpenter report[24] questioned hiring practices of head athletic trainers based on possible gender bias, the Eason et al study[21] highlighted the importance of female athletic trainers identifying both male and female role models and mentors within the athletic training context. The identification of male and female role models and mentors is an important factor for female athletic trainers balancing workplace issues such as gender discrimination.[25] The sex of the mentor was not as important as the demonstration of professional behavior and support of professional development by the mentor. Mazerolle et al[25] found that female athletic trainers felt that it was important to have mentors during the initial socialization into the profession, but also the opportunity to serve as a role model for young female undergraduate or graduate athletic training students.

Eason et al[21] also found that mentors had the ability to positively or negatively affect female athletic trainers' perceptions of work-life balance. The female athletic trainers depicted specific mentors and the impact those mentors had on their perceptions of work-life balance and professionalism. Women who had female mentors who effectively balanced their work and family responsibilities were more optimistic regarding their own abilities to maintain work-life balance. Conversely, women who saw their mentors or role models struggle not only felt that attaining work-life balance was a stretch, but also had a stronger desire to change clinical settings or leave the profession entirely. They referred explicitly to role models and mentors who attained career success at the expense of their personal lives, and the female athletic trainers in the study did not want to make the same sacrifice for their own careers. Unfortunately, the impact of role models and mentors is not always a positive. Repetitive negative learning experiences exhibited by role models and mentors may adversely affect a learner's development of professionalism.[9] Medical residents have revealed that it is not uncommon for clinician-teachers to utter negative and contemptuous comments about the medical profession, leaving them feeling unenthusiastic and pessimistic about the profession they chose.[9]

Curiously, the majority of females in the Eason et al study[21] expressed their wishes to see more females balancing their personal and professional lives to serve as role models and mentors, regardless of their own career aspirations. These women wanted to see peers achieving success in work-life balance and expressed their beliefs that these kinds of role models and mentors may have the ability to affect the retention of other female athletic trainers. As more females remain in the profession who are effectively managing motherhood, the more likely they are to mentor others to do the same and at the very least impart an appreciation of the skills necessary to be successful assuming both roles. In spite of female athletic trainers' desire to see more mothers serving as role models and mentors, many participants were choosing to leave their current clinical roles or the athletic training profession entirely, fundamentally contradicting their own requests to have more mentors and role models.

Importance of Mentors and Role Models for the Novice Clinician

For the novice athletic trainer, the initial introduction and orientation to their diverse roles can be an overwhelming experience. The novice needs a period of guidance and direction in order to acclimate to their environment and responsibilities. Have you ever taken a moment to reflect on all of the "soft skills" you use in your daily practice as an athletic trainer (or will use in the future)? Where did you learn how to present findings to a supervising physician, negotiate salary, or pack for a week-long road trip? Where did you learn to supervise athletic training students, or talk to parents of an injured athlete? You should hopefully realize that being an athletic training professional involves much more than the skills you will learn in the classroom. In your own reflections perhaps you were reminded of an individual you have worked with in your career or learned from during your education. With recent discussions regarding entry-level master's programs for athletic training education and a push regarding the importance of transition to practice, mentoring and role modeling need to be included in the discussion. Additionally, a mentor and role model can help ensure that a novice clinician is indeed following the best practices as established by the NATA.

A recent study by Clines et al[26] provides evidence that graduate assistant athletic trainers are selecting their positions, in part, based on the availability of mentorship. What is compelling, however, is that the graduate assistant athletic trainers emphasize that the support they desire is linear peer-to-peer role-modeling relationships as opposed to the mentorship received from a hierarchal relationship with an experienced professional. The results from Clines et al[26] do not downplay or suggest a hierarchal relationship is not important in professional growth or development, but they do suggest that once certification is gained, peers provide a more favorable, colloquial, and supportive relationship. This is not unique, as most individuals become more comfortable with their skills as they become immersed in their professional culture, which is often fostered by peers and practicing professionals.[21] Comradeship between graduate assistant athletic trainers may result from a shared understanding of each other's roles and provide a foundation for their relationship.

Head Athletic Trainers as Mentors and Role Models

A recent study conducted by Mazerolle et al[27] found that head athletic trainers informally encourage work-life balance through role modeling. Head athletic trainers in the study[27] discussed the value of being a strong role model for their staff members regarding work-life balance. They talked about the importance of retaining their own personal work-life balance strategies and implementing those strategies into their daily lives. The ability to model a balanced lifestyle was an important factor in the head athletic trainers' ability to promote work-life balance for his or her staff. Interestingly, head athletic trainers in the Mazerolle et al study[27] also described how their own mentors had been positive influences on their philosophies regarding work-life balance, echoing the thoughts of female athletic trainers employed in the D-I setting who felt that mentors balancing family and work responsibilities had the potential ability to shape perceptions of work-life balance and enhance retention of female athletic trainers.

As we have previously discussed, there are differing opinions regarding how culture is created within an organization, but most researchers agree that leaders of an organization and managers within a department have a relatively significant influence on establishing culture through a top-down perspective. Individuals employed in the position of supervisor are the gatekeepers to establishing a work environment that enhances a family-friendly atmosphere and ensures their employees achieve work-life balance. It is important for leaders to have a clear vision to establish values and underlying assumptions that will guide their organization.

Aside from the organizational benefits, there is research that indicates that leaders who serve as mentors can also benefit from these relationships, that it is not just the protégés who gain all the advantages. Certain benefits experienced by the mentor include improved job performance, career revitalization and success, recognition by others, a sense of personal fulfillment, increased job satisfaction, and organizational commitment.[28-30] Though this area needs to be further examined in general, it does appear that head athletic trainers who are able to mentor their employees on establishing work-life balance are able to reap the rewards of practicing what they preach.

HOW CAN AN ORGANIZATION SUPPORT MENTORING PROGRAMS?
Establish clear objectives
1. What do you expect from the mentor?
2. What do you expect from the protégé?
3. What should the mentor and protégé expect from you?
Support from the top
1. Do others within the organization model effective mentoring?
2. Garner resources if necessary.
Thoughtful matching process
1. Base on program objective.
2. Consider physical proximity.
3. Ensure consistency and transparency.
4. Include some similarity.
5. Give mentors and protégés input into the match.
High-quality mentors
1. Select mentors carefully.
2. Help protégé identify blind spots.
3. Effective mentors should push protégé to excel.
4. Effective mentors should want to mentor.
(continued)

HOW CAN AN ORGANIZATION SUPPORT MENTORING PROGRAMS? (CONTINUED)
Thank your mentors
1. Do not make mentoring a chore; show your appreciation.
2. Offer incentive to your mentors as way to show their value.
Provide training
1. Provide your definition of mentoring.
2. Ensure expectations, responsibilities, and objectives are clear.
Ongoing interactions, support, and accountability
1. Schedule meetings at regular intervals.
2. Be accessible in case mentor or protégé has any questions.
3. Be receptive and listen in case problems arise.
Evaluation
1. Collect data at regular intervals.
2. Collect qualitative and quantitative data to show potential impact.
3. Evaluation needs to tie back to objectives.

SUMMARY

This chapter serves as an introduction to the concepts of mentoring and role modeling. Every athletic training career is unique and may have different characteristics. We do know however that attrition is an issue within our profession as individuals continue to depart. One way to conceivably impede the emigration from the profession is to expose young professional athletic trainers to more role models and mentors. It also becomes imperative to expose our athletic training students to both male and female mentors that will impart the career and professional advice they need, but also mentors who can demonstrate the reality of managing work-life balance. We need to show our athletic training students that working as an athletic trainer can be a feasible and sustainable option for individuals of all life stages.

ACTIVITIES FOR REINFORCEMENT

Questions for Review

1. What is the difference between a mentor and a role model?
2. What factors make a mentoring relationship successful?
3. Why is mentoring important in the athletic training profession?
4. What are the stages or phases of a mentoring relationship?

Case Vignettes

Case #1

Eric is the program director of an athletic training program with a low certification exam pass rate. He has read a lot recently about how mentoring may increase academic and career success of individuals. There are currently 25 students enrolled in Eric's program, with 12 students each in the sophomore, junior, and senior classes. Additionally, there are more than 40 preceptors at close to 20 clinical sites. Eric would like to try to create a more formal relationship between his students and their clinical preceptors as well as potentially create peer role modeling among his students. Eric would like to bring his idea to the head of the department to encourage departmental support.

1. What might be the academic advantages of establishing a formal mentoring program?
2. Are there any benefits to organizing peer role modeling groups among the undergraduate students?
3. When speaking to the head of the department, what key points should Eric address when referring to the benefits of a mentoring program?
4. When speaking to the head of the department, what support should Eric ask for?
5. If Eric is able to establish a formal mentoring program, what characteristics should he look for when pairing mentors with mentees?

Case #2

Elizabeth, a mother of 2, has been working at a large urban secondary school for 10 years. She chose to work at this setting because she felt as though it would provide her with the best opportunity to balance a personal and professional life. During her undergraduate experience she didn't have any female preceptors that had children and graduated feeling that she could never be a mom and an athletic trainer at the collegiate level. Elizabeth is very happy in her situation at the high school but does wonder if she would have been able to succeed in another clinical setting. She has the opportunity to supervise athletic training students from a local college and makes a point to tell them (regardless of their gender) that they can work at whatever clinical setting they want and have a balanced lifestyle if they are surrounded by good people. She doesn't want her students to feel as though they missed out on any opportunities.

1. Would you describe Elizabeth as a role model or mentor to the athletic training students she supervises?
2. How did Elizabeth's preceptors negatively influence her perceptions of work-life balance during her undergraduate career?
3. Do you think having a female preceptor with children successfully managing her personal and professional roles might have affected Elizabeth's career path?
4. Do you think the gender of a role model or preceptor matters when it comes to work-life balance perceptions? What about other career influences?

Discussion Questions

1. What factors do you believe are most important in a mentoring relationship?
2. What are the most important things a person can do to foster a mentoring relationship?
3. What do you believe to be the most important outcomes of a mentoring relationship?

REFERENCES

1. Levinson D, ed. *The Seasons of a Man's Life.* New York, NY: Alfred A. Knopf Inc; 1978.
2. Kram KE. *Mentoring at Work: Developmental Relationships in Organizational Life.* Glenview, IL: Scott, Foresman and Company; 1985.
3. de Tormes Eby LT, Allen TD, Hoffman BJ, et al. An interdisciplinary meta-analysis of the potential antecedents, correlates, and consequences of protégé perceptions of mentoring. *Psychol Bull.* 2013;139(2):441-476.
4. DuBois DL, Portillo N, Rhodes JE, Silverthorn N, Valentine JC. How effective are mentoring programs for youth? A systematic assessment of the evidence. *PSPI.* 2011;12(2):57-91.
5. Butch L. Mentorship program designed to advance women in academic surgery. *Bull Am Coll Surg.* 2009;94(10):6-10.
6. Sambunjak D, Straus SE, Marusic A. Mentoring in academic medicine: a systematic review. *JAMA.* 2006;296(9):1103-1115.
7. Allen TD, Eby LT, Poteet ML, Lentz E, Lima L. Career benefits associated with mentoring for protégés: a meta-analysis. *J Appl Psychol.* 2004;89(1):127-136.
8. Ragins BR, Kram KE. The roots and meaning of mentoring. In: *The Handbook of Mentoring at Work: Theory, Research, and Practice.* Thousand Oaks, California: SAGE Publications Inc; 2007:3-15.
9. Kenny NP, Mann KV, MacLeod H. Role modeling in physicians' professional formation: reconsidering an essential but untapped educational strategy. *Acad Med.* 2003;78(12):1203-1210.
10. Reuler JB, Nardone DA. Role modeling in medical education. *West J Med.* 1994;160(4):335-337.
11. Johnson WB, Rose G, Schlosser LZ. Student-faculty mentoring: theoretical and methodological issues. In: Allen TD, Eby LT, eds. *The Blackwell Handbook of Mentoring: A Multiple Perspectives Approach.* Oxford, England: Blackwell; 2007:49-69.
12. Pitney WA, Ehlers GE, Walker SE. A descriptive study of athletic training students' perceptions of effective mentoring roles. *IJAHSP.* 2006;4(2):1-8.
13. Pitney WA, Ehlers GG. A grounded theory study of the mentoring process involved with undergraduate athletic training students. *J Athl Train.* 2004;39(4):344-351.
14. Levy LS, Sexton P, Willeford KS, et al. Clinical instructor characteristics, behaviors and skills in Allied health care settings: a literature review. *Athl Train Ed J.* 2009;4(1):8-13.
15. Laurent T, Weidner TG. Clinical instructors' and student athletic trainers' perceptions of helpful clinical instructor characteristics. *J Athl Train.* 2001;36(1):58-61.
16. Pitney WA, Ilsley P, Rintala J. The professional socialization of certified athletic trainers in the national collegiate athletic association division I context. *J Athl Train.* 2002;37(1):63-70.
17. Pitney WA. The professional socialization of certified athletic trainers in high school settings: a grounded theory investigation. *J Athl Train.* 2002;37(3):286-292.
18. Clark PG. Values in health care professional socialization: implications for geriatric education in interdisciplinary teamwork. *Gerontologist.* 1997;37(4):441-451.
19. Mazerolle SM, Gavin KE. Perceptions of female athletic trainers' on motherhood in the athletic training profession. *J Athl Train.* 2013;48(5):678-684.
20. Leonard JC, Ellsbury KE. Gender and interest in academic careers among first- and third-year residents. *Acad Med.* 1996;71(5):502-504.
21. Eason CM, Mazerolle SM, Goodman A. Motherhood and work-life balance in the Division I setting: impact of mentors on the female athletic trainer. *J Athl Train.* 2014;49(4):532-539.
22. Straus SE, Chatur F, Taylor M. Issues in the mentor-mentee relationship in academic medicine: a qualitative study. *Acad Med.* 2009;84(1):135-139.
23. Kahanov L, Eberman LE. Age, sex, and setting factors and labor force in athletic training. *J Athl Train.* 2011;46(4):424-430.
24. Acosta RV, Carpenter LJ. Women in intercollegiate sport. A longitudinal, national study, thirty-five year update, 1977-2012. 2012.
25. Mazerolle SM, Borland JF, Burton LJ. The professional socialization of collegiate female athletic trainers: navigating experiences of gender bias. *J Athl Train.* 2012;47(6):694-703.
26. Clines SH, Mazerolle SM, Eason CM, Pitney WA. Perceptions of support networks during the graduate assistant athletic trainer experience. *J Athl Train.* 2014. In press.
27. Mazerolle SM, Goodman A, Pitney WA. Achieving work-life balance in the national collegiate athletic association division I setting, part I: the role of the head athletic trainer. *J Athl Train.* 2015;50(1):82-88.
28. Allen TD, Poteet ML, Burroughs SM. The mentor's perspective: a qualitative inquiry and future research agenda. *J Voc Behav.* 1997;51:70-89.
29. Bozionelos N. Mentoring provided: relation to mentor's career success, personality, and mentoring received. *J Voc Behav.* 2004;64:24-46.
30. Eby LT, Durley JR, Carr SE, Ragins BR. The relationship between short-term mentoring benefits and long-term mentoring outcomes. *J Voc Behav.* 2006;69:424-444.

11

Healthy Habits and Choices for Athletic Trainers

Christianne M. Eason, MS, ATC

OBJECTIVES

After reading this chapter, the reader will be able to do the following:
1. Conceptualize the meaning of "healthy lifestyle" and all of its components.
2. Explain why physical activity and healthy eating habits are positive components of a healthy lifestyle.
3. Understand the relationship between stress and job satisfaction.
4. Recognize the negative effects stress can have on the body.
5. Critique their own lifestyles and assess their level of healthy behaviors.

INTRODUCTION

The word *health* comes from *hale*, which means wholeness, being whole sound or well. The World Health Organization defines health as "a state of complete physical, mental, and social well-being and not merely the absence of disease or infirmity."[1] Health really is the ability to achieve individual potential in all 5 dimensions including physical, emotional, social, mental, spiritual, and environmental. Wellness on the other hand is the ability to achieve the highest level of health possible in each dimension. Table 11-1 provides a definition for each of the 6 dimensions of health.

Currently, very little research exists on the health habits of athletic trainers. One recent study indicated that less than half of the certified athletic trainers in the study met the minimum guidelines for exercise as set forth by the American College of Sports Medicine (ACSM).[2] There are many suggestions on how organizations may help to increase health behaviors among their employees and include: promote preventative care (vaccines), encourage exercise, emphasize education, on-site health clinics, implement incentive programs, provide healthy food options, be

Mazerolle SM, Pitney WA.
Workplace Concepts for Athletic Trainers (pp 179-190).
© 2016 Taylor & Francis Group.

TABLE 11-1
DIMENSIONS OF HEALTH

DIMENSION OF HEALTH	DEFINITION
Physical	Body size and functioning
Social	Productive interactions with others and personal network
Mental	The ability to make responsible decisions and think clearly
Emotional	The ability to express emotions and maintain self-confidence
Environmental	An appreciation of the external environment around you
Spiritual	Having a sense of purpose and meaning to your life

mindful of mental health, and recommend behavioral resources.[3] While there are currently no studies examining how physical activity levels are associated with burnout, a 1984 study did find a positive correlation between stress and burnout.[4] With concerns related to retention within the field of athletic training and our knowledge of how burnout may affect career longevity,[5,6] the concept of healthy behaviors, specifically the ability to manage life stress, becomes a crucial piece to the retention discussion. Athletic trainers are health professionals and should be considered healthy behavior role models because it is assumed that they will apply their education and professional knowledge to their own lives and lifestyles.

This unfortunately is not always the case, as many athletic trainers find it hard to balance time between their work lives and their personal lives. Often athletic trainers put the needs of others ahead of their own. Fatigue and need for recovery may mean that athletic trainers find it difficult to overcome conceivable barriers that stand in the way of achieving a healthy lifestyle. This is especially true of behaviors that actively promote health, such as healthy eating and physical activity, which typically require more organization, effort, and planning than the more negative health behaviors. An understanding of spillover lets us know that work has the potential to impact non-work life in terms of time, strain, and behavior.[7] For example, work may affect the time individuals have for family and friends, which may cause strain even when they are at home, which in turn influences their behavior at home. Fatigue from work may lead to limited resources for other roles and activities, such as exercise. Each of these aspects of spillover has the ability to influence the extent to which individuals engage in healthy and unhealthy behaviors. Individuals who are inactive at work may be physically inactive in their personal lives. Additionally, overworked individuals may lack the time to exercise and may place less importance on healthy behaviors if they are experiencing stress at work. Conversely, it is possible that healthy behaviors are used as methods of coping. In recent years, with a growing interest in health psychology and work-life balance, there is a growing interest in how health behaviors may affect job outcomes and vice versa.

The purpose of this chapter is to present information on healthy behaviors (specifically healthy eating and physical activity), discuss the impact of stress and how it may relate to job satisfaction, and present what we know about athletic trainers and healthy behaviors. The goal is that athletic trainers reading this chapter will be reminded of the importance of making their health a priority and to reinforce the effort that many are already making.

HEALTHY EATING

Food—the plants and animals we consume
Nutrition—the scientific study of food and how food nourishes the body and influences health

Proper nutrition can help us improve our weight, prevent certain diseases, achieve and maintain healthy weight, and maintain our energy and vitality. The study of nutrition encompasses how we consume, metabolize, digest, and store nutrients and how those nutrients affect our bodies. It also studies factors that influence our eating patterns and makes recommendations about the amount we should eat of each type of food. As athletic trainers, nutrition is something we cover in our undergraduate curriculum and pass along to the athletes that we work with. Additionally, it is common for athletic trainers to work with registered dieticians to enhance the health of athletes. It is important that we are practicing what we preach so to speak and that we take in the proper nutrition for our own needs as nutrition is one of several factors contributing to wellness. Tables 11-2 through 11-4 provide a quick visual review of some important nutritional concepts.

Good nutrition and eating habits are associated with lower stress levels and better overall health.[8] While links between stress stemming from the workplace and eating have been largely overlooked by the research, there is a large amount of literature examining general stress-induced eating. Conner and Armitage[9] reported that most research looking into the general effects of stress reported an increase in food intake, though the majority of the studies focus on animal research, laboratory studies, or stress from exams. There is some conflicting evidence as Stone and Brownell[10] found that stress led to reduced eating among individuals of normal weight. Individual differences in responses to stress are likely the explanation for such conflicting results.

PHYSICAL ACTIVITY

Engaging in regular exercise and reducing sedentary behavior is necessary for the health of adults.[11] Numerous studies have shown that physical activity has widespread benefits on health and disease prevention. Evidence supporting the physical and mental health benefits of physical activity and exercise continue to amass at an augmented rate. In their review of the literature, Penedo and Dahn[12] found that regular and moderate physical activity can decrease risk of coronary heart disease, obesity, cancer, cardiovascular disease, and arthritis. Additionally, they reported that engaging in regular physical activity can also benefit emotional well-being.

Calculate your maximum heart rate (MHR):
Moderate intensity is a heart rate from 50% to 70% of MHR.
Vigorous intensity is a heart rate from 70% to 85% of MHR.

Each component of physical fitness conceivably affects some aspect of health. There are substantial quantitative data on the relationships between fitness and health, with most data focusing on body composition and cardiorespiratory fitness. Higher levels of cardiorespiratory fitness and muscular fitness are each associated with lower risks for poorer health.[13,14]

TABLE 11-2
CALORIES PER GRAM OF VARIOUS NUTRIENTS

NUTRIENT	KCAL PER GRAM
Carbohydrates	4
Alcohol	7
Fats	9
Protein	4

TABLE 11-3
OVERVIEW OF VITAMINS

	FAT-SOLUBLE VITAMINS	WATER-SOLUBLE VITAMINS
Type	Vitamin A, D, E, and K	Vitamin C, the B vitamins
Storage in the body	Able to store in adipose tissue	Cannot store large amounts
Consumption requirements	Do not need to consume RDAs every day	Need to consume RDAs on daily or weekly basis
Dietary sources	Found in variety of fat-containing foods: meats, dairy, oils, nuts, seeds	Abundant in many foods: whole grains, fruits, vegetables, meats, dairy
Toxicities	More likely due to storage capabilities. Megadosing is possible	Rarely occurs when consumed in diet. Can acquire toxic levels through supplements
Deficiencies	Deficiencies may sometimes develop (especially in people with diseases that prevent normal absorption of fat or those who consume little fat)	Symptoms of deficiency and disease can result rather quickly because of lack of storage

RDA: recommended daily allowance.

TABLE 11-4
OVERVIEW OF MINERALS

TYPE	NAMES	CHARACTERISTICS
Major minerals	Calcium, phosphorous, sodium, potassium, chloride, magnesium, sulfur	Needed in amounts > 100 mg/d Amount present in the human body is > 5 g
Trace minerals	Iron, zinc, copper, manganese, fluoride, chromium, molybdenum, selenium, iodine	Needed in amounts < 100 mg/d Amount present in the human body is < 5 g

TABLE 11-5 OVERCOMING OBSTACLES TO PHYSICAL ACTIVITY[41]	
OBSTACLES	**POSSIBLE SOLUTIONS**
Lack of time	Identify available time slots. Identify at least 3 30-minute time slots you could use for physical activity.
	Add physical activity to your daily routine. (Walk or ride your bike to work or shopping, walk the dog, exercise while you watch TV, park farther away from your destination, etc).
	Select activities requiring minimal time, such as walking, jogging, or stair climbing.
Social influence	Explain the importance of physical activity to friends and family. Ask them to support your efforts.
	Invite friends and family to exercise with you.
	Develop new friendships with physically active people.
Lack of motivation or energy	Convince yourself that if you give it a chance, physical activity will increase your energy level; then, try it.
	Invite a friend to exercise with you on a regular basis.
	Join an exercise group or class.
Lack of resources	Select activities that require minimal facilities or equipment, such as walking, jogging, jumping rope, or calisthenics.
	Identify inexpensive, convenient resources available in your community (community education programs, park and recreation programs, worksite programs, etc).

Though the health benefits make it clear that physical activity should be a part of any healthy lifestyle, it can often be challenging to incorporate it into daily life. Brownson et al[15a] conducted a study on 1818 United States adults and found that the 4 most commonly reported barriers to exercise were lack of time, feeling too tired, already getting enough exercise at work, and having no motivation to exercise. While this study was not specific to athletic trainers, there are connections that can be made as to why athletic trainers may not be meeting ACSM exercise guidelines. Table 11-5 illustrates some possible solutions to overcoming obstacles to physical activity.

STRESS AND ITS IMPACT

The physical and mental impacts of stress have long been established. In the most basic terms, stress is the mental and physical response of our bodies to the changes and challenges in our lives. A stressor is any physical, social, or psychological condition or event that causes our bodies to adjust to the situation. A stressor that causes negative effects in the body is referred to as *distress* while a stressor that causes positive effects on the body is referred to as *eustress*. An example of eustress would be physical activity because it causes the body to adjust to changes but results in positive health benefits. When we think of stress, we do, however, typically think of distress. Distress may contribute to mental disability and emotional dysfunction that could manifest in the following ways:

- Lost work productivity
- Difficulties in relationships
- Misuse of drugs and other substances
- Displaced anger

Distress has also been shown to affect individuals in multiple physical ways. Highly stressed individuals are at greater risk for the following:

- Cardiovascular disease: Stress accounts for approximately 30% of the attributable risk of myocardial infarction.[15b]

- Impaired immunity: Psychoneuroimmunology analyzes the relationship between the mind's response to stress and the immune system's ability to function effectively.

- Diabetes: One of the major functions of stress hormones (epinephrine and cortisol) is to raise blood sugar.

- Obesity: Higher levels of stress increase the amount of cortisol released in the body, causing weight gain.

Other physical manifestations of stress include the following:

- Hand tremors and sweaty hands and feet
- Diarrhea, gassiness, constipation, and an increased urge to urinate
- Stomachache, nausea, "butterflies"
- Tightness in chest, heart pounding, palpitations
- Backache, muscle cramps, neck stiffness
- Dry mouth, jaw pain, grinding teeth
- Blushing, oily skin
- Tension headaches, migraines, dizziness

There is evidence to suggest that maintaining a healthy lifestyle during distressing times may reduce some of the negative effects of stress on the body and the accelerated aging that comes with it.[16] Researchers examined whether exercising, sleeping well, and a healthy diet could reduce the effects of stress and aging at the cellular level among 239 women, ages 50 to 65.[16] To determine the effect of stress on the cells, researchers measured the length of telomeres, which are protective "caps" at the end of chromosomes. Each time a cell divides, telomeres shorten slightly and divide, and the length is believed to be a measurement of a cell's aging. Their results showed that major stressful life events were linked to a shortening of the telomeres, but that healthy behaviors had a mitigating influence. That is, women who engaged in more healthful behaviors experienced a smaller decline in telomere length for each stressful event that occurred during the year of the study. Additionally, they found that women who ate poorly, exercised less, and slept less had more telomere shortening, even with comparable levels of stress. This study highlights the importance of promoting healthy living, particularly under times of stress.

While the physical manifestations of stress are well established in the literature, the relationship between stress and job satisfaction is not as well understood. The notion of job satisfaction influencing stress and vice versa is not a contemporary idea. A 1989 study conducted among nurses found that level of dissatisfaction with work environment significantly predicts the degree of stress experienced.[17] The mechanism for this relationship comes from the work-stress literature, as described in the stress-control model,[18] which links job satisfaction and stress outcomes. Additionally, employee stress and dissatisfaction at work can become the catalysts for negative health outcomes.[19]

In recent years a number of studies have begun to examine the extent to which work stress predicts health behavior.[18,20-23] In these studies, however, it is not possible to distinguish the effects of work stressors and general life stressors. Nonetheless, when employee samples are used it is probable that their stress perceptions do encompass work issues. Studies examining employees typically show that stress has a negative effect on a wide range of health behaviors. One study found that high perceptions of stress were associated with less frequent exercise, higher-fat diets, and more cigarette smoking.[21] Research that focuses specifically on the effects of work stress on health behavior often draw on the job strain model, which suggests that strain is predicted by a combination of job demands and job control.[18,23] The model suggests 4 types of job based on different combinations of control and demands. A "high-strain" job is high in demand but low in control and is likely to predispose employees to poor physical and psychological well-being. A "low-strain" job is a combination of control high and low in demand. The "active" job is high in demand and control, and the "passive" job is low both in control and demand. The active job may lead individuals to develop barriers at work and at home, while the passive job may lead to learned helplessness and reduced activity. This theoretical framework suggests that high-strain jobs may lead to increased stress-relieving behaviors such as smoking or drinking and may reduce the health behaviors of healthy eating and exercise. Active jobs may lead to similarly active lifestyles, while passive jobs may lead to passive lifestyles.

Worksite health promotion programs have made an attempt to confront this issue by implementing stress-management programs. However, in a critical review of stress-management programs, no evidence was found that these pre-packaged stress-management programs are effectively implemented in organizations.[24] A later review also found that stress-management programs were not consistently beneficial to employees.[25] The most consistent benefit to employees appears to be reducing subjective feelings of emotional distress. These findings highlight the importance of managing stress within the organization, but indicate that programs established by the organization may not be the most beneficial way to manage stress. Perhaps the focus should be on skills that can be taught in order to help manage or alleviate stress.[26]

Recognizing the importance between the healthy lifestyle and stress relationship, the American Heart Association recently posted a list of 10 positive healthy habits individuals may want to develop in order to protect themselves from the harmful effects of stress:[27]

- **Use family and friend support networks:** A regular dose of friendship is great medicine. Being able to share emotions and have others share with you is a great way to relieve stress.

- **Take part in regular physical activity:** Regular physical activity may help relieve mental and physical tension. Physically active adults have lower incidence of depression and loss of mental function.

- **Laugh often:** Don't be afraid to laugh out loud at something that you find funny. Laughter makes us feel good.

- **Embrace things you are able to change:** It is never too late to learn a new skill or set a new goal. This applies for personal and work roles.

- **Slow down:** Allow enough time to get the most important things accomplished without having to rush.

- **Give up bad habits:** Blood pressure may be increased through too much alcohol, caffeine, or cigarettes. Take enjoyment in the things you enjoy, but do so in moderation. If you smoke, quit.

- **Get plenty of rest:** Make it a goal to get 6 to 8 hours of sleep each night.

- **Get organized:** Use "to-do" lists and prioritize tasks.

- **Practice giving back:** While time can be at a premium, volunteer when you can. Helping others can make you feel good and appreciate the things you have.

- **Try not to worry:** Though easier said than done, the world won't end if your kitchen is messy.

HEALTH BEHAVIORS AND JOB SATISFACTION

Generally, people who are satisfied with their jobs have been shown to be happier both mentally[28] and physically.[29] What is unclear, however, is the direction of the relationship between health and job satisfaction. In other words, does job satisfaction facilitate health, or does health facilitate job satisfaction? While not able to definitively state a relationship one way or the other, Peterson and Dunnagan[22] did find that demographic variables are better able to discern job satisfaction than health behaviors. This indicates that there is merit in the belief that job satisfaction promotes health, but that healthy behaviors do not automatically promote job satisfaction. These findings are supported by Karasek,[18] who found job factors to be the next strongest set of predictors of health and illness after age.

There are those out there that suggest workplace health promotion programs will increase employees' job satisfaction, but the research is mixed. With recent focus on obesity issues in this country, workplace health promotion has become more popular within American organizations. Health promotion programs are typically composed of fitness classes, nutrition and weight management programs, stress management classes, and smoking cessation interventions. An online search would reveal things such as desk treadmills, which supposedly allow employees to be active during the workday while still being productive. A review of literature from the mid-1990s reported that formal measures of job satisfaction have shown little difference between fitness program participants and control groups, but that workers generally maintain a belief that participation in the programs will improve their satisfaction and morale within their organization.[30] A study by Peterson and Dunnagan[22] assessed the impact of participation in a health promotion program and engagement in healthy behaviors on job satisfaction among full-time university employees. They found significant differences in job satisfaction based on regular exercise behavior but no differences in job satisfaction based on health promotion programs at work. The results suggest that health promotion programs do not significantly affect job satisfaction, but involvement in regular physical activity may.

While health promotion programs are often used by organizations, there is evidence to suggest that the psychosocial environment may be more predictive of job satisfaction and healthy behaviors of employees. The psychosocial environment refers to the culture and climate of the organization. Some examples of psychosocial workplace environments include respect for work-life balance, policies in place to recognize and reward good performance, valuing the wellness of employees, zero tolerance for harassment, bullying, and discrimination, and encouraging employee feedback. Bosma et al[19] conducted a large-scale study to investigate occupational, lifestyle, and social influences on health in a civil service population. Their results suggested that the psychosocial environment in the workplace is an excellent venue for understanding the relationship between health and work outcomes. This is supported by Stansfeld et al,[31] who found that positive work characteristics in civil servants were found to be related to greater overall well-being and lower levels of psychiatric disorder.

Using the same data set, Marmot et al[32] found that psychosocial factors in the work environment, such as job characteristics, satisfaction, and design, were important in the etiology of coronary heart disease. This link between coronary heart disease and work was found to be associated with low job control. The recommendation of the authors was that greater attention to work environment design may be one important way to reduce negative health outcomes. In support of this, North et al[33] reported that psychosocial work environment is a strong predictor of absences from sickness. They concluded that increased levels of support and control at work may have beneficial effects in regards to health and well-being of employees and increased productivity.

The premise of worksite health promotion programs, though popular, do not necessarily improve health, engagement in healthy behaviors, or increase job satisfaction. There is, however, evidence to indicate that an alternative relationship exists between health and job satisfaction.

That is, increased job satisfaction through changes in the organization and psychosocial constructs of the work environment may markedly improve health outcomes. Specifically, that means employee health may be improved through the adoption of healthy lifestyle practices and through organizational promotion of positive psychosocial factors in the workplace. Instead of attempting to increase job satisfaction through promoting healthy lifestyles, organizational leaders should be thinking of how to improve health through job satisfaction.

HEALTHY BEHAVIORS, WORK-LIFE BALANCE, AND ATHLETIC TRAINING

Anecdotally, with issues related to work-life balance, it would seem as though athletic trainers have a difficult time finding the time for exercise and to prepare healthy food options for themselves. There is, however, very little known about the health habits of athletic trainers. In fact minimal research exists regarding the physical activity of athletic trainers. We do know that inflexibility and lack of control over schedules and hours worked and travel are causes of discord between athletic trainers' work and personal lives.[34] Knowing that, it would not be hard to speculate that some athletic trainers may feel as though they do not have enough time to take care of themselves.

A concern with not being able to maintain work-life balance is always the development of burnout. Athletic trainers, like many other health care professionals, are susceptible to burnout due to their prolonged exposure to stressful job settings and stressors.[35] In addition to the potential exposure for burnout, athletic trainers are likely to have decreased perceptions of their own wellness.[35] Health is not defined solely as a lack of illness, but as mental, emotional, social, and physical well-being.[1] Because of burnout's potential to drastically affect the mental and physical health of those experiencing the phenomenon, it will affect the health and wellness of an individual. Some of the common health-related symptoms of burnout include anxiety, depression, headache, and poor appetite.[36] Job-related symptoms of burnout include low productivity and increased absenteeism.[36] Among the athletic training population, long work hours and high levels of stress may lead to job burnout and subsequently result in a decline in quality of life and health.[37]

While the literature examining healthy behaviors in athletic training is limited, there are a few recent studies that have examined the concept. A recent study using the Perceived Wellness Survey reported that male and female athletic trainers did not differ in overall scores of perceived wellness, but men did report greater emotional but lower social well-being than women.[35] While perceived wellness and health and fitness habits should not be compared directly, Groth et al[2] found that decreased physical activity in athletic trainers was associated with decreased perceived wellness scores in males and females. They found that only 41% of athletic trainers met the ACSM guidelines for exercise.[2] In terms of nutritional habits, Groth et al[2] reported that athletic trainers were not following nutritional recommendations. No athletic trainers in their study met the daily reference intake for all 5 food groups during a typical week. However, their alcohol and tobacco consumption was less comparable to the general population. Of their sample, 47% of the females were considered overweight or obese and 74% of the males were considered overweight or obese according to body mass index measurements.[2] Cuppett and Latin[38] reported that the physical activity of athletic trainers varied by employment setting and that women scored higher than men in overall daily activity. This could explain the higher body mass index measurements observed by Groth et al.[2]

There is some indication that engaging in healthy behaviors, specifically physical activity, may actually serve as a strategy to manage job stress and promote work-life balance. A recent study by Mazerolle et al[34] found that exercise is one strategy that female athletic trainers working in the Division I (D-I) setting use to balance their work and personal lives. Many of the female athletic trainers in their study found it important to work out and expressed that it gave them the personal time they needed to de-stress and rejuvenate. Other studies within athletic training have found that finding time to get away is an important attribute in creating work-life balance,[39] and exercise has been found to be a stress reduction strategy.[40]

SUMMARY

As health care providers, athletic trainers should be role models for healthy behaviors. While more research is needed in this area, we recommend that athletic trainers eat a healthy diet, participate in physical activity regularly, and get plenty of sleep in order to establish a better work-life balance. While it may seem that the time it takes to do these things may increase the imbalance, the reality is that these activities may help reduce the negative effects of stress. It is important to prioritize yourself and limit the distress in your life.

ACTIVITIES FOR REINFORCEMENT

Questions for Review

1. What is meant by the phrase *healthy lifestyle*?
2. What are the dimensions of health that one must attend to in order to live a healthy lifestyle?
3. What are the negative effects of stress on one's body?
4. What is the relationship between stress and job satisfaction?

Case Vignette

Case #1

Megan has been working as an assistant athletic trainer at a small D-I college for 3 years. She enjoys her job, but lately feels like she has no time for herself. When she was in college she made exercise a priority, though eating healthy in the dorms was always a challenge. Lately she feels like the most exercise she gets is walking to the practice fields instead of taking the golf cart. This lack of exercise in her life is really starting to bother her and is becoming a source of stress. She also feels that with the hectic practice schedule there is no time to go food shopping so she is constantly grabbing take-out on her way home.

1. If Megan continues to feel stressed regarding her lack of exercise, how might the stress manifest itself physically, mentally, and in relation to her job performance?
2. What advice would you give Megan to incorporate more physical activity into her life?
3. Would you describe the athletic training profession as a "high-strain," "low-strain," "active" or "passive" job? Does your answer depend on the clinical setting? Why or why not?
4. If you were a head athletic trainer, how could you help ensure that the members of the sports medicine staff had adequate time to achieve a healthy lifestyle? Do you believe this is the responsibility of the head athletic trainer?

Discussion Questions

1. What component of a healthy lifestyle do you believe is most important? Explain.

2. What do you believe is the most common source of stress for athletic trainers in the college and secondary school environment?

3. What advice would you give to an athletic trainer to help him or her reduce stress?

REFERENCES

1. World Health Organization. *Constitution of the World Health Organization*. New York, NY: World Health Organization; 1946.
2. Groth JJ, Ayers SF, Miller MG, Arbogast WD. Self-reported health and fitness habits of certified athletic trainers. *J Athl Train*. 2008;43(6):617-623.
3. Lastowka L. 8 ways to promote wellness in the workplace. http://www.ncbi.nlm.nih.gov/pmc/articles/PMC 3655756/. Updated 2014. Accessed October 1, 2014.
4. Etzion D. Moderating effect of social support on the stress-burnout relationship. *Appl Psychol*. 1984;69(4):615-622.
5. Jourdain G, Chênevert D. Job demands-resources, burnout and intention to leave the nursing profession: a questionnaire survey. *Int J Nurs Stud*. 2010;47(6):709-722.
6. Hunt V. Dangerous dedication: burnout a risk in profession. *NATA News*. 2000;November:8-10.
7. Staines G. Spillover versus compensation: a review of the literature on the relationship between work and nonwork. *Hum Relat*. 1980;2(33):111-129.
8. Baum A, Posluszny D. Health psychology: mapping biobehavioral contributions to health and illness. *Annu Rev Psychol*. 1999;50:137-163.
9. Conner C, Armitage CJ. *The Social Psychology of Food*. 1st ed. Philadelphia, PA: Open University Press; 2002.
10. Stone AA, Brownell KD. The stress-eating paradox: multiple daily measurements in adult males and females. *Psychol Health*. 1994;9(6):425-436.
11. Garber CE, Blissmer B, Deschenes MR, et al. American College of Sports Medicine position stand. Quantity and quality of exercise for developing and maintaining cardiorespiratory, musculoskeletal, and neuromotor fitness in apparently healthy adults: guidance for prescribing exercise. *Med Sci Sport Exer*. 2011;43(7):1334-1359.
12. Penedo FJ, Dahn JR. Exercise and well-being: a review of mental and physical health benefits associated with physical activity. *Curr Opin Psychiatry*. 2005;18(2):189-193.
13. Barlow CE, LaMonte MJ, Fitzgerald SJ, Kampert JB, Perrin JL, Blair SN. Cardiorespiratory fitness is an independent predictor of hypertension incidence among initially normotensive healthy women. *Am J Epid*. 2006;163(2):142-150.
14. Blair SN, Cheng Y, Holder JS. Is physical activity or physical fitness more important in defining health benefits? *Med Sci Sports Exerc*. 2001;33(Suppl 6):S379-S399.
15a. Brownson RC, Baker EA, Housemann RA, Brennan LK, Bacak SJ. Environmental and policy determinants of physical activity in the United States. *Am J Public Health*. 2001;91(12):1995-2003.
15b. Yusuf S, Hawken S, Ounpuu S, et al. Effect of potentially modifiable risk factors associated with myocardial infarction in 52 countries (the INTERHEART study): case-control study. *Lancet*. 2004;364:937-952.
16. Puterman E, Lin J, Krauss J, Blackburn EH, Epel ES. Determinants of telomere attrition over 1 year in healthy older women: stress and health behaviors matte. *Mol Psychiatry*. 2015;20(4):528-535.
17. Hipwell AE, Tyler PA, Wilson CM. Sources of stress and dissatisfaction among nurses in four hospital environments. *Br J Med Psychol*. 1989;62(71):79.
18. Karasek R. Lower health risk with increased job control among white collar workers. *J Organ Behav*. 1990; 11:171-185.
19. Bosma H, Marmot MG, Hemingway H, Brunner E, Stansfeld SA. Low job control and risk of coronary heart disease in Whitehall II (prospective cohort) study. *BMJ*. 1997;314(7080):558-565.
20. Jones F, Kinman G, Payne N. Work-stress and health behaviors: A work-life balance issue. In: Jones F, Burke RJ, Westman M, eds. *Work-Life Balance: A Psychological Perspective*. New York, NY: Psychology Press; 2012: 185-216.
21. Ng DM, Jeffrey RW. Relationships between perceived stress and health behaviors in a sample of working adults. *Health Psychol*. 2003;22(6):638-642.
22. Peterson M, Dunnagan T. Analysis of a worksite health promotion program's impact on job satisfaction. *J Occup Env Med*. 1998;40(11):973-979.
23. Karasek RA. Job demands, job decision latitude, and mental strain: implications for job redesign. *Admin Sci Quart*. 1979;24(2):285-308.

24. Pelletier KR, Lutz R. Healthy people-healthy business: a critical review of stress management programs in the workplace. *Am J Health Promot.* 1988;2:5-19.

25. Murphy L. Stress management in work settings: a critical review of the health effects. *Am J Health Promot.* 1996;11:112-135.

26. Herzberg F. One more time: how do you motivate employees? *Harv Bus Rev.* 1987:109-120.

27. American Heart Association. Fight stress with healthy habits. http://www.heart.org/HEARTORG/Getting Healthy/StressManagement/FightStressWithHealthyHabits/Fight-Stress-with-Healthy-Habits_UCM_307992 _Article.jsp. Updated June 12, 2014. Accessed July 28, 2014.

28. Ilgen DR. Health issues at work: opportunities for industrial/organizational psychology. *Am Psychol.* 1990;45 :252-261.

29. Spector PE, Jex SM. Relations of job characteristics from multiple data sources with employee affect, absence, turnover intentions and health. *J Appl Psychol.* 1991;76:46-53.

30. Shephard RJ. Worksite health promotion and productivity. In: Kaman RL, ed. *Worksite Health Promotion Economics: Consensus and Analysis.* Champaign, IL: Human Kinetics; 1995:147-173.

31. Stansfeld SA, North FM, White I, Marmot M. Work characteristics and psychiatric disorder in civil servants in London. *J Epidemiol Community Health.* 1995;49(1):48-53.

32. Marmot MG, Bosma H, Hemingway H, Brunner E, Stansfeld S. Contribution of job control and other risk factors to social variations in coronary heart disease incidence. *Lancet.* 1997;350:235-239.

33. North FM, Syme L, Feeney A, Shipley M, Marmot M. Psychosocial work environment and sickness absence among British civil servants: the Whitehall II study. *Am J Pub Health.* 1996;86:332-340.

34. Mazerolle SM, Ferraro EM, Eason CM, Goodman A. Factors and strategies that contribute to work-life balance of female athletic trainers employed in the NCAA Division I setting. *Athl Train Sprt Health Care.* 2013;5(5):211-222.

35. Naugle KE, Behar-Horenstein LS, Dodd VJ, Tillman MD, Borsa PA. Perceptions of wellness and burnout among certified athletic trainers: sex differences. *J Athl Train.* 2013;48(3):424-430.

36. Kania ML, Meyer BB, Ebersole KT. Personal and environmental characteristics predicting burnout among certified athletic trainers at National Collegiate Athletic Association institutions. *J Athl Train.* 2009;44(1):58-66.

37. Hendrix AE, Acevedo EO, Hebert E. An examination of stress and burnout in certified athletic trainers at Division I-A universities. *J Athl Train.* 2000;35(2):139-144.

38. Cuppett M, Latin RW. A survey of physical activity levels of certified athletic trainers. *J Athl Train.* 2002; 37(3):281-285.

39. Mazerolle SM, Pitney WA, Goodman A. Strategies for athletic trainers to find a balanced lifestyle across clinical setting. *Int J Athl Ther Train.* 2012;17(3):7-14.

40. Dixon MA, Bruening JE. Perspectives on work-family conflict in sport: an integrative approach. *Sport Manag Rev.* 2005;8:227-254.

41. Centers for Disease Control and Prevention. Overcoming barriers to physical activity. http://www.cdc.gov/ physicalactivity/everyone/getactive/barriers.html. Updated February 16, 2011. Accessed July 28, 2014.

Principles of Effective Communication for Athletic Trainers

Stacy E. Walker, PhD, ATC

OBJECTIVES

After reading this chapter, the reader will be able to do the following:

1. Appreciate the importance of effective communication.
2. Use basic communication skills.
3. Identify the communication skills needed to provide patient-centered care.
4. Engage in communication with other health care providers.
5. Employ basic strategies to resolve conflict in the workplace.

INTRODUCTION

Regardless of where an athletic trainer is employed, he or she must have good communication skills. Effective communication is an essential skill for all health care providers. Demonstrating effective communication skills is part of professionalism, which is one of the foundational behaviors of professional practice for athletic trainers.[1] A respect for others and a commitment to equality regardless of social, cultural, or ethnic background is essential for effective communication.[2] Competent health care providers recognize that quality of communication between patient and clinician is critical and has the power to also hurt as well as heal.[3] For example, patients who are dissatisfied with the communication with their health care provider report decreased adherence to their medication.[4] Communication is effective when together patients and health care providers exchange information while enabling patients to actively participate in their care.[5] In order for this process to be effective, communication between the clinician and patient must be a 2-way process whereby the patients understand the information provided by the clinician and the clinicians integrate the information gleaned from their patient into plans of care.[5] Health care practice includes

Mazerolle SM, Pitney WA.
Workplace Concepts for Athletic Trainers (pp 191-203).
© 2016 Taylor & Francis Group.

the sensitivity to know what information should be provided to clients/patients but also how that information should be delivered.[3]

Communicating a home exercise program to a patient is a perfect example of the importance of communication. Imagine a patient who has left the hospital with home exercise instructions following a total knee replacement. Without proper patient education, the patient might arrive back home and wonder which specific exercises to do, how often to do them, and how vigorously. This uncertainty can affect recovery and patient outcomes. Performing too little exercise could lead to muscle atrophy and joint stiffness whereas too much exercise could result in being painful, sore, and swollen.

In addition to patients, athletic trainers interact daily with other health care providers, coworkers, athletic directors, parents, and administrators. Imagine a situation in which an athletic trainer fails to use direct language when discussing an injury report and return-to-play status of an athlete. Vague language such as "He is getting better" or "I think she could make it through a practice" does not communicate the return-to-play status. If the coach interprets these statements as positive, meaning the athlete can return to play, yet the athletic trainer meant "they are improving but they are not ready," this could prove problematic for many reasons. First, the coach now has lost some trust in what the athlete trainer says. Second, the athlete could return to play earlier than he or she should and this could lead to further injury. One characteristic of a quality athletic trainer is communication.[6] Athletic trainers must be able to discuss medical and work-related information and interact with a wide variety of individuals in a manner they can understand.[6] Too much medical jargon could confuse a parent and/or administrator as they may not be familiar with such medical terms. However, it is professional to use medical jargon when discussing patient care decisions such as return to play with other health care providers. The athletic trainer must be able to collaboratively discuss and plan patient care decisions with other health care providers. In working collaboratively with other health care professionals, athletic trainers must communicate in a responsible manner that supports a team approach to the treatment and management of their patients.[7] In addition to other health care providers, athletic trainers communicate with coworkers, administrators, and athletic directors on a variety of issues such as medical insurance, budgetary issues, and return-to-play decisions.

This chapter is designed to provide basic communication information and strategies for clear and effective interactions with patients, other health care providers, and coworkers, regardless of your workplace setting. The content is designed to assist you in communicating effectively to avoid miscommunications that could adversely affect your patients as well as your relationships with patients, coworkers, administrators, and athletic directors. Armed with other valuable information in this textbook, you also should be equipped with the communication skills to prevent and/or address issues such as workplace discrimination, workplace bullying, and managing work-life balance issues.

COMMUNICATION

For the purposes of this chapter, communication refers to transferring information from one person to the other. This section will focus on some basic communication skills for athletic trainers. All of these skills can be used when communicating with patients, coworkers, and other health care providers. It's important to remember that both verbal and nonverbal communication are often communicated and interpreted together. When we verbally communicate with someone we speak to them either in person or through some other media such as a phone or computer. Nonverbal communication is wordless information such as body language (eg, facial expressions, gestures, eye movement), tone of voice, and body posturing. You communicate verbally and nonverbally constantly with your peers, preceptors, and patients. Regardless of who you are communicating with, it is important to be cognizant of some basic communication skills.

> It's important to remember that both verbal and nonverbal communication are often communicated and interpreted together. When we verbally communicate with someone, we speak either in person or through some other media such as a phone or computer.

Basic Communication Skills

Nonverbal Communication

An important part of communication is nonverbal such as your body language, tone of voice, and eye contact. Most individuals already possess a wealth of knowledge and experience in nonverbal communication from everyday interactions.[8] Nonverbal communication can be planned or can be subconscious or spontaneous. For example, upon entering a room a person could consciously smile and present a warm greeting. Other times nonverbal communication is subconscious and not planned such as when we are surprised by someone or something that has been said. You want to portray nonverbal communication that is consistent with your intent. For example, if you say "I am listening" but are faced away from a person looking at a computer screen or phone and avoiding eye contact, that individual will not feel you are listening.

> The most important information exchanged during conflicts and arguments is often communicated nonverbally. Nonverbal communication is conveyed by emotionally driven facial expressions, posture, gesture, pace, tone, and intensity of voice.

Your body position is important to consider when interacting with an individual. Open body posturing consisting of either standing or sitting and leaving the trunk and body open conveys openness and willingness. On the other hand, crossing the arms can be interpreted as defensiveness or resistance. In addition to open body posturing, you want to at times lean forward toward the other person to convey you are listening. Nodding and warm facial expressions are other positive methods of nonverbal communication. A tone of voice that is a relaxed tone and soft volume will be interpreted quite differently from a high-pitched, loud tone. Another consideration is the location where the communication occurs. Individuals can react differently to what is being communicated based on location.[9] Depending on the need for the communication, the athletic training clinic may be appropriate or if privacy is needed a physician's examination room or an office could be used. While this might not seem like nonverbal communication, planning the location sets the tone for the conversation. For example, if a patient needs to discuss a sensitive issue such as feeling depressed, he or she will feel safe speaking with you in a private location vs out in the open in the athletic training clinic. Table 12-1 offers some examples of nonverbal communication to display and avoid during conversations. Different aspects of nonverbal communication together convey a message to the other person. You can show you are attentive to the other person by having a direct gaze (eye contact), leaning in, and nodding.

TABLE 12-1
NONVERBAL COMMUNICATION DOS AND DON'TS

DOS—THINGS TO DISPLAY

Eye contact
Warm, relaxed tone of voice
Encouragement (nods, gestures)
Leaning in
Sitting with an open posture at the same level
Smiling and looking concerned

DON'TS—THINGS TO AVOID

Crossing arms
Facing away from the individual
Looking away from individual
Excessive nodding
Anxious tone of voice

Nonverbal communication cues can play 5 roles:

1. Repetition: They can repeat the message the person is making verbally.

2. Contradiction: They can contradict a message the individual is trying to convey.

3. Substitution: They can substitute for a verbal message. For example, a person's eyes can often convey a far more vivid message than words do.

4. Complementing: They may add to or complement a verbal message. A boss who pats a person on the back in addition to giving praise can increase the impact of the message.

5. Accenting: They may accent or underline a verbal message. Pounding the table, for example, can underline a message.

Listening

Communication involves listening to another individual or individuals. Patient satisfaction is related to listening. Patients who feel their health care provider is listening to them report better patient satisfaction.[10] Listening requires your attention directly to that person. If you catch yourself thinking of what to say next or what question to ask next, you may not be focusing on the person in front of you. Imagine if you needed to address a conflict with a coworker. You approach in a private manner but he or she is avoiding eye contact and seated facing away from you. This is an obvious sign of not listening. Body language such as eye contact, nodding, and leaning forward all indicate to the other person you are listening. Interrupting, avoiding eye contact, and facing away from the individual all will make him or her feel that you are not listening. Remember, sometimes people just want to be heard and do not necessarily require a response.

Active listening tips:

1. Pay attention: eye contact and nonverbal cues they are giving off.
2. Show you are listening: nod or smile, use simple gestures by saying "yes" or "go on."
3. Provide feedback—ask him or her to clarify or summarize.
4. Do not interrupt the speaker; allow him or her to finish.

Asking Open-Ended Questions

Open-ended questions require the other person to expand and explain a situation. These questions are not answered with a "yes" or "no." They are questions that let the patient's point of view guide the discussion. Questions such as, "How can I help you today?" or "How have you been since your last treatment?" or "How do you think we can resolve this problem?" are questions that provide information from the other person's perspective. Follow-up questions are often asked to find out further information and ensure understanding. Short bouts of silence can be used to encourage continued sharing of information. When speaking to a parent or a patient about their condition, it's important to understand their needs and expectations. A great question to ask is, "how is this injury/illness affecting you at home, school, or work?"

Clarifying

A clarifying question is one that helps you to gain more information and understanding. These questions are asked to elicit more information to further understand the situation. When asking these questions, ask for specific examples and admit if you do not understand something. You could even paraphrase or summarize the information you learn from a clarifying question to further your understanding. Here is a list of some general clarifying questions:

1. Did I hear you say _____?
2. What criteria did you use to _____?
3. Could you help me understand _____?
4. Could you give an example of how you _____?

A more specific example would be a situation in which a patient has been prescribed antibiotics (example could also be a rehab set of exercises). You want to inquire as to how the patient is doing and if he or she is having any trouble with their medication. You ask, "How are the antibiotics going?" Your patient says, "They have been going fine when I take them." A clarifying question would be, "What do you mean 'when I take them'?" This clarifying question helps you further understand if the patient is or is not consistently taking the medication. In the event he or she is not consistently taking the medication, further clarification questions could be used to determine the reasoning. Remember, it is important to avoid leading questions when seeking further information. Leading questions suggest an answer in the question itself. For example, "So you are taking all of your medication, right?"

Empathy

Empathy is the ability to share the experiences and feelings of another person. Empathy is an important part of connecting and building a relationship with someone. When someone is expressing empathy they are trying to connect with and understand the emotional state of another individual. Empathy is different from sympathy. Sympathy is feeling sorrow or pity for an individual. Expressing sympathy could make someone feel you care more about their suffering than actually understanding their emotions and experience. Empathy is expressed through many types of different statements and also through tone of voice, posture, facial expressions, and eye contact as discussed previously. Here is a list of empathetic statements to use:

1. This must be hard news to hear but we will help you get through this.

2. I know you are scared but we can get you more information.

3. Could you tell me what this has been like for you?

4. I can see that you are (angry, frightened, concerned). Can you explain why you feel that way?

5. I can't imagine what this must be like for you.

COMMUNICATING WITH PATIENTS

Effective communication is central to the health of your patients. Poor communication is related to medication adherence[11] and patient satisfaction.[12] Patient satisfaction has also been linked to clinical warmth and listening behaviors on behalf of the health care provider.[10] Poor communication can leave patients uncertain about their diagnosis and prognosis, confused about results of diagnostic tests, and unsure about further management plans.[13]

Athletic trainers interact with their patients daily for evaluative, management, and planning of diagnostic or treatment interventions. We all want the best care for our patients and part of providing the best care is establishing a relationship or partnership with patients. Providing *patient-centered care* establishes a partnership among practitioners, patients, and families to ensure decisions respect the patients' needs and preference as well as solicit input.[14] Patients are actively engaged in shared decision making that occurs between the clinician, patient, and possibly other parties such as family or other health care providers.[15] Providing patient-centered care is one of the Institutes of Medicine (IOM) 5 core competencies for all health care professionals. A part of providing patient care is clear communication. Poor communication between the patient and athletic trainer can affect rehabilitation adherence.[16]

When speaking with patients, it's important to build and continue to build a relationship. Depending on the situation, friends or family may even be included in the shared decision-making process. Whether communicating just with the patient or also with their friends and family, the building of this relationship is ongoing.[17] Moreover, one's cultural background is a key consideration. There is no one way to treat any racial and ethnic group. It is felt that it's impractical for physicians and nurses to learn aspects of every culture that could influence the medical encounter. Instead, a patient-centered approach, treating the patient as an individual, is recommended regardless of culture.[14]

In addition to all of the aforementioned communication strategies (eg, listening, paraphrasing), there are other elements of communication to consider when interacting with a patient. You want to begin the interaction by listening to his or her opening statement and inquire as to any other reasons or concerns for speaking with you. As you are listening, pay attention to your body language (Are you maintaining eye contact? Are you leaning forward?), and ask open-ended questions to obtain a further understanding of your patient. At certain points you may need to clarify information with specific questions often answered in "yes" or "no." Once you get a further understanding of the patient's concern or situation, paraphrasing or summarizing what you have learned will convey to the patient you are listening and processing the information he or she is providing. This paraphrasing in turn provides the patient with an opportunity to clarify and/or share further information. During your conversation use common language and non-medical jargon that your patient understands. Also remember not all patients are aware of or understand their conditions and may be ashamed to acknowledge that they do not understand the medical information you are providing regarding their condition and may not ask for help.[14] In addition to asking clarifying questions to ensure they understand the information you are providing, you could even use pictures or diagrams. These visuals provide focused information that could help you determine the degree of patient comprehension.[14] Once you feel you have a clear understanding of your patient and his or her condition, you may begin to develop a preliminary diagnosis or treatment plan. During this time, you may also educate your patient on the rehabilitation process as this could influence the patient's motivation to adhere to a rehabilitation protocol.[16] When applicable, encourage your patient to share in the decision-making process regarding care and ask questions. Once agreement and plans have been outlined, closure to the encounter is needed to summarize information as well as discuss any follow-up that may need to occur.

Athletic trainers often encounter patients with various injuries and illnesses. Each patient is unique. One important consideration is the patient's mindset, experiences, and history. A first-degree ankle sprain could be viewed as a minor injury by a college-aged athlete who has suffered previous sprains. For a high school student with little history of injuries, a first-degree ankle sprain could be viewed as "bad news" and be scary. In medicine, bad news refers to the moment when a physician provides significant information about a diagnosis, prognosis or treatment to patients and their families[18] that is interpreted by the patient to have a negative effect on the present and future. Many athletic trainers practice in settings where patients participate in sports at the high school, college or professional level. For many of those patients, bad news could be being unable to return to play for a short or long period of time, sustaining a season- or career-ending injury or a major illness. While as a student, athletic trainers learn how to evaluate an ankle sprain, the evaluation of that ankle occurs on a patient with different needs and concerns. How this information is perceived depends on factors such as expectations, previous experiences, and general personality. Your patient may feel various emotions such as shock, horror, anger, disbelief, and denial.[19] No two patients react the same way, and it's important to understand what your patient values when planning their care.

SEGUE

One method for learning and evaluating communication with patients is using the SEGUE framework:[20] **S**et the stage, **E**licit information, **G**ive information, **U**nderstand the patient, and **E**nd the encounter. This framework helps break down the communication into distinct parts and allows practice in a step-by-step fashion. The SEGUE is a research-based checklist used to teach and evaluate communication skills. This framework is the most widely used method of teaching and evaluating communication skills in medical schools in the United States and Canada.[20] The SEGUE employs a checklist (Table 12-2) that you or an instructor can use to evaluate your communication with a patient. While the checklist details specific behaviors or information-gathering techniques, it does allow freedom for individual style. For example, greeting the patient can be accomplished in varying styles depending on the clinician's personality. Items are coded yes if they are accomplished at least one time during the patient encounter and no if they are not. Items marked with an arrow (→) distinguish them as a form or process. Detailing the coder training is beyond the scope of this textbook but additional information can be found elsewhere.[20,21]

EFFECTIVE COMMUNICATION IN THE WORKPLACE

Athletic trainers, regardless of the setting, interact with a variety of individuals each day. Patients and their family members, other health care professionals, co-workers, and coaches all communicate with athletic trainers. Communication with each of those different individuals requires knowledge of basic communication skills as described earlier as well as the perspective of each individual to determine what information to share and how to share it. For example, different information and language will be used when discussing a possible tibial stress fracture with the patient vs the consulting physician.

All athletic trainers want to provide patient-centered care. Communicating effectively with other health care providers is part of that care. One barrier to effective communication is the

TABLE 12-2 **SEGUE Checklist**	
SEGUE STEP	**BEHAVIORS TO DEMONSTRATE**
Set the stage	• Greet patient appropriately. • Establish reason for visit. • Outline agenda for visit. • Make a personal connection with patient. • Maintain patient's privacy.
Elicit information	• Elicit patient's view of the health problem and/or progress. • Explore signs and symptoms. • Discuss any previous treatments. • Discuss lifestyle issues and prevention strategies. • Avoid leading questions. • Give patient the opportunity to talk. • Listen to patient. • Check or clarify information.
Give information	• Explain rationale for diagnosis. • Teach patient about his or her own condition. • Encourage patient to ask questions. • Adapt to patient's level of understanding (eg, medical jargon).
Understand the patient	• Acknowledge patient's accomplishments/challenges. • Acknowledge waiting time. • Express caring, empathy. • Maintain respectful tone.
End the encounter	• Ask if there is anything else to discuss. • Review next steps with patient.
Adapted from Makoul G. The SEGUE framework for teaching and assessing communication skills. *Patient Educ Couns.* 2001;45(1):23-34.	

health care setting. Health care occurs in complex settings where patient care is provided by multiple individuals in the same setting and/or at other locations. This mobility makes it difficult to sometimes locate or contact staff and they may not be updated on the status of patients.[22] In addition, interruptions and last-minute changes in schedule or coverage of athletes could be a barrier to effective communication. These could serve as distractions when normally communication would have occurred.

Communication is directly related to patient safety with communication errors being second only to human error in sentinel events.[23] A sentinel event[24] is an unexpected occurrence involving death or serious physical (loss of limb or function) or psychological injury, or the risk thereof.

	TABLE 12-3 ESSENTIAL COMPONENTS OF **SBAR**
SBAR STEP	**WHAT TO DO**
Situation	• Identify yourself and your role, then describe the situation. • Patient's name, age, gender, and main reason for your call.
Background	• Provide a succinct history of the patient pertinent to this situation. • Provide the patient's diagnosis, current signs and symptoms, and any other pertinent information such as vital signs, medications, lab results, diagnostic findings, current therapy being provided.
Assessment	• What is the current situation? • What is your assessment of the situation?
Recommendation	• What is your recommendation in this situation and what do you need from the other health care provider (referral for specialist, x-rays, medication, continue therapy)?

Adapted from Institute for Healthcare Improvement—SBAR technique for communication: A situational briefing model. http://www.ihi.org/resources/Pages/Tools/SBARTechniqueforCommunication ASituationalBriefingModel.aspx.[26]

It has been found that effective communication between nurses and physicians require decisions about *what* to report, *how* to call (if on the phone), and *how* to structure the information, and this must not be left to chance.[25]

*S*ituation-*B*ackground-*A*ssessment-*R*ecommendation (SBAR)

To structure such information, one very common tool used is the SBAR. The SBAR[26] provides a strong predictable mode of communication and can be used between health care providers when discussing patient care.[27] SBAR in particular is also often used during a patient "hand-off."[28] A hand-off is when patient(s) are transferred or handed off from one individual or team of physicians to another.[29] This tool has been used in emergency situations[30] as well as nonemergency situations such as preoperative briefings[31] and in a rehabilitation setting.[32]

Health care is hierarchical, with athletic trainers serving under the direction of a physician. Expressing concerns to a physician or other health care providers requires assertion. When using the SBAR, use assertive language and avoid hinting that a problem may occur. Saying "Well, it's possible they have a fracture" or "I think this patient has a fracture and needs an x-ray" sends 2 different messages. Table 12-3 displays the essential steps of the SBAR.

Conflict Resolution

Even when trying to effectively communicate, misunderstandings and miscommunication occurs. People will not always agree with each other's decisions and actions and this can result in conflict. Failure to address conflict can result in hurt feelings and potential loss of relationship. When conflict does occur, it needs to be addressed and resolved. If you feel you need to address a conflict with a person, think through and plan that conversation. Being upset, having an emotional reaction, and confronting someone can result in an argument with no resolution of the problem. Prior to addressing conflict with a person consider the location (eg, in an office, in a hallway, in the clinic with patients present) and mode of communication (eg, face-to-face, email, phone conversation). Optimally, these conversations should occur in private, preferably face-to-face or possibly on the phone depending on the circumstances. Also, consider the person and whether you have a prior relationship with them. It is easier to be upset and not understand the motives of a stranger than that of an individual you already have a relationship with.[33] You want the climate to be calm and to convey to the other person you want to understand his or her point of view.[33] Starting off the conversation with phrases such as "I need your help" or "I need to understand" will convey to the person they are a partner in this conversation.

The following bullet points comprise an abbreviated version of considerations when trying to resolve conflict. They are adapted from the principled negotiation method.[33] This method was designed to arrive at decisions based on merits, look for mutual gains whenever possible, and that the result be fair with mutual gain.

Considerations During Conflict Resolution

- Separate the person from the problem—focus on the problem
- Try to consider the other person's point of view. Why does he or she feel this way?
- Try to look through the eyes of different individuals. How will the situation of a patient unable to return to play look through the eyes of the patient, the coach, parents, family? It's important when negotiating to consider the perspective of other individuals.
- Discuss the other person's perception of events—what do they perceive is the problem?
- Recognize your emotions during the process—are you tensing up, crossing your arms; what is your tone of voice?
- Don't react to emotional outbursts—allow the other person to show emotion.
- Always address fear and anger—acknowledge that the other person is upset, fearful.
- Stop at times and determine if you are really listening to the other person or reacting to what he or she is saying.
- Focus on the present situation—avoid discussing previous problems or concerns.
- Consider there may be multiple solutions to a problem—is there another solution you haven't considered?
- Do not focus on winning or being right—the goal is to resolve the problem with mutual gain.

SUMMARY

There are many considerations when communicating with patients, coaches, coworkers, administrators, and supervisors. Health care settings can be very chaotic and crowded, and an athletic trainer is often navigating diverse employment settings with many individuals to interact with daily. Thus possessing strong communication skills is a necessary attribute for an athletic trainer. Athletic trainers evaluate patients, create plans of care, and revise those plans, and communicating with the patient as well as other health care providers is needed for that process to be successful.

ACTIVITIES FOR REINFORCEMENT

Questions for Review

1. What forms of nonverbal communication do you recall occurring during social interactions you have had in the last 24 hours?

2. Define empathy and identify what verbal and nonverbal communication behaviors are aligned with it.

Engagement Activities

1. Watch videos of other athletic trainers interacting with patients to see their communication styles.

2. Discuss a patient case with your preceptor using the Situation-Background-Assessment-Recommendation (SBAR). Discuss in what situation would he or she use the tool (speaking with physician or other athletic trainer, patient hand-off or other situation) and what information they feel is vital for each section.

3. Once this discussion has occurred, role play the SBAR with your preceptor using current patient cases (http://www.ihi.org/resources/Pages/Tools/SBARToolkit.aspx).

4. Engage in simulations or standardized patient experiences using the Case Vignettes next.

Case Vignettes

Case #1

Lucille is the new athletic trainer for Roosevelt High School. She is currently treating Rusty, a sophomore starting baseball athlete (right fielder), who sustained a first-degree ankle sprain 1 day prior. Because of the swelling and pain, Rusty needs to rest for at least 2 to 3 days prior to returning to play. Lucille walks by Eric's (coach) office and overhears him talking to Rusty. Eric is telling Rusty that his injury isn't that severe and he should be able to practice today. Lucille hasn't met with the athlete, Rusty, yet today, but yesterday had communicated to him, as well as the coach, he would be unable to participate for a few more days. Lucille has had no conflicts with this coach so far.

1. Where and when would it be appropriate to discuss with the coach the undermining of medical decisions?

2. How should Lucille start the conversation?

3. What strategies could Lucille use in discussing the return to play with this patient?

4. Are there any terms or phrases Lucille should avoid?

Case #2

Howard is the new athletic trainer at Adelphi High School. Alice is a senior star soccer player who has college scouts looking at her. She sustained a concussion yesterday and was provided the appropriate care and home instructions. Howard also called her mother, Robin, but was only able to leave a message regarding Alice's care. Alice comes in today and reports she feels fine and would like to participate. Howard explains the return-to-play protocol, but Alice is concerned and calls her mother. Robin comes in to discuss her daughter's playing status. She wants Alice to participate because she is feeling fine and college scouts will be looking at her performance during upcoming practices and games. Alice has a good chance for a full scholarship, and this is the only way Robin can send her to college.

1. How could Howard show Robin he empathizes with her?

2. Robin is upset and frustrated. What are some strategies to stay calm and ensure Robin feels listened to?

3. Robin wants her daughter to play, but it is unsafe for her to play today. How can this conversation be resolved?

4. What are some clarifying statements that would be beneficial during this conversation?

Discussion Questions

1. What are some methods you can use to show you are empathizing with your patients?

2. Thinking about your last patient interaction, what nonverbal characteristics did you display? If you could do that encounter over, what nonverbal characteristics would you display?

3. What are some strategies you will use the next time you are trying to resolve conflict with a colleague?

REFERENCES

1. National Athletic Trainers' Association. Athletic Training Educational Competencies. 5th ed. http://caate.net/wp-content/uploads/2014/06/5th-Edition-Competencies.pdf. Accessed November 28, 2014.

2. von Fragstein M, Silverman J, Cushing A, Quilligan S, Salisbury H, Wiskin C. UK Council for Clinical Communication Skills Teaching in Undergraduate Medical Education. UK consensus statement on the content of communication curricula in undergraduate medical education. *Med Educ.* 2008;42(11):1100-1107.

3. Cavanaugh JT, Konrad SC. Fostering the development of effective person-centered healthcare communication skills: an interprofessional shared learning model. *Work.* 2012;41(3):293-301.

4. Holt E, Joyce C, Dornelles A, et al. Sex differences in barriers to antihypertensive medication adherence: findings from the cohort study of medication adherence among older adults. *J Am Geriatr Soc.* 2013;61(4):558-564.

5. The Joint Commission. *Advancing Effective Communication, Cultural Competence, and Patient- and Family-Centered Care: A Roadmap for Hospitals.* Oakbrook Terrace, IL: The Joint Commission; 2010.

6. Raab S, Wolfe BD, Gould TE, Piland SG. Characterizations of a quality certified athletic trainer. *J Athl Train.* 2011;46(6):672-679.

7. Interprofessional Education Collaborative Expert Panel. *Core Competencies for Interprofessional Collaborative Practice: Report of an Expert Panel.* Washington, DC: Interprofessional Education Collaborative; 2011.

8. Knapp ML, Hall JA, Horgan TG. *Nonverbal Communication in Human Interaction.* 8th ed. Boston, MA: Centage Learning; 2013.

9. Grover SM. Shaping effective communication skills and therapeutic relationships at work: the foundation of collaboration. *AAOHN J.* 2005;53(4):177-82.

10. Henry SG, Fuhrel-Forbis A, Rogers MA, Eggly S. Association between nonverbal communication during clinical interactions and outcomes: a systematic review and meta-analysis. *Patient Educ Couns.* 2012;86(3):297-315.

11. Sleath B, Carpenter DM, Slota C, et al. Communication during pediatric asthma visits and self-reported asthma medication adherence. *Pediatrics.* 2012;130(4):627-633.

12. Phillips LA, Leventhal H, Leventhal EA. Physicians' communication of the common-sense self-regulation model results in greater reported adherence than physicians' use of interpersonal skills. *Br J Health Psychol.* 2012;17(2):244-257.

13. Fallowfield L Jenkins V, Farewell V, Solis-Trapala I. Enduring impact of communication skills training: results of a 12-month follow-up. *Br J Cancer.* 2003;89(8):1445-1449.

14. Markova T, Broome B. Effective communication and delivery of culturally competent health care. *Urol Nurs.* 2007;27(3):239-242.

15. Barry MJ, Edgman-Levitan S. Shared decision making—The pinnacle of patient-centered care. *N Engl J Med.* 2012;366(9):780-781.

16. Granquist MD, Podlog L, Engel JR, Newland A. Certified athletic trainers' perspectives on rehabilitation adherence in collegiate athletic training settings. *J Sport Rehab.* 2014;23(2):123-133.

17. Makoul G. Essential elements of communication in medical encounters: the Kalamazoo consensus statement. *Acad Med.* 2001;76(4):390-393.

18. Warnock C. Breaking bad news: issues relating to nursing practice. *Nurs Stand.* 2014;28(45):51-58.

19. Fallowfield L, Jenkins V. Communicating sad, bad, and difficult news in medicine. *Lancet.* 2004;363:312-319.

20. Makoul G. The SEGUE framework for teaching and assessing communication skills. *Patient Educ Couns.* 2001;45(1):23-34.

21. Schirmer JM, Mauksch L, Lang F, et al. Assessing communication competence: a review of current tools. *Fam Med.* 2005;37(3):184-192.

22. Huang Y, Garrett SK. Defining characteristics of communication quality in culture-changed long-term healthcare facilities. *J Comm Healthcare.* 2012;5(4):227-238.

23. Joint Commission on Accreditation of Health Care Organizations. Root Causes of Sentinel Events, 2004–2013. http://www.jointcommission.org/Sentinel_Event_Statistics/. Accessed August 7, 2015.

24. Joint Commission on Accreditation of Health Care Organizations. 2013. Sentinel event policy and procedures. http://www.jointcommission.org/Sentinel_Event_Policy_and_Procedures/. Accessed November 28, 2014.

25. Krautscheid LC. Improving communication among healthcare providers: preparing student nurses for practice. *Inter J Nurs Educ Scholarship.* 2008; 5; Article 40.

26. Institute for Healthcare Improvement. SBAR Technique for communication: a situational briefing model. http://www.ihi.org/resources/Pages/Tools/SBARTechniqueforCommunicationASituationalBriefingModel.aspx. Accessed August 10, 2014.

27. Pope B, Rodzen L, Spross G. Raising the SBAR. How better communication improves patient outcomes. *Nursing* 2008;38:41-43.

28. Riesenberg LA, Leitzsch J, Little BW. Systematic review of handoff mnemonics literature. *Am J Med Qual.* 2009;24(3):196-204.

29. Solet JD, Norvell JM, Rutan GH, Frankel RM. Lost in translation: challenges and opportunities in physician-to-physician communication during patient handoffs. *Acad Med.* 2005;80(12):1094-1099.

30. Tews MC, Liu JM, Treat R. Situation-Background-Assessment-Recommendation (SBAR) and emergency medicine residents' learning of case presentation skills. *J Grad Med Educ.* 2012;4(3):370-373.

31. Leonard M, Graham S, Bonacum D. The human factor: the critical importance of effective teamwork and communication in providing safe care. *Qual Saf Health Care.* 2004;13(Suppl 1):i85-i90.

32. Boaro N, Fancott C, Baker R, Velji K, Andreoli A. Using SBAR to improve communication in interprofessional rehabilitation teams. *J Interprof Care.* 2010;24(1):111-114.

33. Fisher R, Ury W, Patton B. *Getting to Yes: Negotiation Agreement Without Giving in.* Revised edition. New York, NY: Penguin Group; 2011.

Effective Teamwork

Matthew R. Kutz, PhD, AT, CSCS, CES

OBJECTIVES

After reading this chapter, the reader will be able to do the following:
1. Define and differentiate between groups and teams.
2. Explain the benefits to the workplace and individuals of teamwork.
3. Identify factors that influence teams.
4. Describe how effective teams form and develop in the workplace.
5. Describe characteristics of effective team members.

INTRODUCTION

Teams are one of the most important components to an effective and functional workplace. Perhaps of all the leadership or workplace-related issues that athletic trainers deal with, teams and teamwork is most familiar. Even though the concept is familiar and despite working with coaches who develop and organize teams, there is less overlap into the athletic training workplace than one might expect.

In spite of these differences, there are some similarities that can be extrapolated. Both sports and workplace teams that experience early wins tend to generate greater momentum. Sports teams that practice together experience greater cooperation; likewise, workplace teams that have common experiences may be more likely to cooperate with each other. Finally, many sports teams work to improve their performance by analyzing game films, and workplace teams can improve their performance with frequent debriefs after a task completion. Table 13-1 is a description of the differences between sports team and a workplace team.

Mazerolle SM, Pitney WA.
Workplace Concepts for Athletic Trainers (pp 205-219).
© 2016 Taylor & Francis Group.

TABLE 13-1
DIFFERENCES BETWEEN SPORT TEAMS AND WORKPLACE TEAMS

SPORTS TEAM CHARACTERISTICS	WORKPLACE TEAM CHARACTERISTICS
• Autocratic leadership of the team—head coach	• Diversity of leadership styles
• Clear and established metrics of success—wins vs losses	• Metrics of success are determined by the team
• Clear performance expectations of team members, with unchallenged consequences for poor performance—being benched	• Performance expectations vary and consequences for poor performance can be uncertain
• The task function and purpose of the team has relatively little variability	• Workplace teams are more varied and complex
• Highly externally and internally competitive, even within the team players compete for the coach's attention and playing time	• Internal competition can destroy a workplace team

Ironically, great teams can be a paradox because no team can accomplish anything without the individual effort from its members. Likewise, individual members may not be able to offer significant contributions without team synergy. Along this line, iconic basketball coach Phil Jackson has been credited with saying, "The strength of the team is each individual member, and the strength of each member is the team."[2]

Few things influence workplace morale more than the interpersonal dynamics of teams and workgroups. One of the interesting things about teams is that organizational scientists consider them to be "alive." Shiver and Nesta[3] state that teams are complex organisms that are born, can learn, grow and mature, and develop their own personalities. In fact, team development has been compared to child rearing in that they have different stages of development. Along those lines just as young children can reflect on the parents, a team's performance can be more a reflection of the leader than the individual members. In fact, the health of the organization can often be determined by diagnosing the performance of its teams.

This chapter will discuss the evolving concept of teams as well as the differences between teams and groups. In this chapter there will be a review of types of teams and their importance to a health care organization as well as how teams are an important consideration for the athletic trainer in the workplace now and in the future. Furthermore, the chapter will explain how athletic trainers can contribute value to teams and develop the skills and tools necessary to facilitate effective teamwork.

Evolving Concept of Teams

In Chapter 2 we discussed the evolution of leadership thinking from classical paradigm to organic paradigm. While not as dramatic or obvious, teamwork paradigms have also evolved. During the classical, transactional, and visionary paradigms of leadership, teams were most often considered in terms of how to lead them. Most of the literature was written with the leader in mind and focused on how leaders could develop, maintain, and motivate the teams under their command. In other words, teams and teamwork had a leader-centric perspective. However, with the advent of the organic model of leadership, the concept of team and teamwork began to change. In the contemporary workplace, teamwork is more an issue of how to be a contributing member within a group of co-equals, or a plurality of equal members, and less about team hierarchy. While teams will—and should—always have leaders, the emphasis on this has shifted. Part of the goal of this chapter is to discuss how to be a contributing member of the team regardless of your title or rank within the workplace. It is necessary to realize, however, that all teams are groups, but not all groups are teams.

GROUPS VERSUS TEAMS

A *group* is formed when 2 or more people have a common interest and agree to do something about that interest. Typically groups form either by direct command of someone in authority or self-organize around a common interest. That interest can either be a common passion about something they love or a shared hatred of something they loath. On the other hand, a *team* is a group of people with complementary skills and passions who are committed to a common mission, goals, and approach for which they hold themselves mutually accountable.[4] As opposed to groups, teams tend to include the quality of the interaction within and between the group as part of their success metric. Conversely, groups tend to focus on individual leaders, and/or an assigned task and accountability is usually personal.

In addition to being defined differently, there are other fundamental differences between groups and teams to understand. Typically members of a group work independently of each other whereas members of a team work interdependently—members of groups are typically autonomous—members of teams are usually dependent. Typically when a group is formed little buy-in is needed because their objectives are set for them by an external authority figure. Within the context of team it is necessary that the members have a sense of ownership and often contribute to delineating the roles and purpose of their association. Thus, buy-in is essential for successful teamwork, but not necessarily needed for groups.

Another difference is in how they communicate. Members of groups tend to be very cautious about what they say and how they say it; as autonomous members they may not see or understand the big picture relative to their assignment so comments and suggestions are usually kept to a minimum. On the other hand, team members are encouraged to share their experiences and knowledge with each other so that they can have a better perspective of the big picture. Finally, groups tend to avoid or suppress differing opinions and disagreement and view them as a threat to their task, whereas mature teams see conflict as a part of the creative problem-solving process.

These differences should not be construed or taken to imply that groups are not necessary and that teams are always superior. There are times when groups offer an advantage. For example, groups are extremely effective when something needs to be done quickly or requires an "assembly line" process. Furthermore, groups are easier to assemble when needing interdisciplinary collaboration, especially with large geographical separation. However, generally speaking teams are the more desirable option. Figure 13-1 outlines a few differences between teams and groups.

TYPES OF TEAMS

Describing the different types of teams can be like trying to define leadership; there are so many different ways to classify teams that it can become cumbersome. Previous athletic training literature has described teams as either homogenous or collaborative and interdependent or co-acting.[5] *Homogenous teams* consist of members with similar experiences, backgrounds, or abilities. *Collaborative teams* consist of members who have different backgrounds and experiences. Once a

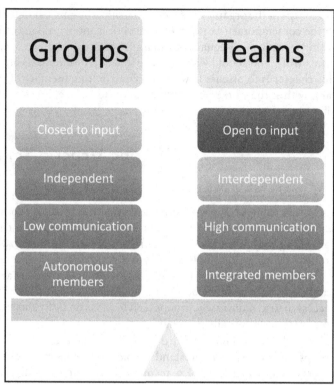

team is determined to be either homogenous or collaborative, they take on additional characteristics such as interdependent or co-acting. *Interdependent teams* rely heavily on each other; and have a high degree of coordination in accomplishing team tasks. *Co-acting teams* are more autonomous and have little coordination when completing their functions and duties. Figure 13-2 is a graphic that highlights the different types of teams and how they are connected.

Once you determine if a team is homogenous or collaborative, interdependent or co-acting, they can then be organized by type. For example, type I would be an interdependent homogenous team whose activity is highly coordinated with all members sharing similar backgrounds and experiences. An example of a type I team may be a team of athletic trainers working within a university's athletic department. The type II team would be a homogenous co-acting team whose activities are autonomous but whose members share similar backgrounds. An example of a type II team might be a committee of athletic trainers from different geographic locations or institutions working together. Type III teams would be interdependent collaborative teams whose members are highly coordinated but with diverse backgrounds. An example of a type III team would be the general sports medicine team that consists of physicians, therapists, athletic trainers, coaches, nutritionists, etc at the same institution working within the same athletic department. Finally, a type IV team or collaborative co-acting team is an autonomous team with diverse backgrounds. An example of a type IV team would be different medical and health care professionals working on a common issue, but retaining autonomy within their discipline. A specific example of a type IV team would be a local Red Cross disaster relief advisory committee.

Descriptive Classification of Teams

There are other ways to describe teams that convey the characteristics of the team. This descriptive classification requires teams be evaluated on 2 dimensions, performance and cooperation. This results in 4 descriptive classifications. Team performance is their capacity to accomplish

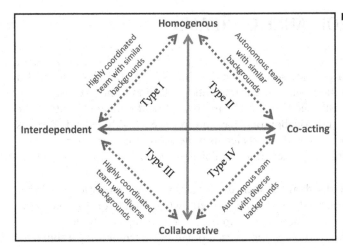

Figure 13-2. Matrix of team types.

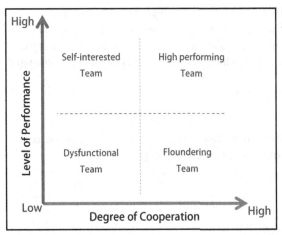

Figure 13-3. The relationship between performance and cooperation.

mutually agreed-on objectives in a reasonable amount of time. Cooperation includes a group's capacity to reduce their individual ambition and participate and interact well with team members. Using these 2 dimensions (Figure 13-3) produces the following 4 types of teams:

1. **High-performing teams** have a high degree of cooperation and a high level of performance. They work well together, complement each other, and accomplish their objectives on time.

2. **Self-interested teams** have a high level of performance and a low degree of cooperation. They accomplish their objectives on time, but spend little time developing relationships or demonstrating empathy toward each other.

3. **Floundering teams** have a high degree of cooperation and a low level of performance. They spend time developing relationships, and demonstrate empathy toward each other, but fail to accomplish their tasks on time.

4. **Dysfunctional teams** have a low degree of cooperation and low level of performance. These teams do not spend any time developing their relationships and fail to perform their assigned duties in a timely manner.

IMPORTANCE OF TEAMS

Within the complex context of health care, many organizations have turned to teamwork (or interdisciplinary collaboration) as a possible solution for the challenges in the changing health care landscape.[3] Increased collaboration between departments, professions, and even organizations can promote synergy, boost cost-effectiveness, and improve patient outcomes. Within the context of athletic training, teams and collaboration have always been highly valued. Perhaps the close association athletic trainers have with sports teams underscores that commitment. This commitment to teamwork places athletic trainers in the unique position to take advantage of the benefits of teams.

Teams are most beneficial when individual members can set aside personal ambition and agendas. Successful team members have learned how to handle their own ambition for the sake of the team's corporate success. When team members mature to the place of being able to do this, they become an indispensable asset in the workplace and to each other and often become a source of great satisfaction to each other.

As we discussed in Chapter 4 the modern workplace is increasingly volatile, uncertain, complex, and ambiguous. As volatility, uncertainty, complexity, and ambiguity increase, required tasks become proportionately more collaborative and require a considerable amount of teamwork. Teamwork is the joint action by a team of people in which individual interests are subordinated for the sake of team unity.[6]

Benefits of Teamwork

When the true spirit of teamwork or collaboration develops on teams, several positive outcomes occur in the workplace. The benefits of teamwork include the following:

- Higher morale
- Increased job satisfaction
- Higher employee retention
- Creative environment
- Shared resources and collaboration
- Enhanced communication
- Attention to ethical behavior and accountability

All of these benefits result in *esprit de corps*. *Esprit de corps* is the feeling of pride, camaraderie, and loyalty among members of a team. *Esprit de corps* within the workplace has a significant influence on culture.

In addition to the benefits of teamwork within the workplace, creating teams offers several advantages over individual effort. Some of those advantages include the following:

- A diversity of perspectives
- Greater sum total of experience
- Synergy
- Strategic thinking
- Shared responsibility
- Ethical checks and balances[5]

This list is by no means exhaustive; there are certainly several advantages to the workplace and the individual when teams and teamwork are priority. However, this does not mean that everything is easier on teams. There are situations and circumstances when teams and teamwork is not ideal or at the very least difficult. Working on teams in developing teamwork requires intentional effort, which may have barriers from time to time.

Barriers to Teamwork

There are several barriers to teamwork; among the most common are groupthink and social loafing. *Groupthink* occurs when members of a team assume the other members either already know or share a similar opinion. When this happens team members tell themselves, "I'm not going to, 'state the obvious,'" which can undermine some of the benefits of teamwork identified earlier. A second phenomenon that can occur on teams that hinders their development and attainment of goals is social loafing. *Social loafing* is when a particular member or members of the team fail to contribute their best effort because other members on the team are perceived as harder working or have more at stake. These 2 phenomena can be devastating to a team and they should be guarded against vigilantly.

Other barriers to teams and teamwork include the fact that team development takes time, teams that do not move toward teamwork will naturally move toward becoming bureaucratic, and sometimes it takes longer for teams to make decisions. Team members must resist the temptation to make a quick decision without the input of others. However, there are times when an individual can handle a situation more efficiently, especially in an emergency situation. Determining when a team or individual decision is preferable can be challenging. Finally, conflicts between different personality types are always a risk to the *esprit de corps* of a team.

FUNCTIONS OF TEAMS

Teams have both task and maintenance functions.[7] *Task functions* are activities directly related to accomplishing the directives of the team. Task functions include the following:

- Initiating activities
- Seeking information
- Giving information
- Elaborating concepts
- Coordinating activities
- Summarizing ideas
- Testing ideas
- Evaluating effectiveness
- Diagnosing problems

Effective teams know which members are best suited to complete specific tasks. In the contemporary workplace, responsibility for facilitating the team is shared between team members based on their strengths, as the importance of these tasks varies throughout the lifecycle of the team. Completing these task functions in the right sequence and at the right time is essential to the team's success. On the other hand, if a team focuses solely on its task functions—and neglects other functions—it is likely that tension will build. For example, if a team meets only to "diagnose problems" or pass along information, it is unlikely that cohesion and the necessary maturity to set aside personal agendas will develop. Therefore, it is necessary for the team to also perform maintenance functions.

Maintenance functions are equally as important and include activities that satisfy the interpersonal dynamics between team members. To state it rather simply, teams must also have fun and know when it is appropriate—or necessary—to relate interpersonally—and not just over an agenda or tasks. Maintenance functions include the following:

- Supporting others
- Following others' leads
- Gatekeeping communication
- Setting standards
- Expressing member feelings
- Testing group decisions
- Consensus building
- Harmonizing conflict
- Reducing tension

When teams engage in maintenance functions, it increases the sense of cooperation and unity,[6] which is essential to team effectiveness.

Creating Team Effectiveness

Effective teams are diverse, share a common interest, are creative, and often self-managed. Understanding and championing diversity is one of the most important elements of a healthy workplace. Diversity is not limited to ethnic, cultural, or gender differences. The essence of diversity is about ideas, and ideas are shaped by experience. Inviting people to participate on teams with different experiences and backgrounds is important. Parker[8] identified 4 styles of diversity among team members: the contributor, the collaborator, the communicator, and the challenger. Each of these 4 styles represents diversity relative to how they contribute to the team. *Contributors* are data driven; they supply the team with data and information necessary to perform their tasks and typically adhere to high standards of performance. *Collaborators* are team members who have the capacity to see the big picture and see past and through obstacles. They are the ones who encourage and motivate other members to join in the effort to accomplish the team's goal. The *communicators* are the team's listeners. They facilitate the group processes, participate in maintenance functions, and make sure the appropriate information is disseminated to the right people. Finally, the *challengers* are the team members who look for weaknesses and threats to the current course of action. They tend to question everything the team does in an attempt to make sure that the team is staying true to its mission and purpose. In all likelihood an individual member may assume more than one of these styles; and though challengers need not be antagonistic—although sometimes they are—it is important for the other members of the team not to view challengers as negative or pessimistic.

In the case of a co-acting team, which is a team with different backgrounds and experiences, perhaps even from different departments or organizations, it is necessary to have a fifth style, the integrator. *Integrators* are members who help diffuse conflicts that arise from the different perspectives and experiences.[9] Integrators usually have an interdisciplinary background and a peacekeeping mindset.

DEVELOPING MATURE TEAMS

Teams mature over time. No team is fully mature when it is formed; maturity takes time. Mature teams go through a multiple-phase process where performance gradually increases. The first phase consists of confusion, followed by dissatisfaction, which is followed by resolution, and eventually maturity.

Most confusion on the team consists of understanding individual's roles and functions. Most teams, at their onset, have questions about each other, each other's experiences and expertise, and their own roles and capacity to contribute. This confusion naturally leads to frustration and may

TABLE 13-2
CHARACTERISTICS OF MATURE TEAMS
1. All members contribute what they are thinking.
2. Decisions and actions are made on consensus, not a vote.
3. A member's value is judged by the merit of the idea and not on personal issues.
4. Appropriate priorities are reflected as time spent on the different agenda items.
5. Members understand, know, and appreciate each other.
6. Members are objective about approaching their goals and tasks.
7. Rewards and criticisms are shared.
8. Information is fed to all members.
9. Individuals are respected as members of the team regardless of contribution.
Adapted from Gangel K. *Team Leadership: Using Multiple Gifts to Build a Unified Vision.* Chicago: Moody Publishers; 1997.

require outside intervention at the onset. Once the confusion is settled performance improves, but confusion is exchanged for dissatisfaction.

Team members' dissatisfaction is not with their role per se, but in the trust dynamic. It is at this phase where people say to themselves, I know what I'm supposed to do and I know what you're supposed to do, but I'm not convinced that you're able to do it yet. They then subconsciously—sometimes overtly—require the other members of the team to prove they can do their job. This dissatisfaction is simply a manifestation of trust that hasn't yet been earned. Once that trust is earned the team makes a dramatic shift to resolution where another increase in performance is realized. It is when a team reaches the resolution phase that they truly become self-governing and interdependent and any outside interaction can be reduced or eliminated.

A team that has reached resolution is clear on the roles of each team member, convinced the other members are capable and willing to perform their functions, and have earned the trust of their fellow members. After a few successful tasks, the team moves into the final stage of maturity.

Maturity is when a team's performance has no ceiling, team members are comfortable with each other and confident in everyone's ability to perform. This confidence is often manifested in team members' willingness to subordinate their own agendas for the sake of the team and even promote other team members ideas before their own. In a phrase, a mature team is earmarked by their willingness to "defer to each other." Table 13-2 is a list of characteristics of mature teams.

BUILDING TEAMS

Many people consider teambuilding exercises some of the more valuable techniques for improving workplace dynamics.[10] Furthermore, research has demonstrated that teambuilding programs can improve group processes.[11] Interdisciplinary teams respond particularly well to teambuilding programs because it helps educate team members on the ability and capacity of professionals whom they might not otherwise know or interact with.

One of the most effective ways to build teams is to encourage team members to seek feedback from each other as well as external members—being careful not to violate the trust of team members. Other important elements of teambuilding include intentionally discussing errors, critically reflecting on successes and failures, and willingness to experiment with new ways of doing things.

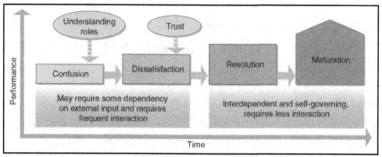

Figure 13-4. Process of team maturation. (Reprinted with permission from Kutz M. *Leadership and Management in Athletic Training: An Integrated Approach*. Baltimore, MD: Lippincott, Williams, and Wilkins; 2010.)

These types of conversations need to become a priority of workplace administrators so that they will allow and even facilitate these discussions.

A great way to build teams is to get them out of the traditional workplace and into a different environment and ask them to accomplish a task that is not related to the reason they were formed. In other words, ask them to work together on something fun that is not necessarily related to a task function. Many teambuilding programs support the maintenance function of the team.

Examples of teambuilding exercises that have been demonstrated to be successful are outdoor challenges, including survival-type exercises or ropes courses, and even rowing. Asking team members to reflect on how these outdoor or physical challenges contribute to teamwork is an important part of the teambuilding debrief. Common teambuilding games used by athletic trainers include "trainer Olympics," where athletic trainers compete against each other or in groups to perform common athletic training tasks for speed and accuracy. Such tasks might include ankle taping, mixing the perfect batch of sport drink, firemen carry relays, or cooler carry relay races. Other activities athletic trainers can do to bond as a team include getting out of the athletic training room from time to time and putting their skills to use in other venues; for example, volunteering at a community road race, medical or humanitarian mission, or Special Olympics. In essence, teams should be provided opportunities to relate together outside of their traditional team roles removed from their traditional setting. Teambuilding exercises can be extremely structured or flexible; the important thing is that they are always fun and that the team be allowed to critically reflect on the teambuilding activity. Figure 13-4 outlines the process a team goes through as it develops maturity.

MANAGING TEAM CONFLICT

All teams experience conflict. The issue for effective teams is not the absence of conflict, but the capacity and willingness to resolve conflicts quickly. Resolving conflicts quickly is a hallmark of a mature team. *Conflict* arises when 2 or more individuals perceive that their goals or values are in opposition.[12] Colquitt and colleagues describe 5 responses to conflict based on assertiveness or the degree of concern for one's own outcomes and cooperation, which is the degree of concern for others' outcomes.[12] The 5 behaviors are competing, avoiding, accommodating, collaborating, and compromising.

The *competing* behavior occurs when individual team members demonstrate high concern for their own outcome and a low concern for others' outcomes. This is often characterized as a win-lose situation. Typically this response to conflict should be avoided, as it typically signals and unbalanced distribution of power. The *avoiding* behavior is characterized by low concern for personal outcomes and low concern for other's outcomes, and is often characterized as a lose-lose situation.

Those who participate in avoidance behaviors are typically thought of as, "simply not caring." Avoidance behavior as a conflict management strategy is particularly problematic, especially in athletic training. One of the biggest concerns is that it undermines clear and open communication, which is essential for a successful team. Other consequences of avoidance behavior include carrying around unresolved issues, lowering individual and team morale, having low self-esteem, losing credibility, and undermining creativity. It is necessary to know some warning signs of avoidance behaviors, such as delaying inevitable conflict, hoping that someone will just "go away," or just waiting until the problem "resolves itself." Athletic trainers must make every effort to cope with conflict by means other than avoidance. *Accommodating* behavior is characterized as high concern for others' outcomes and low concern for personal outcomes. Accommodating is often referred to as a lose-win situation. Typically accommodating behavior implies that the issue at hand is really not important to one of the parties. A *collaborating* response is characterized as high concern for personal outcomes combined with high concern for others' outcomes. Collaborating is called the win-win situation, and is typically the goal of mature and well-functioning teams. Collaboration is celebrated as the most desirable outcome of conflict; however, it is also considered the most difficult to attain. Teams who strive to resolve conflict through collaboration usually end up returning to the proverbial "drawing board" to reframe the problem and solution. This can take time and energy from the team, but in the end is typically worth it. The last response to conflict is compromise. *Compromising* is when all of the different sides represented concede something they think is necessary or important. Compromise is the most common form of conflict resolution,[10] but may not be perceived as a win-win for the team.

Sources of Conflict

Sources of conflict on a team can be many and varied. Research and scholars tend to divide sources of conflict into 2 groups: structural and personal. Structural or organizational sources are caused by workplace design and hierarchy. Interpersonal sources are when conflict is a result of different ideas and goals between individuals within the workplace.

Structural Sources

Structural (also called organizational) sources of conflict include things like specialization, interdependence, sharing resources, goal differences, authority relationships, and jurisdictional ambiguity.

Specialization can cause conflict when jobs are highly specialized and employees become experts in a certain task. The reason this can cause conflict is that there are times when other members of the team have no idea how to perform a task. This can lead to inconsistencies and breakdowns in communication and trust. An example of how specialization may affect athletic training is to divide athletic trainers into different groups, such as faculty and clinicians. It is possible that this sort of structural separation—while easy to justify—has unintended consequences, such as mistrust between the 2 units and development of different goals and values, which can cause gridlock. Furthermore, consequences associated with specialization could arise if a particular athletic trainer did all the anterior cruciate ligament (ACL) rehabilitation and another only shoulder rehabilitation. While interdependence is a goal of mature teams, it can also be a source of tension within young teams, especially when people fail to deliver. This can slow down the rest of the team and can result in conflict. Perhaps one of the most common structural sources of conflict occurs when team members are required to compete for resources. Obviously, this tension is exaggerated when resources become scarce and teams feel they have to race with each other to acquire them. While teams need leadership, there are times when the authority structure within the team results in conflict. Typically conflict occurs when someone resents another's position or simply does not like being told what to do. Likewise, it is possible to have an autocratic boss, which also facilitates conflict. Finally, jurisdictional ambiguity, which is when a particular team or department does not have the authority or information necessary to handle a particular situation, often attracts conflict. Basically, it comes down to not knowing who is ultimately responsible for a particular issue or can manifest when one department or division blames another instead of taking responsibility. Jurisdictional ambiguity can be escalated by specialization; within athletic training this might become problematic if clinicians and faculty assume the "other" is handling a given situation.

Interpersonal Sources

Interpersonal sources of conflict include things like divergence in skills, personalities, perceptions, conflicting values and ethics, communication, and cultural differences. Divergence in skills is typically seen when experienced workers are required to work with new or unskilled coworkers. This is especially problematic when deadlines are not extended or expectations changed to accommodate a learning curve. The more skilled or experienced workers tend to draw premature judgments about their new or young colleagues' capacity and ability, which can lead to conflict. Within the context of athletic training education, divergence is particularly problematic, especially when Board of Certification (BOC) certification is the only criteria considered necessary. For example, graduate assistant athletic trainers, while novices, can be expected to perform at a high level almost immediately by clinical staff. Sometimes when a newly certified athletic trainer fails to perform as well as a seasoned athletic trainer, their competency is unfairly called into question. Furthermore, upperclassmen often participate in clinical education side-by-side with underclassmen. The differences in competency can cause frustration for all parties. Likewise, clinical athletic trainers and faculty may experience divergence when faculty enters the clinical arena after a long layoff—and they may be rusty—or when clinicians enter the classroom with little or no teaching experience.

While diversity is a virtue in the workplace certain personalities may find it difficult to mix with others. For example, a Type A personality—characterized by hard-driving, high-intensity, decisive characteristics—may find it difficult to work with a Type B personality, which typically is characterized as lower intensity and displaying a slower pace and steady workflow. Misaligned perceptions can also cause conflict, especially when one group is expecting a certain outcome that is never realized.

Another common source of interpersonal conflict is when values and ethics collide. Values are important components of the interpersonal dynamic. Examples of conflicting values could be between the sexes or generations. For example, female workers may value a more reasonable work day so that they can get home to their families, where male workers might not appreciate that and expect evenings to be sacrificed for the sake of the team. Likewise, older generations tend to value loyalty—or at least define it in terms of longevity; whereas younger generations define loyalty in terms of intensity of effort. An older member of the team may not consider someone loyal until he or she has worked in the same job for several years, whereas younger members consider them loyal because they add hours and work on weekends; something the older generation might hesitate to do. Relative to ethics, everyone has them; the conflict often is over when they should be applied and to what extent. For example, certain people are convinced that anything legal is by default also ethical, whereas others believe there are situations that a certain action can be unethical despite being legal.

Communication is often referenced as a source of conflict when teams are not functioning well. The human language, including body language is heavily nuanced. Messages are lost or distorted because one of the involved parties—the giver of the message or the receiver of the message—mishandles the message. Sometimes the message is simply articulated incorrectly and other times the receiver of the message misconstrues what was said. In either case conflict is inevitable. There are also natural barriers to communication such as geographic distance, and technology (email) that can distort messages. Finally, cultural differences, while generally considered an asset, can lead to conflict. When cultural differences lead to conflict it is rarely because one group is being purposefully intolerant of another group. Typically conflict that stems from cultural differences is from one group's lack of understanding of another culture.

Summary

Teamwork is extremely important within the health care context and specifically between athletic trainers. Understanding and developing concepts specific to teamwork is an important task that athletic trainers must engage in regardless of their position within their organization or professional status. Within the past few decades, the concept of the team has evolved from a leader-centric dynamic to a more holistic interaction between peers. With this change it is important to distinguish between groups and teams. Groups form when 2 or more people have a common interest and agree to do something together. Teams transcend groups; while they do have common interests they also incorporate a high level of accountability within their cooperation. Knowing the type of team you are on is necessary to working efficiently on a team. Teams can be classified according to their level of performance and degree of cooperation. Mature teams are comfortable with each other's contribution and mature team members are comfortable with the other members' level of accountability and ability to contribute. Another aspect of mature teams is their willingness to manage conflict by identifying and dealing effectively with the sources of conflict.

Activities for Reinforcement

Questions for Review

1. Consider different groups or teams you are part of (eg, athletic training student's club, extra-curricular clubs, quiz bowl team, intramural sports teams, or colleagues at clinical sites). Using Figure 13-2 (matrix of team types), what type of team do you think you are? Explain why.

2. Using the same teams/groups (identified above) as a reference, explain where you are on the process of team maturation (see Figure 13-4).

   a. What strategies can you take to further mature?

3. Identify several task functions of the sports medicine team and discuss how they are different from the maintenance functions of the same team.

4. Which interpersonal sources of team conflict do you believe are most difficult to overcome? Why?

5. Which structural sources of conflict do you feel a good leader should be able to alleviate? Explain why.

6. Give an example of a team that you have been a part of that successfully overcame adversity.

7. What type of team is easiest for you to be a part of. Why?

8. How does your personality ease or contribute to team conflict?

Case Vignettes

Case #1

Sally has 12 years of experience as an athletic trainer (with 8 years as an assistant at a major Division 1 [D1] university), but is in only her fourth year as the athletic trainer at a newer, very large local high school. Her athletic director recently informed her of a new school levy being voted on in the community, which is sure to pass, and will combine the athletic programs of 2 high schools that competed against each other in the community league. John is a 20-year veteran of that other—older—high school, which includes several league and regional championships. John has a staff of 2 part-time assistants and several student assistants. Sally and John are being asked to work together once the schools merge, with Sally as the head athletic trainer and John and his staff as "assistants." Because of his seniority in the school system, John will make a higher salary than Sally. Furthermore, John is a little upset at what he has called "the politics" behind the decision for Sally to be "head athletic trainer," especially given his seniority, his experience leading a staff, and the number of championships his school has won. Sally does not understand John's frustration because she does not consider John's role to be subordinate to hers, rather she views their roles as equal. Sally desperately wants to move forward professionally and in the best interest of the school, the community, and the athletes they serve. She is not sure how to help John understand her perspective or work together. One of her biggest concerns is creating the type of athletic training team she envisions will be necessary to meet the needs of the student-athletes—who may hold onto old alliances—after the levy is passed.

1. What type of team will this new sports medicine team be?

2. What types of things can Sally begin to do before the levy is passed to develop her new team?

3. Should Sally be concerned about John's attitude?

4. Are John's concerns justified? Why or why not?

5. Should the higher administration get involved with helping Sally or John resolve any team formation issues?

6. What would you do if you were in Sally's situation?

7. What would you do if you were in John's situation?

Case #2

Chris is the head athletic trainer at Local State College (LSC) and Sean is the athletic training program director for LSC. Each is the "boss" in his respective department; while the departments overlap they are clearly autonomous in organizational structure. Occasionally Chris will teach a class in the athletic training education program where he is supervised and evaluated by Sean. Likewise, Sean occasionally provides athletic training clinical services to LSC's athletic department where he is supervised and evaluated by Chris. Chris and Sean have worked together for several years and have had no real conflicts to speak of; in fact they get along very well and have always resolved any conflicts between them immediately. Recently LSC has decided to hire an additional athletic training faculty member who will have a 60% teaching load and 40% clinical service load; and Sean was invited to chair the search committee. Naturally he invited Chris to serve on the committee. Furthermore, another faculty member from the athletic training department (who is very familiar with Chris and Sean) and one of the head coaches (who knows Sean by name only) from the athletic department were asked to serve on the committee as well. At their initial meeting the committee got off to a great start, but once applications started to come in a very clear division was forming based on qualification of candidates. Chris and the head coach clearly favored candidates with a strong clinical background and paid little attention to candidates' research interests or teaching backgrounds. On the other hand, Sean and the other faculty member strongly favored candidates with a solid research agenda and strong teaching experience and paid little attention to clinical experiences. When deciding on qualified candidates to interview, there was a clear impasse.

1. What is/are the source(s) of conflict between these team/group members?

2. Is this search committee a group or a team? Why do you think so?

3. Does the sole responsibility to resolve any conflicts rest with Sean, or should it be shared between Chris and Sean? Why or why not?

4. Is it important to have 100% consensus before a decision is made? What might be the advantages and disadvantages of waiting for 100% consensus?

5. How might you suggest that this issue be resolved?

Discussion Questions

1. Is there a relationship between teamwork and leadership? Explain.

2. Think about the teams you have been on and explain the various roles (eg, captain, motivator) you have observed. How have these various roles worked together to lead to effective teamwork?

3. What barriers to teamwork are likely the most difficult to deal with?

REFERENCES

1. Birle P. *Chicago Bulls*. La Jolla, CA: MVP Books; 2013:15.
2. Shiver J, Nesta C. Building a successful leadership team. In: Rubino LG, Esparza SJ, Chassiakos TSR, eds. *New Leadership for Today's Health Care Professionals: Concepts and Cases*. Jones & Bartlett: Burlington, MA; 2014.
3. Katzenbach J, Smith D. The discipline of teams. *HBR*. 1993;71:111-120.
4. Kutz M. *Leadership and Management in Athletic Training: An Integrated Approach*. Baltimore, MD: Lippincott, Williams & Wilkins; 2010.
5. Nelson D, Quick J. *Understanding Organizational Behavior*. Belmont, CA: Cengage; 2011.
6. Lassey WR. Dimensions of leadership. In: Lassey WR, Fernandez RR, eds. *Leadership and Social Change*. La Jolla, CA: University Associates; 1976:10-15.
7. Parker G. *Team Players and Teamwork*. San Francisco, CA: Jossey-Bass; 1990.
8. Maier N. Assets and liabilities in group problem-solving: the need for an integrative function. *Psych Rev*. 1967;74:239-249.
9. Stephan E, Mills W, Pace W, Ralphs I. HRD in the Fortune 500: A survey. *Train Dev J*. 1988;42:26-42.
10. Salas E, Dickinson T, Tanenbaum S, Converse S. *A meta-analysis of team performance and training*. Naval training system Center technical reports. Orlando, FL: United States Government; 1991.
11. Colquitt J, Lepine J, Wesson M. *Organizational Behavior*. New York, NY: McGraw-Hill; 2011.

14

Time Management in Athletic Training

Jennifer Doherty-Restrepo, PhD, LAT, ATC

OBJECTIVES

After reading this chapter, the reader will be able to do the following:

1. Apply time management strategies to improve professional and personal success.
2. Organize surroundings to improve time management.
3. Use time-saving technology.
4. Implement prioritization systems and time-categorization systems to more effectively use time.
5. Design time-blocking and appointment-setting strategies to more effectively use time.
6. Recognize and confront challenges to time management.

INTRODUCTION

Today's society is time dependent with a seemingly ever-increasing pace of life, thereby demanding effective time-management skills. We must be able to adapt to the faster pace of life to cope with time pressure.[1] We are pressured to not only multitask, but also do things at a faster pace.[1] We often strive to meet the demands of school, work, family, and personal responsibilities but frequently feel there is not enough time to successfully complete all of our necessary tasks.[2]

Given the complexity of today's health care system, with an increasing emphasis on efficiency and effectiveness, health care professionals must effectively manage their time.[3,4] Athletic trainers are multi-skilled health care professionals that provide prevention services, emergency care, clinical diagnosis, therapeutic intervention, and rehabilitation of injuries and medical conditions in the physically active population.[5] Unfortunately, the athletic training profession is often characterized by long and inflexible work hours, which have been linked to job burnout[6,7] and work-life

Mazerolle SM, Pitney WA.
Workplace Concepts for Athletic Trainers (pp 221-234).
© 2016 Taylor & Francis Group.

conflict.[7,8] Concerns over long work hours and work-life conflict have led athletic training students and athletic trainers to change their jobs and, in some instances, even their career path.[7,9] Athletic trainers who have more control over their schedules are able to achieve better work-life balance.[10,11] Research supports that effective time management positively affects our perceived control of time, job satisfaction, productivity, physical health, and psychological well-being.[12-14] We, as athletic training students or athletic trainers, must identify and use effective time-management approaches to promote professional success and personal satisfaction.

TIME MANAGEMENT

Time may be defined as that "thing" measured in seconds, minutes, hours, days, years, etc.[15] It may further be defined as the measureable period during which an action, process, or condition exists or continues.[15] Time is a non-spatial continuum that is measured by events that succeed one another from the past through the present and on to the future.[15] Activities are carried out using time, most of which are time bound.[16] For example, the Board of Certification (BOC) application process is time bound in that it must be completed within 1 year once started. Another example: An AT has only 3 minutes to stop a nosebleed during a wrestling match. Ultimately, there are only 24 hours in a day and 7 days in a week to complete all of our activities and to meet all of our responsibilities. The optimal use of time is imperative because it is limited in supply.

There is no consensus in the literature on the definition of time management. Time management is considered the process of controlling time to achieve multiple tasks within a limited time.[16] Actions geared to the effective use of time to achieve specific, goal-oriented activities are considered time-management behaviors.[12] Time-management strategies are categorized as a combination of time assessment, planning, and self-monitoring behaviors, all of which should lead to more perceived control of time and better well-being.[12,17] The following sections will discuss the aforementioned time-management behaviors in more detail and present various time-management strategies.

> Effective time management requires organization, planning, and self-discipline.

TIME MANAGEMENT STRATEGIES

Time Assessment

To effectively manage our time, we must become aware of and assess how we use our time. Self-awareness of time use, attitudes, and perceptions affect our acceptance of tasks and responsibilities within our capabilities.[16] The first step toward developing and implementing effective time-management strategies is to create an environment that supports effective time management. Such an environment starts with a well-organized work space and an effective filing system for quick and easy retrieval of important documents.[16,18] To assess your environment relative to time management, answer the following questions: Is my workspace organized? How much time do I spend organizing myself, or my materials, in preparation for work? Do I use computer-based time management tools to help me get organized?

While we get organized, we also need to determine if we are using our time effectively. Keep a time log for 1 to 2 weeks. Keeping a time log makes an abstract concept of time more concrete and enables us to detect "time-wasters."[18] "Time-wasters" include unimportant tasks, socializing,

	TABLE 14-1
	TEN COMMON TIME-WASTERS AND POTENTIAL SOLUTIONS

TIME-WASTER	POTENTIAL SOLUTION
Commuting	Enjoy listening to music or an audio book
	Quiet self-reflection
	Read (if using public transportation)
	Call a friend or family member (using hands-free technology)
Disorganization	Clean and organize workspace
	Develop filing system for papers, electronic files, and emails
Email	Check no more than 3 to 4 times per day
	Disable auto-alerts for new mail
	Develop an organized filing system for saved messages
	Delete unwanted messages at first pass
	Identify and discard junk mail
Meetings	Arrive on time
	Bring work to complete if others are not punctual
Paperwork	Handle papers once
	Develop an organized filing system
Physical interruptions	Close your door
Procrastination	Identify and rectify reasons for procrastination
	Break large projects down into smaller tasks
Repetitive activities	Set auto-alerts on electronic calendar/task list
Telephone calls	Check messages and return calls 1 to 2 times per day
Waiting	Complete small, quick, and easy tasks

poor communication, incomplete information, leaving tasks unfinished, and long meetings.[16,18] To identify if you are using your time effectively, answer the following questions: "How much time do I spend on "time-wasters"? "Do I complete easier, less-important tasks before working on more important tasks?" "Do I decide to socialize rather than get my work done?" "Do I procrastinate?" Refer to Table 14-1 for a list of common "time-wasters" and potential solutions.

During our time assessment, we should be able to identify when and where we are most productive. To determine when you are most productive, answer the following question: Am I an "early morning riser," an "afternoon peaker," or a "night owl"?[3] Once you have identified your most productive time of day, you need to guard this prime time on your schedule and complete your most important tasks.[3,18] While assessing our time, we should be able to identify where we are most productive and work there.[3] To determine where you are most productive, answer the following question: Do I work best in my home office, at the library, in a coffee shop, by the pool, or elsewhere? Regardless of when or where you work best, you still must avoid "time-wasters" and procrastination. While assessing our time, we also should be able to recognize "hidden time" that is lost while waiting or commuting and complete small, quick, and easy tasks during this time.[3] For example, if a professor is running 15 minutes late to class, you can book a flight home for the holidays or get some reading done for the next class.

Effective time management requires organization, and there are various time management tools available to help us get organized. Word processors, such as Microsoft Office, have task lists and folders that are easily compiled and managed. An athletic training student can easily create a folder for each course, thereby organizing important documents by course for quick and easy retrieval. Microsoft Outlook has a task list that is easy to prioritize and includes reminder alerts for upcoming meetings or due dates for task completion. We can synchronize our email accounts with our smartphone for quick and easy access to all of our email correspondence. Various online time management tools are available as well at http://www.rememberthemilk.com, http://toodledo.com, and http://todoist.com. Given the various tools at our disposal, we can easily create an organized, and mobile, work environment that supports effective time management. Effective time management dictates that we get organized and give priority attention to important tasks, which requires planning.

Planning

Effective time-management strategies require planning. Planning is defined as a set of mental and behavioral processes that combine cognitive, emotional, and motivational resources to reach desired goals.[19] In demanding and dynamic professions, such as athletic training, planning involves setting goals, prioritizing goals, establishing a routine, and coping with distractions from achieving goals.[20] Proper planning leads to more perceived control of time and better overall well-being.[4,12,17] The following sections will discuss the following planning techniques in more detail: goal setting, prioritization, routinization, and coping with distractions.

> Effective time management behaviors include setting goals, establishing priorities, creating a routine, and minimizing distractions.

Goal Setting

A goal is something we are trying to do or achieve.[15] Goal setting gives us focus and helps us channel our time more effectively, which is critical in time management.[16] We should develop goals that are specific, measurable, attainable, realistic, and timely (SMART) (Figure 14-1).[21] We are more likely to achieve a specific goal than a general goal. For a goal to be specific, we must answer the 6 "W" questions (Table 14-2): *Who?, What?, Where?, When?, Which?,* and *Why?*[21] An example of a general goal would be "Increase my grade point average (GPA)." We can turn this into a SMART goal by saying "Increase my GPA from a 3.3 to a 3.7 within 1 academic year by studying a minimum of 3 hours a day to improve my chances of being accepted to graduate school."

A SMART goal incorporates concrete criteria for measuring our progress toward achieving a goal.[21] To determine if our goal is measureable, ask questions such as: *How much? How many?,* and *How will I know when I achieved my goal?* Measuring our progress toward a set goal will help us reach our predetermined targets and will provide us with a sense of achievement, thus motivating us further to achieve our goals. A SMART goal is attainable. When we identify goals that are most important to us, we are able to formulate a plan to achieve those goals.[21] This plan may involve the development of abilities, skills, or attitudes necessary to achieve our goals. SMART goals are realistic in that we are willing and able to work toward achieving them.[21] Only we can determine if a goal is realistic and how high we can aim to achieve our goals. A high goal is frequently easier to accomplish than a low goal because we may be more motivated to reach higher, more important, goals.[21] Finally, a SMART goal is timely in that it is time bound. Establishing a time frame, or due date, creates a sense of urgency, provides motivation, and allows us to monitor our progress in achieving our realistic and attainable goal.[21]

We should set both short- and long-term goals. Short-term goals are those that are achievable in 1 to 3 years, whereas long-term goals are those that are achievable in 5 to 10 years.[22] One strategy

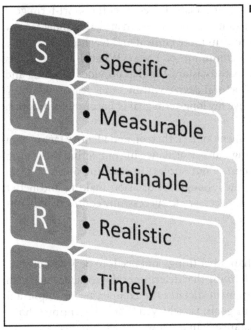

Figure 14-1. Criteria for creating SMART goals.

TABLE 14-2	
THE 6 "W" QUESTIONS FOR FORMULATING A SPECIFIC GOAL	
Who?	Who is involved in achieving this goal?
What?	What do I want to accomplish?
Where?	Where is the location or place of this goal?
When?	When do I want to accomplish this goal? Set a time frame.
Which?	Which things are required for me to accomplish this goal? Which things may prevent me from accomplishing this goal?
Why?	Why do I want to accomplish this goal? Provide specific reasons, purpose, or benefits.

for establishing long-term goals is to write down 10 long-term goals every day for 1 week, then identify the goals that are consistently represented on the daily lists.[23] Next, write out the steps required to achieve the long-term goals and include them in our short-term goals. For example, I am a novice runner and I have a long-term goal of running a full marathon (26.2 miles) before I turn 45 (in 6 years). To achieve this long-term goal, I have set various short-term goals to prepare me for a full marathon. Some of my short-term goals include running 5 miles 4 times a week for 3 months, running 10 miles twice a week for 1 year, running a half marathon each year leading up to the full marathon. Another example, when I graduated with my undergraduate degree in athletic training, I set the long-term goal of becoming a program director of an accredited athletic training program. To reach this long-term goal, I had to set various short-term goals to obtain the necessary education and experience to fulfill the responsibilities of a program director. One of my short-term goals was to obtain an athletic training graduate assistantship that provided autonomous clinical experience, teaching opportunities, and funding for the completion of my graduate degree within 2 years. Upon completion of my graduate degree, I set the short-term goal of obtaining a full-time split appointment as an assistant athletic trainer in athletics and a faculty member in an athletic training education program to gain more clinical and teaching experience as well as program administration experience for a minimum of 1 year. When I achieved this goal, I set another short-term goal of securing a graduate assistantship that provided teaching and accreditation-related experiences while pursuing a doctoral degree within 3 to 5 years. Obtaining these short-term goals enabled me to ultimately achieve my long-term goal of becoming a program director.

We must periodically review our goals for achievement, or lack thereof, and identify factors that facilitate or inhibit our goal achievement.[24] Reviewing our performance in completing short-term goals allows us to make necessary adjustments to ensure our success in reaching our long-term goals.[3] Reviewing our list of long-term goals promotes thoughtful decision making and better enables us to protect and prioritize the time and effort necessary to successfully complete both our short- and long-term goals.[3]

Prioritization

A priority is something that is more important than other things and needs to be accomplished or dealt with first.[15] Prioritizing is a component of planning that determines the sequence in which tasks should be completed.[25] Effective time management dictates the completion of important tasks, or those that are most relevant to achieving our goals, be achieved first.[26] Oftentimes, however, priorities are set based on the path of least resistance.[16] In other words, easy or pleasant tasks are completed first, thereby delaying the completion of more challenging, important, or urgent tasks.[25]

There are various methods to help us prioritize tasks, such as conducting an *ABC* Analysis, applying the *Pareto Principle*, and keeping a to-do list. The *ABC Analysis* prioritizes goals in the following order: *A—Tasks that are urgent and important, B—Tasks that are important but not urgent,* and *C—Tasks that are neither urgent nor important.*[16] Priority is given to those tasks categorized as A or B. Research suggests that the most successful people spend 65% to 80% of their time on tasks that are "important but not urgent" (category B).[16] The typical person spends only 15% on "important but not urgent" (category B) tasks while spending 50% to 60% on "urgent but not important" (we could consider this category D) tasks.[16] "Urgent but not important" tasks include addressing interruptions or handling other peoples' priorities. The aforementioned categorization of goals may be put into a matrix with 4 quadrants (listed in order of priority): Quadrant 1—Tasks that are important but not urgent, Quadrant 2—Tasks that are urgent and important, Quadrant 3—Tasks that are urgent but not important, and Quadrant 4—Tasks that are neither urgent nor important (refer to Tables 14-3 and 14-4 for examples). Time-management experts suggest that we should block time in our weekly schedule to complete activities in Quadrant 2 (tasks that are "urgent and important"); however, most of our time should be spent on activities in Quadrant 1 (tasks that are "important but not urgent") because they will lead to achieving our long-term goals.[3]

To ensure we achieve our goals, we may apply the *Pareto Principle* to prioritize our tasks. The *Pareto Principle*, also known as the 80/20 rule, was developed by Vilfredo Pareto, an Italian economist, in 1895.[16] This principle states that 20% of our activities are vital while 80% are trivial. Oftentimes the vital 20% are the most difficult tasks;[16] however, they will contribute the most to achieving our goals. To apply the *Pareto Principle*, we would review our list of tasks or our calendar of activities and categorize each as vital or trivial to achieving our goals. Then, we would organize our schedule and plan our time accordingly to focus on the vital tasks and activities required to achieve our goals.

Keeping a to-do list that prioritizes tasks in order of importance is another effective time-management technique. There are 2 steps in preparing an effective to-do list.[16] First, write down all the steps necessary to complete a task and develop concrete action plans that specify when, where, and how the task will be completed or the goal achieved.[25] Larger tasks should be broken

TABLE 14-3

EXAMPLE PRIORITIZATION OF TASKS FOR AN ATHLETIC TRAINING STUDENT

	URGENT	NOT URGENT
Important	*Quadrant 2* Study for tomorrow's exam Case report due in 3 days	*Quadrant 1* Preceptor evaluation due in 3 weeks Update resume Submit internship application for next semester
Not Important	*Quadrant 3* Routine phone calls Interruptions	*Quadrant 4* Checking Facebook Posting to Twitter Watching ESPN

TABLE 14-4

EXAMPLE PRIORITIZATION OF TASKS FOR AN ATHLETIC TRAINER

	URGENT	NOT URGENT
Important	*Quadrant 2* Patient emergency National presentation due in 3 days Budget due tomorrow	*Quadrant 1* Interacting with patients Completing injury reports Networking Review long-term goals
Not Important	*Quadrant 3* Routine phone calls Insurance billing Staff interviews Interruptions	*Quadrant 4* Checking email Routine paperwork Committee meeting Time wasters

down into smaller action steps, which should take no longer than 2 hours to complete.[24] Second, prioritize each task or action step using the *ABC Analysis* or *Pareto Principle*. The to-do list is then completed in order of importance. A daily, weekly, or monthly to-do list allows us to plan our time to complete important tasks. Time-management experts recommend spending 10 to 15 minutes at the end of each day to plan and prioritize tomorrow's to-do items.[18] Being able to check off items on our to-do list highlights our progress in achieving our goals and provides self-reinforcement for planning further accomplishments.[18]

Routinization

Effective planning leads to the development of a routine. A routine is a regular way of doing things in a particular order.[15] Routines provide a sense of predictability, familiarity, and time control thus decreasing the thinking time needed for time management.[4] To establish a routine, we can use "schedule blocking," which includes recurring, horizontal appointments on our calendar that entails doing the same activity at the same time of day.[24] Horizontal "scheduling blocking" builds momentum and maximizes achievement.[27] We can also use a color-coding scheme to prioritize tasks and activities on our calendar to keep us focused on achieving our goals. For example, red items are important and cannot be changed whereas green items are less important and may be modified. Refer to Table 14-5 and Figure 14-2 for examples of an athletic training student's weekly calendar that demonstrates horizontal "schedule blocking" and a color-coding scheme.

Coping with Distractions

A distraction is something that makes it difficult to think or pay attention.[15] The average person switches tasks every 3 minutes, and, once sufficiently distracted may require up to an average of 30 minutes to resume the original task.[24] Research suggests that unplanned tasks are rated more urgent and important, and are completed to a higher degree than planned tasks.[25] Therefore, one must plan by setting goals, prioritizing goals, and establishing a routine to minimize distractions. Unplanned tasks, or distractions, evolve from a variety of sources. Email is a potential distraction. Time management experts suggest that we check email only 3 to 4 times throughout the day[3] and that we handle email items only once.[24] Visual and auditory distractions should be minimized while we are working on important, urgent, or vital tasks. To promote productivity, we should turn off visual and auditory interruptions such as auto-alerts for incoming email or text messages.[3,24] If turning visual or auditory auto-alerts is not an option, then we cope with distractions by applying the *"if-then"* rule.[25] *If* someone interrupts us unexpectedly, *then* we can politely and succinctly respond by making an appointment to discuss the issue later. To monitor our progress in achieving our goals, we can calculate the percentage of tasks completed on our to-do list each day.[25] This provides a precise and objective measure of our productivity, which can assist in minimizing distractions and re-focusing our efforts on important tasks that will allow us to achieve our goals.

Self-Monitoring

Self-monitoring our time-management behaviors requires discipline. Self-discipline is the ability to make ourselves do things that should be done.[15] Relative to time management, self-discipline involves our motivation to complete a task despite distractions. Qualities associated with discipline include hard work and perseverance; whereas the absence of motivation, tending to interruptions, and procrastination signify a lack of discipline.[24] If we are not disciplined, we will find ourselves engaged in activities that do not contribute to achieving our goals and we will waste time reorienting ourselves to the original task(s) and goal(s). Therefore, we need to identify our lapses in discipline and address our tendencies to procrastinate or to attend to interruptions. To do this, we need to monitor our activity while completing a task and keep a log of how we use our time. Be honest.

As an example, consider a situation whereby your supervisor, the director of a sports medicine clinical, has assigned you to write a report on the evidence to support the use of instrument-assisted soft-tissue mobilization in treating patellar tendinosis. The report is important as it may influence the care plans for patients, as well as the allocation of continuing education funds for clinicians. You estimate that it will take 1 week to write the report after conducting a search for evidence and assessing its quality. Using horizontal scheduling, you block 2 hours of writing time in the morning (since you discovered that you are most productive in the morning) to go to the library (since you identified the library as your most productive location) every day the week prior to the due date set by the supervisor. During each 2-hour writing block, you should ask yourself: How long did it take for me to get organized so that I could start writing? How much time did I actually spend writing? How much time did I spend on distractions (such as checking email) or interruptions (such as answering a colleague's question)? Did I procrastinate by completing quick, easy, smaller tasks before I started writing during my 2-hour block? Procrastination, attending to distractions/interruptions, and a lack of discipline contribute to ineffective time management, thereby reducing our productivity.[24]

TABLE 14-5

SAMPLE 5-DAY CALENDAR USING BLOCK SCHEDULING AND A COLOR-CODING SCHEME

	MONDAY	TUESDAY	WEDNESDAY	THURSDAY	FRIDAY
7 am	Wake-up	Wake-up	Wake-up	Wake-up	Wake-up
8 am to 10 am	Modalities class	Read/Study for Modalities class	Modalities class	Read/Study for Modalities class	Modalities class
10 am to 12 pm	Orthopedic assessment class	Read/Study for Orthopedic Assessment class	Orthopedic Assessment class	Read/Study for Orthopedic Assessment class	Orthopedic Assessment class
12 pm to 1 pm	Lunch	Lunch	Lunch	Lunch	Lunch
1 pm to 2 pm	Check/Reply to emails	Check/Reply to emails	Check/Reply to emails	Check/Reply to emails	Check/Reply to emails
2 pm to 6 pm	Clinical education	Clinical education	Clinical education	Clinical education	Clinical education
6 pm to 7 pm	Dinner	Dinner	Dinner	Dinner	Dinner
7 pm to 8 pm	Watch TV and check/reply to emails	Watch TV and check/reply to emails	Watch TV and check/reply to emails	Watch TV and check/reply to emails	Watch TV and check/reply to emails
8 pm to 9 pm	Workout	Workout	Workout	Workout	Workout
9 pm to 10 pm	Relax and plan for tomorrow	Relax and plan for tomorrow	Relax and plan for tomorrow	Relax and plan for tomorrow	Relax and plan for tomorrow
10 pm	Bedtime	Bedtime	Bedtime	Bedtime	Bedtime

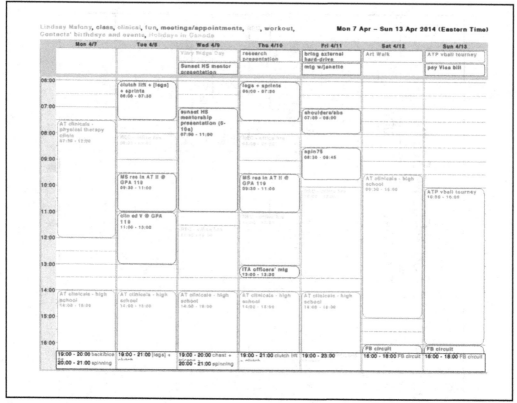

Figure 14-2. A sample 7-day calendar using block scheduling and a color-coding scheme.

We should all periodically reevaluate our habits of procrastination, attending to distractions/interruptions, and lack of discipline to ensure we have adequately addressed these issues for the betterment of our time management. Likewise, regularly monitoring whether we are completing our tasks, or achieving our goals, is important. If we are failing to achieve our goals, self-monitoring will allow us to modify our behaviors and/or goals.[23] Are we procrastinating? Are we getting distracted? Are our goals unrealistic? An important life survival skill is to realize when we can get away with "good enough" and when we need to re-prioritize to put forth our best effort.[23] Are we overcommitted? Self-monitoring will allow us to identify how we use our time, which will provide us with the necessary feedback to refocus and reprioritize our efforts while limiting distractors and interruptions.[12,16]

> Self-monitoring of time-management behaviors requires discipline and honesty.

Personal Time

Through self-monitoring, we may identify the need to incorporate personal time into our schedule to establish work-life balance. Research suggests that time for personal rejuvenation is necessary for an athletic trainer to remain committed to the profession.[28] This personal time allows us to engage in personal interests, such as hobbies, and to spend time with family and friends. An effective way to achieve time for personal rejuvenation is to set boundaries, which may require learning to say "no."[29,30] Setting boundaries involves the creation of a relatively stable schedule, which requires acquiring some control over our schedule.[29] For example, an athletic training student can discuss (negotiate) a schedule with his or her preceptor that maximizes clinical learning yet affords adequate time to meet other responsibilities (including some personal time).

To maintain our boundaries and time for personal rejuvenation, we may need to say "no" to additional responsibilities. For example, the program director just sent an email to all students looking for volunteers to assist with a 4-hour high school student aide workshop scheduled for next week. We need to carefully look at our schedule, our weekly responsibilities, and our to-do list prior to answering the email. It may be tempting to please the program director by volunteering to help, but, we have 2 exams and a group project due next week. Therefore, we (should) say "no" to this opportunity but look forward to volunteering for future events. It may feel difficult to set boundaries or to say "no" to a program director, preceptor, or boss; however, it is an effective time management strategy that can positively affect professional and personal satisfaction and overall well-being.

> Setting boundaries is an important and effective time-management strategy for maintaining good work-life balance.

Personality Traits

Self-monitoring also involves the examination of our personality traits. Research suggests that certain personality traits are antecedents of effective time management, namely conscientiousness and emotional stability.[25,31-33] A conscientious individual is very careful about doing what he or she is supposed to do and is concerned with doing things correctly.[15] An emotionally stable individual is calm and secure, not depressed, hostile, or neurotic.[31] Conscientiousness and emotional stability are positively related to task completion[31,32] and negatively related to procrastination.[33] Conscientious individuals are expected to complete more tasks because they are committed to doing what needs to get done, they avoid distractions, and they deal effectively with distractions.[25] Emotionally stable individuals are expected to possess better problem-solving skills, to effectively overcome obstacles, and to remain focused through task completion.[25] We can examine our personality traits to determine if we are conscientious, calm, and secure. If not, we should develop and implement effective time-management strategies to help us plan, prioritize, and routinize our time to focus on important tasks that will allow us to achieve our goals.

SUMMARY

In a review of literature conducted by Claessens et al,[12] the positive effects of time management are duly noted. Their research suggests that college grades and study habits are positively affected by effective time-management behaviors. Furthermore, time-management behaviors are positively related to perceived control of time, job satisfaction, and health while negatively related to tension and psychological distress. With effective time-management skills, you will be more self-disciplined in knowing when and how to most efficiently complete tasks, which will ultimately increase your productivity.[16] You will become more organized as a result of effective time management and better able to accomplish tasks leading to goal attainment. With efficient and effective time-management behaviors, important tasks are completed on time thereby improving productivity and reducing stress.[16] Your peers, and supervisors, will recognize your productivity level as you complete your work on time (or early), which will boost your morale and confidence.[16] Effective time-management behaviors will help you achieve better work-life balance, thereby giving you more time, and energy, to fulfill school, work, family, and personal responsibilities.[16]

ACTIVITIES FOR REINFORCEMENT

Questions for Review

1. Why is it important to assess the way in which you manage your time before you start implementing time management strategies?

2. What is a time waster? Give three examples.

3. What is a smart goal and why is goal setting necessary?

Case Vignettes

Case #1

Kelly is an athletic training student who just started her last semester of an accredited professional athletic training program. She is going to have a busy semester because of the following: (1) her final research project is due at the end of the semester (first week of May), (2) she will be taking the Board of Certification (BOC) exam in April, and (3) as president of the student organization she is responsible for planning the end-of-the-year party to honor the graduating students. Only 1 week into the semester, Kelly is already feeling overwhelmed and highly stressed.

1. What should Kelly do to feel less overwhelmed and stressed?

2. Kelly just received a phone call from her program director. The program director has asked Kelly to serve on the Athletic Training Program Advisory Board to help develop a 5-year strategic plan. The program director thinks it is important to gain a student's prospective while developing the strategic plan and has expressed that she values Kelly's input. Should Kelly say yes? Why or why not?

3. If Kelly says yes, what are the potential advantages and disadvantages?

4. If Kelly says no, what are the potential advantages and disadvantages?

5. Regardless of Kelly's answer, how can she cope with her decision?

Case #2

Kyle and Jeremy are life-long friends and graduate athletic training students. They attend the same program, they share an apartment, and they are working together to complete their capstone project. Their capstone project is a semester-long assignment that requires them to develop and implement an injury-prevention education program for parents and coaches in the community. It is the third week of the semester and Kyle just realized that their outline of the education program is due in 2 days. He and Jeremy have not even begun to discuss their capstone project.

1. What should be Kyle and Jeremy's first course of action? Why?

2. Kyle works best in the morning while Jeremy works best at night. How can they work together to be productive?

Discussion Questions

1. Select one of the following goals: (1) *I want to pass the BOC exam on my first attempt*, (2) *I want to be admitted to the graduate program of my choice*, or (3) *I want be employed within 1 month of graduation*. Discuss whether your selected goal is a short- or long-term goal. Is it a SMART goal? Why or why not?

2. Using one of the aforementioned goals, develop a to-do list (that spans a minimum of 3 months) of tasks/activities necessary to achieve your goal. Apply the *Pareto Principle* to identify the 20% of tasks/activities that are vital to achieving your goal. Discuss how you determine whether a task/activity was vital or trivial.

3. Identify 3 to 5 "time-wasters" or ways in which you procrastinate. Discuss methods you employ to reduce "time-wasters" and/or procrastination.

Engagement Activities

1. Keep a time log for 1 week (Monday through Sunday) noting all of your activities and the amount of time you are engaged in each activity. Examine your time log to (1) identify the time of day during which you are most productive, (2) identify the time of day during which you are easily distracted, (3) calculate how much time you were engaged in productive work, and (4) calculate how much time you spent on "time-wasters."

2. Create a monthly calendar using horizontal schedule blocking. Include the following items at a minimum: class time, clinical education time, study time, personal time (eg, exercise, book club, walk the dog), and scheduled time for to-do items.

3. Create a list of SMART goals including 10 short- and 3 long-term goals. Discuss with a class-mate how each of your goals is specific, measurable, attainable, realistic, and timely.

4. Create a to-do list for the semester. Prioritize the to-do list using either the *ABC Analysis* or the *Pareto Principle* technique.

REFERENCES

1. Garhammer M. Pace of life and enjoyment of life. *J Happiness Stud.* 2002;3(3):217-256.
2. Macan T, Gibson JM, Cunningham J. Will you remember to read this article later when you have time? The relationship between prospective memory and time management. *Pers Indiv Differ.* 2010;48:725-730.
3. Gordon C. Recapturing time: a practical approach to time management for physicians. *Postgrad Med J.* 2014;90(1063):267-272.
4. Waterworth S. Time management strategies in nursing practice. *J Adv Nurs.* 2003;43(5):432-440.
5. National Athletic Trainers' Association. Profile of athletic trainers. www.nata.org. Updated 2014. Accessed July 27, 2014.
6. Pitney WA. Organizational influences and quality-of-life issues during the professional socialization of certi-fied athletic trainers working in the National Collegiate Athletic Association Division I setting. *J Athl Train.* 2006;41(2):189-195.
7. Mazerolle SM, Bruening JE, Casa DJ, Burton LJ. Work-family conflict, part II: job and life satisfaction in National Collegiate Athletic Association Division I-A certified athletic trainers. *J Athl Train.* 2008;43(5):513-522.
8. Mazerolle SM, Bruening JE, Casa DJ. Work-family conflict, part I: antecedents of work-family conflict in National Collegiate Athletic Association Division I-A certified athletic trainers. *J Athl Train.* 2008;43(5):505-512.
9. Mazerolle S. Undergraduate athletic training students' influences on career decisions after graduation. *J Athl Train.* 2012;47(6):679-693.
10. Pitney WA, Mazerolle SM, Pagnotta KD. Work-family conflict among athletic trainers in the secondary school setting. *J Athl Train.* 2011;46(2):185-193.
11. Mazerolle SM, Pitney WA. Examination of work-life balance among athletic trainers in the clinical rehabilita-tion setting. *Athl Train Sports Health Care.* 2012;4(6):257-264.
12. Claessens B, van Eerde W, Rutte C. A review of the time management literature. *Pers Rev.* 2007;36(2):255-276.
13. Chang A. The mediating effects of time structure on the relationships between time management behaviour, job satisfaction, and psychological well-being. *Aust J Psychol.* 2011;63(4):187.
14. Häfner A, Stock A. Time management training and perceived control of time at work. *J Psychol.* 2010;144(5):429-447.
15. Merriam-Webster Dictionary. http://www.merriam-webster.com. Updated 2014. Accessed July 27, 2014.
16. Odumeru JA. Effective time management. *Singaporean J Bus Econ Manag Stud.* 2013;2(1):9-17.
17. Macan TH. Time management: test of a process model. *J Appl Psychol.* 1994;79(3):381-391.

18. Pagana K. Teaching students time management strategies. *J Nurs Educ.* 1994;33(8):381-383.
19. Friedman SL, Scholmich EK. *The Developmental Psychology of Planning: Why, How, and When Do We Plan?* Mahwah, NJ: Lawrence Erlbaum Associates; 1997.
20. Claessens BJ. Planning behavior and perceived control of time at work. *J Organ Behav.* 2004;25(8):937.
21. Top achievement. http://topachievement.com/. Accessed July 27, 2014.
22. Christie S. *Effective Time Management Skills for Doctors.* Nottingham: Developmedica; 2009.
23. Chittenden EH, Ritchie CS. Work-life balancing: challenges and strategies. *J Palliat Med.* 2011;14(7):870-874.
24. Chase J. Time management strategies for research productivity. *West J Nurs Res.* 2013;35(2):155-176.
25. Claessens BJ. Things to do today . . . : a daily diary study on task completion at work. *Appl Psychol.* 2010;59(2):273.
26. Covey SR, Merrill AR, Merrill RR. *First Things First.* New York, NY: Simon & Schuster; 1994.
27. Lakein A. *How to Get Control of Your Time and Your Life.* New York: Signet Books; 1976.
28. Pitney WA. A qualitative examination of professional role commitment among athletic trainers working in the secondary school setting. *J Athl Train.* 2010;45(2):198-204.
29. Mazerolle S, M., Pitney W, Goodman A. Strategies for athletic trainers to find a balanced lifestyle across clinical settings. *Int J Athletic Ther Train.* 2012;17(3):7-14.
30. Mazerolle S. Assessing strategies to manage work and life balance of athletic trainers working in the National Collegiate Athletic Association Division I setting. *J Athl Train.* 2011;46(2):194-205.
31. Barrick MR. Personality and performance at the beginning of the new millennium: what do we know and where do we go next? *Int J Select Assess.* 2001;9(1-2):9-30.
32. Judge TA. Relationship of core self-evaluations traits—self-esteem, generalized self-efficacy, locus of control, and emotional stability—with job satisfaction and job performance: a meta-analysis. *J Appl Psychol.* 2001;86(1):80-92.
33. van Eerde W. A meta-analytically derived nomological network of procrastination. *Pers Indiv Differ.* 2003;35(6):1401-1418.

SUGGESTED READINGS

Covey SR, Merrill AR, Merrill RR. *First Things First.* New York, NY: Simon & Schuster; 1994.
Vanderkam, L. *168 Hours: You Have More Time Than You Think.* New York: Penguin Group; 2010.
Vanderkam L. *What the Most Successful People Do Before Breakfast.* New York: Penguin Group; 2012.
Vogel A. Work smarter, not harder: applying the principles of interval training to your career. *Idea Fitness Journal.* 2013;10(7):96-105.

15

Emotional Resilience in Athletic Training

William A. Pitney, EdD, ATC, FNATA

OBJECTIVES

After reading this chapter, the reader will be able to do the following:

1. Define emotional resilience.
2. Explain why emotional resilience is important in one's life.
3. Identify the traits of emotionally resilient people.
4. Explain how resilience is developed or acquired.
5. Describe how emotional resilience is measured.

INTRODUCTION

Health care professionals generally, and athletic trainers specifically, work in demanding practice environments. Whether dealing with an angry coach, a concerned parent, perturbed patient, or difficult co-worker, you are likely to experience stress and strain, conflict and consternation, anxiety and adversity. Thus, one must prepare to address and overcome hard times in order to have a fulfilling and successful career.

Overcoming adversity and coping effectively with stress are partially based on the extent to which one is emotionally resilient. Individuals who develop emotional resilience are able to prepare for and contend with emotionally challenging experiences and skillfully deal with tough times.[1]

In this chapter I will begin by defining emotional resilience and provide a historical context. I will then create a case for its importance and discuss the attributes that resilient people possess as well as the steps we can take to become resilient health care providers.

Mazerolle SM, Pitney WA.
Workplace Concepts for Athletic Trainers (pp 235-246).
© 2016 Taylor & Francis Group.

EMOTIONAL RESILIENCE DEFINED

Emotional resilience, also known as psychological resilience, is defined in many ways. It has been described as the ". . . ability of an individual to adjust to adversity, maintain equilibrium, retain some sense of control over their environment, and continue to move in a positive manner."[2(p3)] Emotional resilience is also identified by many as a "protective mechanism that operates in the face of negative stressors."[3(p262)] Additionally, resilience has been defined as the ability to navigate changes successfully and maintain good mental health by being psychologically flexible.[4]

Imagine, as an athletic trainer, having a team practice time or a physician consultation changed and needing to negotiate that stress in relation to the rest of your schedule. You may miss a dinner with the family, have to reschedule your own appointments, or miss a workout because of the change. Being frustrated, angry, and discouraged will not change the outcome, and will likely lead to increased stress on your part. Being psychologically flexible and positive about this or similar circumstances can allow you to steer a positive career path. This is not saying you must always accept last-minute changes and "give in" to all demands; indeed you may have to strategically negotiate times when you will not be flexible as it relates to similar situations. However, the premise with emotional resilience is that even if you have to say "no" to such an additional request, you do so with a positive attitude and sense of purpose to negotiate your boundaries around your work schedule.

EMOTIONAL RESILIENCE
Emotional resilience is the ability to positively adjust to an adverse, stressful or difficult situation and maintain one's good mental health.

HISTORICAL OVERVIEW

Researchers have a long and storied history of empirically investigating factors associated with emotional resilience.[5] The initial investigations of resilience were with the psychosocial coping literature related to child development.[6] For example, in the 1970s, research focused on adaptive patterns of individuals diagnosed with schizophrenia. This early research focused on intellectual processing that helped individuals cope with adversity.[7] Moving into the 1980s, attention was turned to understanding resilience among those who were socioeconomically disadvantaged, those dealing with chronic illness, and the personal qualities of resilient children.[5] Since this time, researchers have examined how individuals have adapted to challenging personal experiences such as the mental illness of their parents,[8] or devastating personal experiences such as homelessness, natural disasters. and war.[7] More recently, researchers have also explored the way in which one's social environment (eg, social groups, families, colleagues) influences one's level of resilience.[7]

The emotional resilience literature has primarily concentrated on victims, patients, and underserved populations; only recently has professional resilience been examined.[6] Because, as Hodges and colleagues point out, health care work environments such as nursing have been described as tumultuous and resembling war, the topic of resilience has a great deal of application to athletic training. The profession of athletic training has been characterized as extremely challenging with a great number of occupational stressors.[9] If a professional can effectively cope with the stress of the work environment, she can be successful in her role. The need for resilience, however, goes beyond one's professional role as it can also benefit health and general well-being.[10]

WHY IS EMOTIONAL RESILIENCE IMPORTANT?

Our demanding work environments are sometimes structured in a manner that creates a perfect storm for stress. Whether stress is the result of a health care team of athletic trainers that are understaffed, dealing with difficult coaches, working long hours, and lacking administrative support; or perhaps an athletic trainer is dealing with work-life imbalance, lack of opportunities for growth or promotion, or a poor salary, or perhaps a combination of any of these issues—stress tends to creep into the workplace and can have some devastating results.

Stress can negatively affect our physical and emotional well-being. The American Institute of Stress[11] explains that stress is linked to heart attack, stroke, hypertension, immune system disturbances, and even autoimmune diseases such as rheumatoid arthritis. From an emotional angle, stress has been linked to depression and burnout,[12] including its components of increased emotional exhaustion, depersonalization, and reduced personal accomplishment.[13] These emotional and physical consequences take their toll on employees. Indeed, emotional exhaustion has been found to lead to reduced quality of care performance in nurses,[14] and stress is associated with job dissatisfaction, absenteeism, and intent to leave an organization.[15]

These negative outcomes are costly in many ways for organizations and individuals alike. Consider, for example, the cost for the physical and emotional health care for the employee, the cost associated with poor patient care outcomes, and the cost associated with needing to hire employees who decide to leave. The associated costs and negative outcomes have prompted actions to facilitate emotional resilience. Perhaps the best known efforts are with the United States military, which has studied emotional resilience programs for soldiers.[16]

In deployed soldiers, emotional resilience has been shown to inhibit the development of post-traumatic stress disorder as well as other psychopathology.[17] One critical and noteworthy aspect of resilience is that it is a process that can be learned.[18] Thus, concerted efforts have been made to develop emotional resilience and reap its benefits from both a preventive and treatment perspective. Developing resilience is not a "one-and-done" learning event, however; it must be cultivated throughout a lifetime.[18]

Emotional resilience is not simply an inherent trait; it can be learned or developed.

Programs and efforts to improve emotional resilience must be developed based on an understanding of the attributes of emotionally resilient people, as well as how some of these traits are developed and encouraged. Efforts to improve resilience are addressed in 2 ways: 1) at the individual level—identifying what we can individually focus on to help ourselves be resilient, and 2) at the organizational level—focusing on what leaders can do to address a health care work setting that promotes resilience. The following sections present information related to these facets.

INDIVIDUAL LEVEL EFFORTS: ATTRIBUTES OF EMOTIONALLY RESILIENT PEOPLE

There is a great deal of research related to the attributes (also known as protective factors) held by individuals who are considered, or consider themselves, to be emotionally resilient, and a great number of attributes have been identified. For example, Earvolino-Ramirez[19] examined lists of protective factors as well as personal characteristics from resilience researchers and identified a

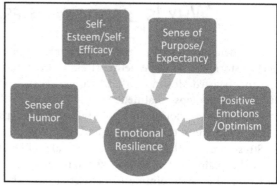

Figure 15-1. Common personal attributes held by emotionally resilient people.

total of 28 attributes. A full explanation of each of these 28 attributes is beyond the scope of this chapter, but focusing on those that are most frequently identified (Figure 15-1) is important.

Self-Esteem/Self-Efficacy

Self-esteem is one's overall sense of his or her self-worth, whereas self-efficacy is defined as one's confidence to address a problem and/or accomplish a task.[20] Positive self-esteem has been correlated with improved coping during stressful situations, whereas negative self-esteem has been associated with unsuccessful coping and an association between self-efficacy and emotional resilience has also been identified.[21]

Sense of Purpose

Having a high sense of purpose and achievement, called expectancy, or self-determination, is a common characteristic among those who are resilient.[19] Believing in your purpose and being determined to achieve it can take you a long way to not being overwhelmed by challenges.[19]

One of my favorite quotes attributed to Native American Chief Seattle relates to this concept and is as follows:

> When you know who you are; when your mission is clear and you burn with the fire of unbreakable will; no cold can touch your heart; no deluge can dampen your purpose. You know that you are alive.

This quote captures the idea that your ability to hold to your sense of purpose is the cornerstone to tolerating and withstanding challenges.

Common traits of emotionally resilient people include a sense of purpose, positive self-esteem, positive emotions, and a good sense of humor.

Positive Emotions

As Tugade et al[22] note, for centuries there has been a tacit belief that positive emotions, such as being cheerful, joyful, and optimistic, result in the ability to withstand negative, stressful experiences. Indeed, positive emotions help build emotional resilience and ". . . multiple, discrete positive emotions are essential elements of optimal functioning. As such, the capacities to experience joy, interest, contentment, and love might be construed as fundamental human strengths that yield multiple interrelated benefits"[23(p228)] such as resolving negative emotions, facilitating emotional well-being, and perhaps improved physiological health.[22]

In order to cultivate our positive emotions, there are 3 strategies that can be used: 1) prolong a positive emotional experience when it occurs, 2) show appreciation for those things you value, and 3) reframe your thoughts to focus on the positive aspects of your experience.[24] Prolonging the positive emotional experience can be performed by simply reflecting on, for example, your pride in helping an injured athlete return to play, your love of working with specific co-workers, or your joy associated with achieving a personal accomplishment such as completing a new credential. Rather than only internalizing these accomplishments, share these positive experiences with a close friend who will celebrate with you and validate your feelings.[24] This, too, will help prolong the experience.

Wilner[24] suggests being grateful and showing appreciation to others—what he calls having an "attitude of gratitude" toward others by findings positive components during distress and expressing one's value to you. For example, if a co-worker goes out of her way to cover an event for you so you can address a personal issue, simply saying thank you, providing a hand-written thank you note, or even a small gift card for coffee can go a long way to making yourself feel good and create positive emotions.

Lastly, reframe how you think about an experience. An emotion typically begins with either an unconscious or conscious assessment of the meaning you attribute to an event, followed by a response tendency (eg, subjective experience, physiological changes, facial expressions, posture).[23] Try to catch yourself when you view an incidence and react negatively. Ask yourself how you can view this situation from a positive angle.

To do this systematically, examine your explanatory style and help yourself reframe an explanation of success and failure from a pessimistic to an optimistic perspective. This will help you develop the skills to overcome adversity and be more resilient.[25] Steinburg and Gano-Overway provide and excellent overview of this process based on the work of Seligman. According to Seligman[26] there are essentially 3 dimensions to explaining our failures: 1) personalization, 2) permanence, and 3) pervasiveness. Personalization relates to whether we find ourselves to be the cause of failure or something/someone external to us. Permanence relates to whether you see the situation as changeable or unchangeable. Lastly, pervasiveness relates to whether the event is viewed as affecting all aspects of our life, or just one part. Table 15-1 presents examples of each dimension and a pessimistic explanation and an optimistic explanation. By understanding the difference, we can catch ourselves when we are pessimistic and reframe our response to an optimistic one. Over time, optimism can be learned and result in a great many benefits, including becoming more resilient.

Sense of Humor

Humor has been implicated as a factor in improving resilience. There are 2 forms of humor that are identified as most conducive to improved resilience. These are self-enhancing and affiliative.[27] Self-enhancing humor is also non-hostile toward others and is associated with being able to laugh at yourself, generally having a "good-natured" view on life. Affiliative humor is described as ". . . a warm and benevolent style involving funny non-hostile jokes and spontaneous witty banter that serves to amuse others, but in a respectful and accepting way."[27(p481)] Both of these forms of humor are associated with stress regulation and positive social outcomes such as relationship building, thus, improve coping with stress during demanding circumstances.

In contrast to the affiliative and self-enhancing forms of humor, which are considered adaptive, 2 other forms of humor exist: self-defeating and aggressive humor, both of which are considered maladaptive.[27] Self-defeating humor is self-deprecating and focuses on putting down oneself to amuse others.[28] Aggressive humor uses either sarcasm or teasing, insults, and ridicule of others in an attempt to be humorous.[29] Maladaptive forms of humor are associated with a failure to regulate

TABLE 15-1
EXPLANATORY STYLE COMPONENTS AND EXAMPLES OF PESSIMISTIC AND OPTIMISTIC RESPONSES

STYLE COMPONENT	PESSIMISTIC RESPONSE	OPTIMISTIC RESPONSE
Personalization Internal vs external	My tape application was terrible; I am really not good at those sorts of skills.	The tape I used was old and perhaps had more tension coming off the role than I thought.
Permanence Changeable vs unchangeable	If my tape procedures are not good by now, they will never be effective.	I am still a young professional with a great deal of time to further develop my skills. I will chalk this up to a good learning experience.
Pervasiveness Global vs specific	I always have difficulty with these sorts of taping procedures	I need to practice this procedure so I can more effectively treat patients.

Note: For these responses, consider a situation whereby a novice athletic trainer who has just started a position as a graduate assistant at a National Collegiate Athletic Association (NCAA) Division I institution is working with a cross country team during pre-season practices. After the conditioning session, an athlete who received a medial longitudinal arch tape procedure reported to the athletic training facility with a huge blister on her arch and heel. The coach is livid with the athletic trainer for causing the blister that will cause the athlete some problems for the afternoon session, and perhaps tomorrow's workout.

stress[28] and are also associated with negative social outcomes such as interpersonal conflict. Thus, always consider the type of humor you use in situations and try to steer clear of maladaptive types.

INDIVIDUAL LEVEL EFFORTS: ACTIVITIES IN WHICH EMOTIONALLY RESILIENT PEOPLE ENGAGE

There are many activities that an individual can engage in to promote his/her own emotional resilience. These include reflecting on your current experiences, continuing to learn, having healthy habits, interacting with others, and rebounding from negative experiences (Figure 15-2).

Reflecting on Your Current Experiences

Reflecting on one's circumstances aids in resilience. Reflection on both your actions and outcomes is a way to further understand your knowledge, skills, abilities, and dispositions. Reflection builds self-knowledge, and you can consider your views on events and whether you need to change to a more optimistic perspective. Reflection allows you to consider your boundaries[1] so you do not overextend yourself into a stressful situation. Reflection also allows for self-discovery[30]—you can learn your strengths, value, worth, and merit and feel positive about yourself, which leads to expectancy and self-efficacy. So, think about your current situation, how you got to that point, and how you can learn from it and move forward in a positive way. Consider your strengths and how you can capitalize on them. Consider your weaknesses and how you can address them.

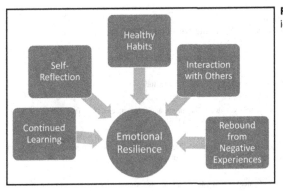

Figure 15-2. Activities that promote emotional resilience.

Continuing to Learn

Positive emotional outcomes can result from engaging in the learning process. In her qualitative investigation on lifelong learning and emotional resilience, Hammond[31] found evidence that learning aided the psychological and mental health of individuals. She argues that learning is about questioning and extending boundaries[31] and this is linked to coping with challenging circumstances and working through problems. Think of a current challenge you have had and take systematic steps to find information that might help you define the problem, learn about how the problem can be addressed, and perhaps how it can be prevented. A great example of this is from my own experience of having to deal with a very difficult individual at work. I constantly had anxiety when needing to communicate with this person. I decided to educate myself about the cause of interpersonal conflict, how to communicate more effectively, and how to understand my blind spots related to the conflict. I read Stone et al's[32] book *Difficult Conversations: How to Discuss What Matters Most* as well as *Decent People, Decent Company: How To Lead With Character at Work and in Life* by Turknett and Turknett.[33] I took on the challenge of learning about the issues instead of trying to simply tolerating the situation. For me at that time, the continued learning made a key difference in my overall well-being.

Having Healthy Habits

Engage in healthy habits such as proper physical activity, good eating habits, and self-care. Physical activity, such as aerobic training, has been found to increase positive mood states. In fact, compared to sedentary individuals, those who exercise regularly have less of a decline in positive affect after experiencing acute stress.[34] Also, self-care practices such as meditation, taking time off for yourself, and simply going for a walk are ways to connect with yourself and calm your mind.[35] To effectively engage in exercise and recover appropriately, proper nutrition is key. Moreover, proper nutrition is essential for ingesting proper levels of vitamins and minerals that aid our cognitive processing, which is necessary to monitor our behaviors and actions in the face of adversity.[30,33]

Besides exercise and eating right, there are other avenues to engage in healthy habits. One's engagement in sports, community service, and creative or artistic activities can also contribute positively to resilience.[7] Interestingly, these strategies overlap with those related to work-life balance. As such, an athletic trainer would be well served to address these factors.

Interacting With Others

Connect with people around you and develop a social support system to help you through tough times, listen to your concerns, offer helpful advice, and call on you to do the same. You have to be willing to accept invitations to go out with friends, allow yourself family time, and act to include

Figure 15-3. The SEARCHERS model for developing emotional resilience.

Self-esteem/Self-Efficacy
See your value in this world and have confidence in yourself and your ability to succeed.

Expectancy
Have a sense of purpose and believe that what you do matters.

Attitude
Adopt a positive outlook. Only you can choose your attitude, so pick a positive one.

Reflection
Think about your situation, how you got to that point, and how you can learn from it and move on; consider how you can look at a situation in a positive way.

Continued learning
Learning can have a positive effect on your confidence, competence, and communication skills, all of which can lead to positive emotional health outcomes.

Healthy Habits
Stay physically healthy. Physical activity, for example, increase positive mood states that impact your attitude.

Engagement with others
Connect with others and develop a social support system so you have people to listen to you and offer you encouragement when you need it.

Reintegration
After experiencing adversity, monitor yourself so you can get back to normal as soon as you feel ready to do so.

Sense of humor
Be willing to find the humor in your life circumstances. This will enhance your coping and moderate your emotional reactions.

others in your life. Share your successes with friends and relish the positive emotions. What we do with our time influences our ability to be resilient and overcome adversity. Having adequate social support from family, friends, and/or colleagues is commonly identified as an important contextual factor.[7,36]

Rebounding from Negative Experiences

After experiencing adversity, monitor yourself so you can get back to a normal personal and professional routine as soon as you feel ready to do so. If you do not feel prepared to reintegrate into the full professional role after a traumatic event or substantial adversity, seek help from a trained counselor to work with you on this aspect of your life.

A Model for Conceptualizing Resilience

Because resilience is dynamic and can be developed, I have summarized the previous factors into the "SEARCHERS" model of emotional resilience (Figure 15-3) as a way to think about how to work toward becoming more resilient in one's career.

The model is not linear, you do not need to follow it one step at a time; nor is it representative of everything you must do in order to be emotionally resilient. Rather, it represents various protective factors, or attributes along with other factors and strategies to deal with work-related challenges found in the resilience literature. These tend to be behaviors or actions of people who are resilient. The model provides a mental viewpoint that can facilitate your thinking so you can make a conscious effort to change your behavior and make yourself more resilient.

Organizational-Related Efforts: Perspectives for Program Leaders

As a current or future leader, I hope you will want to have a medical staff that is committed to maintaining their emotional well-being and be resilient to any stresses and strains associated with their roles. Where should you start to achieve this goal? First, model the personal attributes for your staff as well as the physical well-being and healthy habits. Second, think about how you can use your role to influence the organizational culture. Does your staff support one another? Does a culture of care for one another exist? Beyond personal attributes and activities in which emotionally resilient people engage, other factors have been addressed in programs specifically designed to facilitate emotional resilience.[2] Two are presented here, including: 1) collective efficacy, and 2) positive climate.

Collective Efficacy

Collective efficacy is based on the work of Sampson et al[37] and means that a group, such as an athletic training staff, shares their expectations and mutually agrees on how they will work together to achieve a task larger than themselves—working together to provide high quality of care to their patients. An individual's effort contributes to the success of the whole team. Research by Ross and Gray[38] provided insight into how leaders can build a team's collective efficacy. I have adapted these for use in athletic training settings:

1. Enhance each athletic trainer's knowledge and skill to improve patient outcomes. Promote the importance of continuing education and work with all members of the athletic training staff to identify specific learning outcomes they should address so they can share their new knowledge and skills with the health care team. This will provide a chance to collaboratively share knowledge and skills.

2. Provide performance feedback and action steps to an employee after each evaluation. Link the employee's performance to the group's overall goals.

3. Include the athletic training staff in the decision-making process for the program. Allow individuals to have input on equipment, supplies, professional development programs, etc that will be useful for the health care team.

Positive Climate

A positive climate in which leaders "... empower and support their workforces, by helping them appreciate the meaning of their work..."[2(p27)] facilitates cohesion and improves resilience.[2] Team-building activities can generate a sense of trust among employees and generate confidence in one another, thus enhancing resilience for team members. Also, although these psychological aspects of a positive climate are important, so too is the physical environment. Consider whether the environment is pleasant and bright, or unpleasant and drab. Individuals spend a great deal of time in their work environments and deserve to feel good about their surroundings.

Measuring Emotional Resilience

As health care providers, we need to assess patients initially and then reassess their progress in order to see if our therapeutic intervention is working. We can approach emotional resilience in the same way. There are several ways to measure emotional resilience so you can understand how resilient you are, and whether the previous approaches have worked for you.

Perhaps the most common measure is the 25-item Resilience Scale (RS) and the 14-item Resilience Scale (RS-14) developed by Wagnild and Young.[39] These scales contain items measured on a Likert-like scale from strongly disagree to strongly agree. For the RS-14, scores range from 14 to 98; a score from 14 to 56 indicates very low resilience; a score of 57 to 64 is low resilience; a score of 65 to 73 is moderately low resilience, while a score of 74 to 81 is moderately high; a score of 82 to 90 is high, and 91 to 98 is very high. These resilience scales are copyrighted and approval must be obtained for their use; however, the resilience scale homepage (https://www.resilience-scale.com) offers a personal assessment of your level of emotional resilience.

Another common inventory to measure emotional resilience is the Connor-Davidson Resilience Scale (CD-RISC).[40] This scale consists of 25 items such as I am "able to adapt to change" and I am "not easily discouraged by failure."[40(p78)] The RS, RS-14, and CD-RISC provide options to quantify resilience in order to gain a sense of where an individual is with his or her emotional resilience and whether efforts to improve resilience are working.

Summary

Our mental and emotional health is critical to a long and fulfilling career as athletic trainers. Addressing emotional resilience can ultimately influence one's ability to think clearly, make good decisions, and express emotions. Moreover, emotional resilience can help address change of any sort that makes our lives challenging. Emotional resilience can be improved with individual effort focused on reframing how we view our world and engaging in healthy activities. Organizational leaders can also influence resilience by developing a health care team's collective efficacy and having a positive work climate.

Activities for Reinforcement

Questions for Review

1. What does it mean to be emotional resilient?
2. What are the attributes of emotionally resilient people?
3. What personal strategies can one utilize to become more resilient?
4. What can organizational leaders to do promote emotional resilience?

Case Vignettes

Case #1

Jason is an athletic trainer with a high profile National Collegiate Athletic Association (NCAA) Division I program and is the head athletic trainer for the basketball team. Jason has been in his role for only a year now, and there are 3 weeks left in the season and a high probability of making the NCAA tournament. Jason feels very discouraged because his travel schedule has kept him away from his family more than he would like. Moreover, the coach has called for extra practices on Saturday and Sunday this week because the team didn't perform well last week. The coach has also been very difficult—he has blamed the last 2 losses on Jason because 2 starters injured their ankles. At the conclusion of today's practice Jason saw that it was 8:30 pm already and his day started at 6:00 am Jason started second guessing his decision to take this role. After all, he was perfectly happy in his previous college job and had great colleagues to work with. He also started thinking about whether he was "cut out" for a job like this one. It seemed to him that no matter what he did, the coach berated him because of his incompetence.

1. What advice would you give to Jason about his current situation?
2. What specific strategies might help Jason withstand his current adversity?
3. If you were Jason's supervisor and he shared his feelings with you, how would you help him reframe his thoughts to be more optimistic?

Case #2

Lisa just graduated with her Bachelor of Science degree in athletic training a month ago and just passed her Board of Certification (BOC) exam. She aspires to work in the college setting. She would also like to get a job close to home so she could easily stay connected with her family. Lisa has had a difficult time finding an athletic training job, however. She has applied to 10 different schools, but hasn't had even one interview. She decided to take a part-time "rehabilitation technician" position at the clinic she did her internship with, though she does not find this role very rewarding at all. She fears she will be stuck in the position and will never get a job in the college setting like she hopes.

1. Describe Lisa's explanatory style. Is it conducive to developing resilience?

2. Provide an example of how you might help Lisa change her explanatory style.

3. What specific strategies would you also suggest Lisa use in order to become more resilient and deal with this difficult situation?

Discussion Questions

1. Think about yourself and the characteristics you possess. What traits do you have that align with emotional resilience?

2. Consider a challenge you have dealt with in the last year and explain what strategies you used to cope and adjust to the adversity.

3. Ruminate on a joke you recently heard. What type humor does the joke represent? Is it adaptive or maladaptive?

REFERENCES

1. Waters B. Psychology Today. *10 Traits of Emotionally Resilient People.* May 21, 2013. www.psychologytoday.com/blog/design-your-path/201305/10-traits-emotionally-resilient-people. Accessed November 5, 2014.
2. Jackson D, Firtko A, Edenborough M. Personal resilience as a strategy for surviving and thriving in the face of workplace adversity: a literature review. *J Adv Nurs.* 2007;60(1):1-9.
3. Gooding PA, Hurst A, Johnson J, Tarrier. Psychological resilience in young and older adults. *Int J Geriatr Psychiatry.* 2012;27(3):262-270.
4. Waugh CE, Thompson RJ, Gotlib IH. Flexible emotional responsiveness in trait resilience. *Emotion.* 2011;11(5):1059-1067.
5. Luthar SS, Cicchetti D, Becker B. The construct of resilience: a critical evaluation and guidelines for future work. *Child Dev.* 2000;71(3):543-562.
6. Hodges HF, Keeley AC, Troyan PJ. Professional resilience in baccalaureate-prepared acute care nurses: first steps. *Nurs Educ Perspect.* 2008;29(2):80-89.
7. Herrman H, Stewart DE, Diaz-Granados N, Berger EL, Jackson B, Yuen T. What is resilience? *Can J Psychiatry.* 2011;56(5):258-265.
8. Masten AS, Coatsworth JD. The development of competence in favorable and unfavorable environments: lessons from research on successful children. *Am Psychol.* 1998;53(2):205-220.
9. Reed S, Giacobbi PR Jr. The stress and coping responses of certified graduate athletic training students. *J Athl Train.* 2004;39(2):193-200.
10. Davis MC. Building emotional resilience to promote health. *Am J Lifestyle Med.* 2009;3(1 Suppl):60S-63S.
11. The American Institute of Stress. 50 common signs and symptoms of stress. www.stress.org/stress-effects/. Accessed November 5, 2014.
12. Department of Health and Human Services. National Institute for Occupational Safety and Health. Exposure to stress: occupational hazards in hospitals: 2008. http://www.cdc.gov/niosh/docs/2008-136/pdfs/2008-136.pdf. Accessed November 5, 2014.
13. Montgomery C, Rupp AA. A meta-analysis for exploring the diverse causes and effects of stress in teachers. *Canadian J Educ.* 2005;28(3):458-486.
14. García MG, Calvo JCA. Emotional exhaustion of nursing staff: influence of emotional annoyance and resilience. *Int Nurs Rev.* 2012;59(1):101-107.
15. Pitney WA, Stuart ME, Parker J. Role strain among dual position physical educators and athletic trainers working in the high school setting. *Phys Educ.* 2008;65(3):157-168.
16. Meredith LS, Sherbourne CD, Gaillot S, et al. *Promoting Psychological Resilience in the U.S. Military.* Center for Military Health Policy Research. Santa Monica, CA: RAND Corp.; 2011.

17. Pietrzak RH, Johnson DC, Goldstein MB, Malley JC, Southwick SM. Psychological resilience and postdeployment social support protect against traumatic stress and depressive symptoms in soldiers returning from Operations Enduring Freedom and Iraqi Freedom. *Depress Anxiety.* 2009;26(8):745-751.

18. Cameron F, Brownie S. Enhancing resilience in registered aged care nurses. *Australas J Ageing.* 2010;29(2):66-71.

19. Earvolino-Ramirez M. Resilience: a concept analysis. *Nurs Forum.* 2007;42(2):73-82.

20. Bandura A. *Self-Efficacy: The Exercise of Control.* New York: Freeman; 1997.

21. Dumont M, Provost MA. Resilience in adolescents: protective role of social support, coping strategies, self-esteem, and social activities on experience of stress and depression. *J Youth Adolesc.* 1999;28(3):343-363.

22. Tugade MM, Fredrickson BL, Feldman Barrett LF. Psychological resilience and positive emotional granularity: examining the benefits of positive emotions on coping and health. *J Pers.* 2004;72(6):1161-1190.

23. Fredrickson BL. The role of positive emotions in positive psychology: the broaden-and-build theory of positive emotions. *Am Psychol.* 2001;56(3):218-226.

24. Wilner J. Psych Central. How to maintain and enhance positive emotions. http://blogs.psychcentral.com/positive-psychology/2011/11/how-to-maintain-and-enhance-positive-emotions/. Accessed November 6, 2014.

25. Steinberg G, Gano-Overway LA. Developing optimism skills to help youths overcome adversity. *J Phys Educ Recreation Dance.* 2003;74(5):40-44.

26. Seligman MEP. *Learned Optimism: How to Change Your Mind and Your Life.* New York: Pocket Books; 1990.

27. Kuiper NA. Humor and resiliency: towards a process model of coping and growth. *Eur J Psych.* 2012;8(3):475-491.

28. Besser A, Luyten P, Mayes LC. Adult attachment and distress: the mediating role of humor styles. *Individ Differ Res.* 2012;10(3):153-164.

29. Zeigler-Hill V, Besser A. Humor style mediates the association between pathological narcissism and self-esteem. *Pers Indiv Differ.* 2011;50(8):1196-1201.

30. American Psychological Association. The road to resilience. http://www.apa.org/helpcenter/road-resilience.aspx. Accessed November 6, 2014.

31. Hammond C. Impacts of lifelong learning upon emotional resilience, psychological and mental health: fieldwork evidence. *Oxford Rev Educ.* 2004;30(4):551-568.

32. Stone D, Patton B, Heen S, Fisher R. *Difficult Conversations: How to Discuss What Matters Most.* New York, NY: Penguin Books; 1999.

33. Turknett RL, Turknett CN. *Decent People Decent Company: How to Lead with Character at Work and in Life.* Mountain View, CA: Davies-Black; 2005.

34. Childs E, de Wit H. Regular exercise is associated with emotional resilience to acute stress in healthy adults. *Front Physiol.* 2014;5(161):1-7.

35. Horneffer-Gitner K. Psychology Today. 25 Ways to boost resilience. http://www.psychologytoday.com/blog/design-your-path/201305/25-ways-boost-resilience. Accessed November 6, 2014.

36. McCaan CM, Beddoe E, McCormick K, et al. Resilience in the health professions: a review of recent literature. *Int J Wellbeing.* 2013;3(1):60-81.

37. Sampson RJ, Morenoff J, Earls F. Beyond social capital: spatial dynamics of collective efficacy for children. *Am Sociol Rev.* 1999;64:633-660.

38. Ross JA, Gray P. Transformational leadership and teacher commitment to organizational values: the mediating effects of collective teacher efficacy. *Sch Eff Sch Improv.* 2006;17(2):179-199.

39. Wagnild GM, Young HM. Development and psychometric evaluation of the resilience scale. *J Nurs Measure.* 1993;1(2):165-178.

40. Connor KM, Davidson JR. Development of a new resilience scale: the Connor-Davidson resilience scale (CD-RISC). *Depress Anxiety.* 2003;18(2):76-82.

Financial Disclosures

Dr. Kirk Brumels has no financial or proprietary interest in the materials presented herein.

Dr. Laura J. Burton has no financial or proprietary interest in the materials presented herein.

Dr. Jennifer Doherty-Restrepo has no financial or proprietary interest in the materials presented herein.

Christianne M. Eason has no financial or proprietary interest in the materials presented herein.

Dr. Ashley Goodman has no financial or proprietary interest in the materials presented herein.

Dr. Matthew R. Kutz has no financial or proprietary interest in the materials presented herein.

Dr. Stephanie M. Mazerolle has no financial or proprietary interest in the materials presented herein.

Dr. John T. Parsons has no financial or proprietary interest in the materials presented herein.

Dr. William A. Pitney has no financial or proprietary interest in the materials presented herein.

Dr. Stacy E. Walker has no financial or proprietary interest in the materials presented herein.

Dr. Celest Weuve has no financial or proprietary interest in the materials presented herein.

Index

Printed in the United States
by Baker & Taylor Publisher Services

Printed in the United States
by Baker & Taylor Publisher Services